Contents

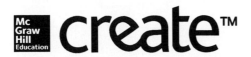

Annual Editions:
Health, 37/e

Eileen L. Daniel

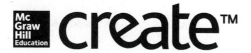

http://create.mheducation.com

ISBN-10: 1259394050   ISBN-13: 9781259394058

Preface

America is in the midst of a revolution that is changing the way millions of Americans view their health. Traditionally, most people delegated responsibility for their health to their physicians and hoped that medical science would be able to cure whatever ailed them. This approach to healthcare emphasized the role of medical technology and funneled billions of dollars into medical research. The net result of all this spending is the most technically advanced and expensive healthcare system in the world.

In an attempt to rein in healthcare costs, the healthcare delivery system moved from privatized healthcare coverage to what is termed "managed care." While managed care has turned the tide regarding the rising cost of healthcare, it has done so by limiting reimbursement for many cutting-edge technologies. Unfortunately, many people also feel that it has lowered the overall quality of care that is being given. Perhaps the saving grace is that we live at a time in which chronic illnesses rather than acute illnesses are our number one health threat, and many of these illnesses can be prevented or controlled by our lifestyle choices. The net result of these changes has prompted millions of individuals to assume more personal responsibility for safeguarding their own health. Evidence of this change in attitude can be seen in the growing interest in nutrition, physical fitness, dietary supplements, and stress management.

If we as a nation are to capitalize on this new health consciousness, we must devote more time and energy to educating Americans in the health sciences, so that they will be better able to make informed choices about their health. Health is a complex and dynamic subject, and it is practically impossible for anyone to stay abreast of all the current research findings. In the past, most of us have relied on books, newspapers, magazines, and television as our primary sources for medical/health information, but today, with the widespread use of personal computers and mobile devices connected to the Internet, it is possible to access a vast amount of health information, any time of the day, without even leaving one's home. Unfortunately, quantity and availability does not necessarily translate into quality, and this is particularly true in the area of medical/health information. Just as the Internet is a great source for reliable and timely information, it is also a vehicle for the dissemination of misleading and fraudulent information. Currently, there are no standards or regulations regarding the posting of health content on the Internet, and this has led to a plethora of misinformation and quackery in the medical/health arena. Given this vast amount of health information, our task as health educators is twofold: (1) to provide our students with the most up-to-date and accurate information available on major health issues of our time and (2) to teach our students the skills that will enable them to sort out facts from fiction, in order to become informed consumers. *Annual Editions: Health* was designed to aid in this task. It offers a sampling of quality articles that represent the latest thinking on a variety of health issues, and it also serves as a tool for developing critical thinking skills.

The articles in this volume were carefully chosen on the basis of their quality and timeliness. Because this book is revised and updated annually, it contains information that is not generally available in any standard textbook. As such, it serves as a valuable resource for both teachers and students. This edition of *Annual Editions: Health* has been updated to reflect the latest thinking on a variety of contemporary health issues. We hope that you find this edition to be a helpful learning tool with a user-friendly presentation. The topical areas presented in this edition mirror those that are normally covered in introductory health courses: Promoting Healthy Behavior Change, Stress and Mental Health, Nutritional Health, Exercise and Weight Management, Drugs and Health, Sexuality and Relationships, Preventing and Fighting Disease, Healthcare and the Healthcare System, Consumer Health, and Contemporary Health Hazards. Because of the interdependence of the various elements that constitute health, the articles selected were written by authors with diverse educational backgrounds and expertise, including naturalists, environmentalists, psychologists, economists, sociologists, nutritionists, consumer advocates, and traditional health practitioners.

Editor

Eileen L. Daniel is a professor of Health Science and Associate Vice Provost for Academic Affairs at SUNY College at Brockport. She earned her doctorate in health education from the University of Oregon and a BS in Dietetics and Nutrition from the Rochester Institute of Technology. She has published over 40 articles in the scientific press and is also the author of *Taking Sides: Clashing Views on Health and Society.*

Editors/Academic Advisory Board

Members of the Academic Advisory Board are instrumental in the final selection of articles for each edition of *Annual Editions: Health.* Their review of articles for content, level, and appropriateness provides critical direction to the editors and staff. We think that you will find their careful consideration well reflected in this volume.

Academic Advisory Board Members

Unit 1

UNIT

Prepared by: Eileen Daniel, *SUNY College at Brockport*

Promoting Healthy Behavior Change

"Those of us who protect our health daily and those of us who put our health in constant jeopardy have exactly the same mortality: 100 percent. The difference, of course, is the timing." This quotation from Elizabeth M. Whelan, ScD, MPH, reminds us that we must all face the fact that we are going to die sometime. The question that is decided by our behavior is when and, to a certain extent, how. This book, and especially this unit, is designed to assist students to develop the cognitive skills and knowledge that, when put to use, help make the moment of our death come as late as possible in our lives and maintain our health as long as possible. While we cannot control many of the things that happen to us, we must all strive to accept personal responsibility for, and make informed decisions about, things that we can control. This is no minor task, but it is one in which the potential reward is life itself. Perhaps the best way to start this process is by educating ourselves on the relative risks associated with the various behaviors and lifestyle choices we make. To minimize all the risks to life and health would be to significantly limit the quality of our lives, and while this might be a choice that some would make, it certainly is not the goal of health education. A more logical approach to risk reduction would be to educate the public on the relative risks associated with various behaviors and lifestyle choices so that they are capable of making informed decisions. While it may seem obvious that certain behaviors, such as smoking, entail a high level of risk, the significance of others such as toxic waste sites and food additives are frequently blown out of proportion to the actual risks involved. The net result of this type of distortion is that many Americans tend to minimize the dangers of known hazards such as tobacco and alcohol and focus attention instead on potentially minor health hazards over which they have little or no control.

Educating the public on the relative risk of various health behaviors is only part of the job that health educators must tackle in order to assist individuals in making informed choices regarding their health. They must also teach the skills that will enable people to evaluate the validity and significance of new information as it becomes available. Just how important informed decision making is in our daily lives is evidenced by the numerous health-related media announcements and articles that fill our newspapers, magazines, and television broadcasts. Rather than informing and enlightening the public on significant new medical discoveries, many of these announcements do little more than add to the level of confusion or exaggerate or sensationalize health issues.

Let's assume for a minute that the scientific community is in general agreement that certain behaviors clearly promote our health while others damage our health. Given this information, are you likely to make adjustments to your lifestyle to comply with the findings? Logic would suggest that of course you would, but experience has taught us that information alone isn't enough to bring about behavioral change in many people. Why is it that so many people continue to make bad choices regarding their health behaviors when they are fully aware of the risks involved? And why do women take better care of themselves than men? Health behaviors such as alcohol, substance abuse, and lack of consistent health care among men, which contributes to men getting sick younger and dying faster than women. We can take vows to try and undo or minimize the negative health behaviors of our past. However, while strategies such as these may work for those who feel they are at risk, how do we help those who do not feel that they are at risk, or those who feel that it is too late in their lives for the changes to matter? For students, college is a place to learn and grow, but for many it becomes four years of bad diet, too little sleep, and too much alcohol. These negative health behaviors affect not only the students' health but also their grades too.

Article   Prepared by: Eileen L. Daniel, *SUNY Brockport*

Crimes of the Heart

It's time society stopped reinforcing the bad behavior that leads to heart disease—and pursued policies to prevent it.

WALTER C. WILLETT AND ANNE UNDERWOOD

Learning Outcomes

After reading this article, you will be able to:

- Explain how changing an area's environment helps to support healthier lifestyles.

- Describe lifestyles conducive to heart health.

- Describe what specific public health measures can contribute to healthy behaviors.

Until last year, the residents of Albert Lea, Mn., were no healthier than any other Americans. Then the city became the first American town to sign on to the AARP/Blue Zones Vitality Project—the brainchild of writer Dan Buettner, whose 2008 book, *The Blue Zones,* detailed the health habits of the world's longest-lived people. His goal was to bring the same benefits to middle America—not by forcing people to diet and exercise, but by changing their everyday environments in ways that encourage a healthier lifestyle.

What followed was a sort of townwide makeover. The city laid new sidewalks linking residential areas with schools and shopping centers. It built a recreational path around a lake and dug new plots for community gardens. Restaurants made healthy changes to their menus. Schools banned eating in hallways (reducing the opportunities for kids to munch on snack food) and stopped selling candy for fundraisers. (They sold wreaths instead.) More than 2,600 of the city's 18,000 residents volunteered, too, selecting from more than a dozen heart-healthy measures—for example, ridding their kitchens of supersize dinner plates (which encourage larger portions) and forming "walking schoolbuses" to escort kids to school on foot.

The results were stunning. In six months, participants lost an average of 2.6 pounds and boosted their estimated life expectancy by 3.1 years. Even more impressive, health-care claims for city and school employees fell for the first time in a decade—by 32 percent over 10 months. And benefits didn't accrue solely to volunteers. Thanks to the influence of social networks, says Buettner, "even the curmudgeons who didn't want to be involved ended up modifying their behaviors."

Isn't it time we all followed Albert Lea's example? Diet and exercise programs routinely fail not for lack of willpower, but because the society in which we live favors unhealthy behaviors. In 2006, cardiovascular disease cost $403 billion in medical bills and lost productivity. By 2025 an aging population is expected to drive up the total by as much as 54 percent. But creative government programs could help forestall the increases—and help our hearts, too. A few suggestions:

Require graphic warnings on cigarette packages. It's easy to disregard a black-box warning that smoking is "hazardous to your health." It's not so easy to dismiss a picture of gangrenous limbs, diseased hearts, or chests sawed open for autopsy. These are exactly the types of images that the law now requires on cigarette packages in Brazil. In Canada, such warning images must cover at least half the wrapping. In 2001, the year after the Canadian law took effect, 38 percent of smokers who tried to quit cited the images. Think of it as truth in advertising.

Sponsor "commitment contracts" to quit smoking. Yale economist Dean Karlan spearheaded a test program in the Philippines in which smokers who wanted to quit deposited the money they would have spent on cigarettes into a special bank account. After six months those who had succeeded got their money back, while those who had failed lost it. Such a program could be run here by public-health clinics and offer greater incentives, such as letting winners divvy up the money forfeited by losers. Even without such an enhancement, says Karlan, "Filipino participants were 39 percent more likely to quit than those who were not offered the option."

Subsidize whole grains, fruits, and vegetables in the food-stamp program. The underprivileged tend to have disastrously unhealthy diets, and no wonder: $1 will buy 100 calories of carrots—or 1,250 calories of cookies and chips. The government should offer incentives for buying produce. The Wholesome Wave Foundation has shown the way in 12 states, providing vouchers redeemable at farmers' markets to people in the SNAP program (the official name for food stamps). "We've seen purchases of fruits and vegetables double and triple among recipients," says president and CEO Michel Nischan.

Set targets for salt reduction. The average American consumes twice the recommended daily maximum of sodium, most of it from processed foods. The result: high blood pressure, heart attacks, and strokes. But New York City is leading a campaign to encourage food manufacturers to reduce added sodium over the next five years. Consumers will barely notice the changes because they will occur so gradually. The FDA should follow New York's lead.

One urban-planning expert advocates a "road diet" in which towns eliminate a lane or two of traffic and substitute sidewalks. "When roads slim down, so do people," he says.

Incorporate physical education into No Child Left Behind. American children may be prepping like crazy for standardized tests, but they're seriously lagging in physical fitness. Regular exercise improves mood, concentration, and academic achievement. It can also help reverse the growing trend toward type 2 diabetes and early heart disease in children and teenagers.

Require that sidewalks and bike lanes be part of every federally funded road project. The government already spends 1 percent of transportation dollars on such projects. It should increase the level to 2 to 3 percent. When sidewalks are built in neighborhoods and downtowns, people start walking. "The big win for city government is that anything built to a walkable scale leases out for three to five times more money, with more tax revenue on less infrastructure," says Dan Burden, executive director of the Walkable and Livable Communities Institute. He recommends a "road diet" in which towns eliminate a lane or two of downtown traffic and substitute sidewalks. "When roads slim down, so do people," he says.

It's all reasonable. But Dan Buettner isn't waiting for any of these measures to surmount the inevitable industry hurdles. This year he's looking to scale up the Blue Zones Vitality Project to a city of 100,000 or more. "If this works, it could provide a template for the government that's replicable across the country," says his colleague Ben Leedle, CEO of Healthways, which is developing the next phase of the project. The challenges will be much steeper in large cities. But with measures like these, we could one day find ourselves growing fitter without specifically dieting or exercising. Finally, a New Year's resolution we can all keep.

Critical Thinking

1. What does a healthy environment consist of?
2. How can communities go about changing their environments to support a healthy lifestyle?
3. What are examples of public health improvements?

Create Central

www.mhhe.com/createcentral

Internet References

American Heart Association
   www.amhrt.org
U.S. National Institutes of Health (NIH)
   www.nih.gov

WALTER C. WILLETT is a physician, chair of the department of nutrition at the Harvard School of Public Health, and coauthor of *The Fertility Diet*. **ANNE UNDERWOOD** is a Newsweek contributor.

Article   Prepared by: Eileen L. Daniel, *SUNY College at Brockport*

American Plague

MICHAEL HOBBES

Learning Outcomes

After reading this article, you will be able to:

- Understand why the per-capita rate of AIDS is higher in the United States than in other developed countries.

- Understand the role needle exchanges play in the prevention of AIDS.

- Have knowledge of the health behaviors that reduce the incidence of AIDS.

So I'm getting AIDS tested the other day in Berlin. I'm sitting in the waiting room and feeling like a Bad Gay, because I've lived here for three years and this is my first time getting tested.

I'm surrounded by all these scared-straight brochures about HIV and AIDS in Germany. Prevalence rates, treatment options, prevention methods, names and addresses of support groups. "Since the start of the epidemic," one of them says, "more than 27,000 people have died of AIDS in Germany."

Wait, that sounds triumphantly low for a country of 80 million people. I pull out my phone and check the Centers for Disease Control and Prevention (CDC) website, which tells me that, in the United States, 636,000 people have died since the epidemic began. That's 23 times higher than Germany, for a country with four times the population.

This makes no sense. Germany has big cities, it has gay men and sex workers and drug users, it has all the same temptations for them to be uncareful that the United States does. How could so many fewer people have died?

Maybe it's a fluke. I visit the Public Health England website and it says 21,000 people have died of AIDS there in total. If the rates were the same as the United States, it would be 128,000.

The further down the Google-hole I go, the more mind-boggling the numbers get. Since the beginning of the epidemic, AIDS has claimed more people in New York City than in Spain, Italy, the Netherlands, and Switzerland *combined*.

The next day I start asking epidemiologists about this divergence. The first thing they tell me is that it is real, even accounting for differences in methodology.[1] Scan the columns on the stats sheets–incidence, prevalence, and deaths–and you find the United States with a two-digit lead going right back to the start of the epidemic. Still now, no matter how much we've learned about how to prevent and treat AIDS, the United States loses more than 15,000 people to it each year. Germany and the United Kingdom lose fewer than 800.[2]

The second thing they tell me is why. AIDS is the same virus no matter what country you're in. But when it arrived in the United States, how it spread, who got it, and why–that's more complicated, and not entirely flattering.

Looking at the data on aids deaths, you see that the virus hit the United States early–and hard. In 1982, the first year of nationwide CDC surveillance, 451 people died of AIDS in America. Just five died in Britain. In 1985, when Germany started reporting, it had 170 AIDS deaths. The United Sates had almost 7,000.

Jonathan Engel, the author of *The Epidemic: A Global History of AIDS,* walks me through the timeline: AIDS first appears in humans in central Africa in the 1950s. A few isolated cases make it from there to the United States and Western Europe, but it fails to catch fire. The virus finally finds a host country in Haiti, ferried to and fro in the veins of guest workers in Africa. By the mid-'70s, Port-au-Prince is a popular tourist and cruise-ship destination–"a gay Bangkok" is how Engel's book puts it–and the virus jumps from male prostitutes to gay American vacationers, to their friends and lovers back home.

Or abroad. One of the first U.K. surveillance reports, from 1983, announces 14 cases of AIDS, then adds: "seven of the cases were known to have had contact with US nationals, suggesting that the present UK situation is simply part of the American epidemic."

But it isn't just that the virus arrived in the United States earlier. As Dr. James Curran, dean of the Rollins School of Public Health at Emory University, points out, Belgium and France had significant central African and Haitian populations; Haiti was a destination for them, too. "But the disease wasn't able to spread through them like it went through American gays," he says.

Which leads to the next factor explaining the larger scale of the HIV epidemic in the United States: the clustering of our high-risk populations. The United States has more people than any Western European country, as well as more mobility, giving rise to larger numbers of and more tightly grouped gay men and intravenous-drug users. Engel's book quotes Frances Fitz-Gerald, writing in *The New Yorker* in 1986, saying "the sheer concentration of gay people in San Francisco may have had no parallel in history."

These clusters were also engaged in riskier behavior. The United States had higher rates of STDs and intravenous-drug use (epidemiologists used to call shooting up "the American disease") before AIDS arrived. All of this, combined with the virus's devious characteristic of being maximally spreadable right after infection, laid the infrastructure for the disease to maraud through one population and jump to others.

The closest thing to a natural experiment on this clustering phenomenon is right in my own backyard. East and West Berlin had the same language, history, and culture—everything but the political and economic structures that allowed gay men to find each other and addicts to find drugs.

"Before the Berlin Wall came down, East Berlin had two gay cafés and two gay bars, for a population of 1.3 million people," says Michael Bochow, a sociologist in Berlin who has been researching HIV in Germany since the beginning of the epidemic. "East Berlin had no bathhouse, no bar with a back room."

Guys in East Berlin were still hooking up with each other—of course they were—but the low labor mobility, combined with the logistical barriers to participating in gay life and getting intravenous drugs, kept clusters from forming.

In 1989, when the Berlin Wall came down, West Germany had about 35,000 people infected with HIV. East Germany had fewer than 500.

I don't want to overstate the case here. This clustering effect is almost inherently unmeasurable (drug use and gayness weren't exactly on the census), and there's no way to know if San Francisco and New York really had higher proportions of gay people than London, Paris, or Berlin. We do know that the virus spread faster through U.S. cities than European ones, but we don't know, may never know, precisely why.

The third explanation for how the HIV epidemic in the United States got so severe so early has to do with intravenous-drug use—and the policies that tried to prevent it. One of the most staggering numbers I came across was that, from the beginning of the epidemic until HIV treatment became widely available in 1996, 124,800 intravenous-drug users were diagnosed with HIV in the United States. In the United Kingdom, it was just 3,400.

Don Des Jarlais, research director of the de Rothschild Chemical Dependency Institute in New York, says HIV in drug users followed a similar trajectory as HIV in gay men. It arrived earlier than in Europe, and it had a more fertile spreading ground thanks to the higher prevalence of drug use.

No one knew how severe the epidemic was among drug users until 1984, when the still-under-development antibody test found that 50 percent of drug users in New York City and Edinburgh and 30 percent in Amsterdam were already infected. (Des Jarlais says genetic tests have since shown that the epidemic in Amsterdam originated in New York.)

Here's where the differences come in. Almost immediately after those first tests, Western European countries installed needle-exchange programs, gave out free syringes, and established opiate-substitution treatment. Germany even got needle vending machines. By 1997, England and Wales were giving out 25 million free syringes per year. Anything to keep the virus from spreading, even if it meant making it a little easier to be a heroin addict that day.

The United States, on the other hand, refused to provide federal funds for needle exchanges or even fund research into whether they were effective. Exchanges were established in some cities—by 1990, New York City was distributing 250,000 syringes a year—but they never achieved the coverage of the countrywide programs in Western Europe.

This sounds like just another episode to file under "Western Europe enlightened, U.S. myopic," but remember how different the context was. The mid-'80s was America's heyday of stigmatizing drug users. This was the era of "Just Say No," Nancy Reagan on "Diff'rent Strokes," McGruff the Crime Dog. America was in the middle of a crack epidemic. All of the negative impacts of that epidemic—the gang violence to prolong it, the War on Drugs to end it—were concentrated in poor, mostly African American communities. Just possessing syringes was illegal in most states. Handing them out in the millions, facilitating one epidemic to end another, seemed like a cruel joke.

"They were saying, 'Why don't you just get rid of drug use from our communities?'" Des Jarlais says. "'You're letting these drugs come in because you don't care about our communities, and now you want to make things worse by giving out syringes.'" This gave national politicians the excuse they needed. The ban on federal funding for needle exchanges wasn't lifted until 2009.

As I'm calling up epidemiologists, hearing these explanations, it feels like something's missing: What about all those public-information campaigns I remember from growing up?

After-school specials, PSAs, the time my Seattle public middle school gave us all a stack of condoms and told us to put them on fruit at home? Did Western European countries implement different, more effective kinds of programs?

Prevention efforts did indeed differ among countries. Germany threw funding at gay community NGOs and gave them carte blanche to devise their own prevention projects. Britain put a John Hurt voice-over on top of Mordor imagery, called it "AIDS: Don't Die of Ignorance," and beamed it to the whole country.

Engel points out that, in the United States, despite Ronald Reagan's sloth-like funding of HIV research and the government's stinginess in supporting NGOs, gay activists were on the streets and in the bathhouses from the earliest stages of the epidemic, condoms in hand, telling people how to protect themselves. At the national level, C. Everett Koop sent a pamphlet to every household in America (literally!), telling them about the disease and achieving the goal, like the British mass campaigns, of scaring us all shitless.

The efforts of gay community groups during this time have been (rightly) lionized in movies like *We Were Here* and *How to Survive a Plague*. Less well known is that intravenous-drug users were also educating each other about how to reduce risks. Drug users started sharing needles with fewer partners, even setting up their own needle exchanges, pilfering clean needles from hospitals, or importing them from Canada. Des Jarlais told me about doctors who used to place boxes of clean syringes around emergency rooms, knowing they'd be taken by drug users and sold or given onward.

The messages and methodologies of these efforts may have differed among the United States, the United Kingdom, and Germany, but their effect appears to be equally decisive. By the mid-'80s, gay men and drug users knew about HIV, they knew about their risks, and they were making changes to reduce them. In all three countries, HIV incidence–the number of people contracting HIV each year–peaked in the mid-'80s, then started to drop as people derisked their sex and drug use.

But for those already infected, none of that mattered; the number of deaths rose steadily through the late '80s and early '90s. The avalanche had been loosed, and there was little anyone–NGOs, doctors, politicians–could do to stop it.

Graphs of aids deaths in almost every developed country look like a wave about to break on the shore. Starting from zero, deaths rise steadily through the '80s, a bit faster in the '90s, then suddenly, around 1995 or 1996, plummet downward.

"That's the beginning of the HAART ERA," says Caroline Sabin, a professor of medical statistics and epidemiology at University College London. She's talking about highly active anti-retroviral therapy, the cocktail of medications that, 15 years after the virus appeared, marked the first truly effective rampart against it.

The next thing you notice about those graphs is that death rates in the United States didn't fall to the same lows as the rest of the developed world. (Check out how great the discrepancy is in the chart.) Sabin points me to a 2013 study that found the United States with four-year HIV mortality rates roughly equal to those in South Africa.

And it's not just the death rates that stayed high. In 2010, the United States had 47,500 new HIV infections. The entire European Union–with a population more than one and a half times that of the United States–had just 31,400.

So what gives? "Keeping people alive is about getting them diagnosed, getting them into care, then making sure they stay in care and on HAART," Sabin says. "And that, unfortunately, is where the U.S. differs from the U.K." It turns out that, just as the AIDS virus seems almost designed to perfectly exploit the weaknesses of the human immune system, treating it seems designed to exploit the weaknesses of our national health care system.

Let's start with diagnosis, the first stage of what epidemiologists call the "cascade of care." An undiagnosed HIV infection is a ticking time bomb for the people carrying it. Each day that goes by, the virus chips away at their immune systems, reducing life expectancies and increasing the cost and chances of complications once they finally get on treatment. They also, crucially, remain more infectious. Up to 50 percent of new HIV infections are transmitted by people who don't know they have it.

Getting an HIV test is, logistically speaking, pretty easy in all three countries. The next stage of the cascade, getting linked to another round of tests and into treatment, is more challenging. In the United Kingdom and Germany, if you test positive for HIV, you'll immediately be referred to an HIV clinic for tests to measure how much of the virus is in your blood and how well your immune system is holding up.

Three-quarters of Brits diagnosed with HIV get to this next stage of care within two weeks, and 97 percent make it within three months. This is not just some nationwide codification of English politeness. Clinics that provide testing are required to get HIV-positive people to the next round of tests or they don't get fully reimbursed. If you screen positive and skip your viral-load test, you'll get a call from the clinic asking why you didn't show up. Some testing centers will walk you straight to the hospital to make an appointment.

In the United States, only 65 percent of people with HIV get linked to a hospital or clinic within three months. A survey in Philadelphia published in 2010 found that the *median* time between diagnosis and treatment was eight months. The effect of the wait can be devastating. A 2008 study found that gay men who had full-blown AIDS before they were diagnosed were 75 percent more likely to die within three years, even if they got on treatment. For people whose viral load is high and T-cell count is low, getting on HAART is like putting on sunscreen after they've already been at the beach for two hours.

The next stage of HIV care is receiving HAART pills and staying on them. People who get medication rapidly and take it consistently aren't just less likely to die of the virus; they're less likely to pass it on. The epidemio-speak term for this is having a "suppressed viral load": The levels of the virus in your blood are so low that tests can't pick them up anymore–and your sex and drug partners are also a lot less likely to.

This is the holy grail of HIV treatment, and arriving there requires at least 90 percent adherence to the pill regimen. If you stop taking the pills then start again, or forget to take them more than once in awhile, the virus could spike or you could develop resistance to the drugs.

In Britain and Germany, two-thirds of people with HIV have a prescription for HAART. In America? Only one-third. Forty-eight percent of Brits with HIV have a suppressed viral load. In the United States, only 25 percent of them do.

The most obvious reason for this gap is cost. In the United Kingdom, HIV treatment is completely free. Some clinics even reimburse you for your bus fare. In Germany, drugs might cost you a co-pay of 5 euros ($7.50), but that's subsidized if you're unemployed or below an income threshold.

Neither the CDC nor the National Institutes of Health tracks the out-of-pocket costs of anti-retrovirals, but Stephanie Cohen of the San Francisco Department of Public Health tells me that someone without insurance and earning too much to qualify for Medicaid could pay as much as $2,000 a month. And that's just the pills. Clinic visits, infections, hospitalizations: The costs of treatment multiply as fast as the virus does without it.

But before we all rush to Twitter to make easy political points about how America is the land of the nothing-is-free, again consider the context. The United States has put tremendous effort and resources ($14 billion per year now) into HIV treatment and has considerable achievements to show for it. Medicaid covers HAART for the poor. The Ryan White Program,

with $2.4 billion in annual federal funding, provides it for the less poor. Some cities, including San Francisco, have better treatment stats than the United Kingdom or Germany.

Consider, too, the scale of the epidemic in the United States. When HAART first became available in 1995, the United Kingdom had around 30,000 people diagnosed with HIV. Germany had 38,000. The United States had 759,000 and more new infections every year than the United Kingdom or Germany had in total. Providing testing, treatment, and follow-up to all those people would have been a Hoover Dam–size investment. One we were not, as a country, willing to make.

It's not just a question of money or political will. In the last two decades, as the United States has put so much effort into filling the cracks in HIV care, the virus has moved into the populations most likely to fall into them.

From its origins as a concentrated, urban epidemic, HIV has migrated resolutely outward and southward. "People test positive and they just go home. Then they come and get tested again," says Susan Reif of Duke University's Center for Health Policy and Inequality Research.

I didn't know it was possible to get a lump in your throat from lists of two-digit numbers, but then Reif shows me the data on HIV in the Deep South versus the rest of the country. HIV prevalence: 2.3 cases per 100,000 people in Vermont; 36.6 in Louisiana. Death rates: 9.6 per 1,000 person-years in Idaho; 32.9 in Mississippi. In 2011, nine of the top ten cities for new HIV infections were in the South. In Louisiana, only 68 percent of people with HIV *saw a doctor* that year.

Meanwhile, in 2012, AIDS dropped off the list of New York City's top ten causes of death for the first time since 1983.

As the geography of HIV has shifted, so have its demographics. Ethnic minorities, rural drug users, and impoverished heterosexuals: The virus has found the people least likely to seek–and have access to–health insurance and specialized clinics.

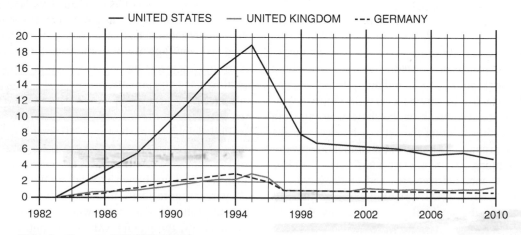

Aids deaths per 100,000 people.

You could drown in the numbers on this if you wanted to, but a study that stuck out to me was one from 2012 that found uneducated black men had an AIDS mortality rate 30 times higher than educated white men. Among uneducated black women, it found that the introduction of HAART barely dropped mortality rates at all. In 2011, AIDS was the ninth-highest cause of death for blacks and twenty-fourth for whites.

Higher levels of stigma, poor infrastructure for treatment in rural areas, abstinence-only education–Reif says they all contribute to the higher rates of diagnoses and deaths. Syringe exchanges are still illegal in almost every Southern state. An estimated 60,000 uninsured or low-income people with HIV live in states that have rejected the Medicaid expansion under Obamacare.

"Each state has a different Medicaid program in terms of whether you're eligible and what your co-pays are," she says. "Some Medicaid programs will only cover a certain number of drugs. So you get five. And you have to pick which five."

Just as explaining the differences between Europe and America requires accounting for the weight of their histories and social structures, so does explaining the differences between the South and the rest of the United States. "The disease burden in the South is high for other diseases, too," Reif says. "A lot of it goes back to institutionalized racism, poverty, the legacy of Tuskegee. There's a lack of trust in health care. The states say they don't have the money [to expand Medicaid]–and there's some truth to that."

No health care system in the world has solved the problem of AIDS. The United Kingdom and Germany have gaps in their cascades, too. They struggle to control costs and reach marginalized populations the same as the States. They just have less margin to reach.

But in trying to explain these numbers, I don't want to excuse them. Some of the reasons the AIDS epidemic has been so devastating in the United States were chosen for us by history. Others we have chosen ourselves.

"At the end of the day, it's best understood as a function of health disparities writ large," says Chris Beyrer, the director of the Johns Hopkins Fogarty AIDS International Training and Research Program. The core difference between the United States and Western Europe, he says, is that "we're a much bigger, much more complex, and much more unjust country."

Critical Thinking

1. Why do minority men have an AIDS mortality rate 30 times higher than white males?
2. What role does lack of national health insurance play in the high rates of AIDS deaths in the United States?
3. What health behaviors play a role in reducing the spread of HIV?

Internet References

Centers for Disease Control and Prevent
  http://www.cdc.gov/hiv/statistics/
National Institutes of Health
  http://aidsinfo.nih.gov/
World Health Organization
  http://www.who.int/topics/hiv_aids/en/

Notes

1. Each country has a slightly different system for reporting HIV cases and AIDS deaths, and epidemiologists are often reluctant to make apples-to-apples comparisons: "It's more like Red Delicious to Granny Smith," one of them told me.

   It's better to think of the surveillance numbers as a range, subject to updates and back-calculations as more data comes in. But still, the differences in measurement are nowhere near enough to account for the gaps among countries. Measuring my income against, say, Oprah Winfrey's would be subject to methodological fuzziness, too–she has capital gains, real estate appreciation, and tax acrobatics–but it's still fair to say she makes more money than I do.

2. I'm comparing the United States with these two countries for the sake of simplicity and because I speak the languages and have access to epidemiologists there. The United Kingdom and Germany are on the high and low side, respectively, of the severity of the AIDS epidemic in Western Europe, but they're not outliers by any means. You could compare the United States with France, the Netherlands, Italy, wherever, and you'd come up with basically the same story.

MICHAEL HOBBES is a human rights consultant in Berlin. He has written for SLATE, PACIFIC STANDARD, and THE BILLFOLD.

Article   Prepared by: Eileen Daniel, *SUNY College at Brockport*

Solve Your Energy Crisis

A Guide to Finding—and Fixing— the Cause of Your Fatigue

CONSUMER REPORTS ON HEALTH

Learning Outcomes

After reading this article, you will be able to:

- Understand the causes of low energy.

- Explain ways to modify sleep habits.

- Describe techniques to enhance energy.

National survey results suggest that "utterly exhausted" may be America's new normal. In one survey, 37 percent of working adults admitted they'd felt fatigued in the previous two weeks. A report by the national Centers for Disease Control and Prevention found that 16 percent of women and 12 percent of men ages 45 to 64 described themselves as wiped out in the prior three months. That's worrisome, because letting fatigue drag on can mess with your mood (and may even boost your risk for depression), as well as with your health, weight, work performance, and sex life.

But there's no need to live in a dog-tired state. "When you find and fix the real cause of your fatigue, you can recover your energy and feel great again," says Martin Surks, MD, program director of the Endocrinology Division at Montefiore and the Albert Einstein College of Medicine. Assuming you're logging 7 to 9 hours of sleep time (and if you aren't, that's what you need to address first), follow these steps, in order, to help you get to the root of your weariness.

Step 1 Improve Your Sleep Hygiene

Sometimes it's not lack of sleep that causes fatigue—it's the lack of refreshing, high-quality slumber. You want to spend the optimal amount of time in deep, restorative sleep and minimize fragmented sleep. (There are several phone apps, such as SleepCycle, that can track sleep quality. The activity monitor Fitbit One does, too.) "Whenever someone is

---

Beverage Boost

What's the best thing to drink when you're feeling zapped? Here, the pros and cons to the most commonly touted liquid energizers.

Water

This should be your first choice. Being dehydrated, even mildly, may lead to fatigue, lack of energy, loss of concentration, and irritability, studies show.

Tea

It has enough caffeine to perk you up but not enough to cause the jitters. Green tea has 24 to 40 milligrams per eight-ounce cup. Black tea has 14 to 61 milligrams.

Coffee

A cup has 95 to 200 milligrams; most adults should have no more than 400 milligrams per day. It takes almost 6 hours for half of the caffeine you consume to be metabolized by your body, so having it too late in the day can disrupt sleep.

Energy Drinks

Energy drink labels don't always list the caffeine count. Our tests showed that they can have more than double the amount in coffee. Some may contain undesirable ingredients such as sugar. If you're looking for a pick-me-up, you're better off with a cup of tea or coffee.

Is There Such a Thing as an Energy Pill?

Many products promise to fend off fatigue and give you some oomph when you're dragging. Do they work? Are they safe? Here's what you need to know:

Vitamin B12 Shots

How they work: B12 helps your body make red blood cells, convert food into fuel, and maintain healthy nerve cells, all of which can have an effect on energy.

   Our take: If you're deficient in vitamin B12, oral supplements have been shown to be as effective as shots, but if you aren't, neither shots nor supplements are likely to raise your energy level.

Armodafinil (Nuvigil) and Modafinil (Provigil)

How they work: These prescription stimulants are FDA-approved for excessive sleepiness due to narcolepsy, sleep apnea, and shift work. They're used off-label to ease fatigue in people with depression, multiple sclerosis, and other conditions.

   Our take: They're costly, and have side effects, such as headaches, severe skin rashes, and tremors. They shouldn't be used in place of getting the sleep you need.

Ginseng

How it works: It's used for fatigue in traditional Chinese medicine, but the exact mechanism is unknown.

   Our take: Short-term use is safe, but it may cause insomnia and blood-pressure changes. Ask a doctor before trying herbal remedies.

Tired? The Health Problems You Need to Check

If you have fatigue and . . .
difficulty concentrating, sleep disruption, loss of pleasure in activities you once enjoyed
It may be . . .
Depression

If you have fatigue and . . .
morning headaches, excessive daytime sleepiness, dozing while driving, loud snoring, you wake up at night gasping for breath
It may be . . .
Obstructive sleep apnea

If you have fatigue and . . .
frequent urination, increased thirst and hunger, blurry vision, irritability, unexplained weight loss
It may be . . .
Diabetes

If you have fatigue and . . .
weight gain, puffiness, cold sensitivity, dry skin or hair, muscle cramps
It may be . . .
Underactive thyroid

If you have fatigue and . . .
loss of appetite, fever, nausea, dark urine, clay-colored slools
It may be . . .
Hepatitis

If you have fatigue and . . .
muscle weakness, shortness of breath, you look pale
It may be . . .
Anemia

experiencing fatigue on a regular basis, they should look at their sleeping habits," says Babak Mokhlesi, MD, director of the Sleep Disorders Center at the University of Chicago. For example, many people believe that a nightcap before bed will help them sleep soundly, but alcohol can cause disrupted sleep. Snoring bedmates, letting pets sleep with you, and bright lights could be causing you to toss and turn at night without your realizing it.

Step 2 Consult Your Doc

If you still feel pooped during the day after two weeks of sleep upgrades, it's time for a visit to your doctor. Fatigue is a symptom (not a condition) of many treatable health problems. "See your primary physician rather than a sleep specialist," Surks says. "He or she can ask questions that will help pinpoint the cause and run tests to rule out a wide range of conditions like depression, diabetes, or hypothyroidism [underactive thyroid]."

Step 3 Review Your Meds

Bring a list of the drugs you take to your appointment or simply toss the pill bottles into a bag (a drug review with your doctor is a smart thing to do every 6 to 12 months anyway). From antidepressants to blood pressure drugs to cholesterol-lowering statins, many common prescription medications can leave you dragging through the day. Drugs can cause fatigue in many ways, including depressing the central nervous system, lowering heart rate, or reducing the body's stores of nutrients, such as magnesium or potassium. If it turns out that you take a potentially energy-draining drug, ask about alternatives.

Step 4 Move a Little More

We know: "Get up and exercise" is the last thing you want to hear when you're beat. But believe us, it's worth a try. Exercise seems to create energy and alleviate fatigue by reducing stress, helping you sleep, and increasing circulation so that your muscles receive more oxygen and nutrients. And you don't have to train for a marathon to see the effects. In a small University of Georgia study, chronically tired couch potatoes embarked on a low- or moderate-intensity exercise routine three times per week for six weeks while a control group didn't exercise. The low-intensity group got the best results: a 65 percent drop in fatigue. The moderate-intensity group improved too, but less so. The researchers think that's because some of those people may have been working out too hard for their fitness level.

Even easier exercise may have a benefit. When researchers at New York City's Hospital for Special Surgery put seniors on a gentle yoga or chair-based exercise routine, 39 percent reported an increase in energy after eight weeks. Research suggests that specially designed routines can ease tiredness for cancer survivors, people with chronic fatigue syndrome, and heart attack survivors.

Step 5 Clean up Your Diet

Stay fueled with regular meals and healthy snacks that are low in fat and packed with fiber (beans, fruits, whole grains, and vegetables). According to a recent Pennsylvania State University study, the more fat people eat at a meal, the sleepier they become afterward. Researchers from Australia and the U.K. found that people felt more alert in the morning after having a breakfast high in fiber and carbohydrates than they did when they had a high-fat or a high-carb, low-fiber meal. Beware of very high-protein diets; some evidence suggests that they can increase fatigue.

Step 6 Reorganize Your Day

Still having trouble after taking steps 1 through 5? You may think you're tired when you're actually tense. One in three people who say they're stressed attribute their fatigue to their mood, according to a survey from the American Psychological Association. "Stress feels like fatigue—you're not in control of your life, it takes longer to do things, and you may have trouble multitasking. It can also interfere with sleep and healthy eating, and leave you without enough time to recharge or relax," says sleep and fatigue researcher David Dinges, PhD, professor in the department of psychiatry at the University of Pennsylvania School of Medicine.

Adding "learn a stress-reduction technique" to your already-crazy to-do list isn't the answer. "Stop and think about what's important to you," Dinges recommends. Saying "no" more often to obligations and activities that aren't high priority gives you more time for the things you enjoy. Those are the ones that will rejuvenate you, he says. Another tip: spend some time each day away from your computer, tablet, or smartphone. "When you feel as if you always have to respond, always have to be in touch, it's hard to relax," he says. "I try to set aside part of the day when I get away from all the electronic noise."

Critical Thinking

1. What health problems are associated with fatigue?
2. Should individuals suffering from fatigue consider taking drugs to boost their energy?

Create Central

www.mhhe.com/createcentral

Internet References

Ace Fitness
   http://www.acefitness.org/acefit/fitness-programs-article/2742/ACEFit-workout-advice-and-exercise-tips
National Sleep Foundation
   http://sleepfoundation.org

Unit 2

UNIT

Prepared by: Eileen Daniel, *SUNY College at Brockport*

Stress and Mental Health

The brain is one organ that still mystifies and baffles the scientific community. While more has been learned about this organ in the last decade than in all the rest of recorded history, our understanding of the brain is still in its infancy. What has been learned, however, has spawned exciting new research and has contributed to the establishment of new disciplines, such as psychophysiology and psychoneuroimmunology (PNI).

Traditionally, the medical community has viewed health problems as either physical or mental and has treated each type separately. This dichotomy between the psyche (mind) and soma (body) is fading in the light of scientific data that reveal profound physiological changes associated with mood shifts. What are the physiological changes associated with stress? Hans Selye, the father of stress research, described stress as a nonspecific physiological response to anything that challenges the body. He demonstrated that this response could be elicited by both mental and physical stimuli. Stress researchers have come to regard this response pattern as the "flight-or-fight" response, perhaps an adaptive throwback to our primitive ancestors. Researchers now believe that repeated and prolonged activation of this response can trigger destructive changes in our bodies and contribute to the development of several chronic diseases. So profound is the impact of emotional stress on the body that current estimates suggest that approximately 90 percent of all doctor visits are for stress-related disorders. If emotional stress elicits a generalized physiological response, why are there so many different diseases associated with it? Many experts believe that the answer may best be explained by what has been termed "the weak organ theory." According to this theory, every individual has one organ system that is most susceptible to the damaging effects of prolonged stress.

Mental illness, which is generally regarded as a dysfunction of normal thought processes, has no single identifiable etiology. One may speculate that this is due to the complex nature of the organ system involved. There is also mounting evidence to suggest that there is an organic component to the traditional forms of mental illness such as schizophrenia, chronic depression, and manic depression. The fact that certain mental illnesses tend to occur within families has divided the mental health community into two camps: those who believe that there is a genetic factor operating and those who see the family tendency as more of a learned behavior. In either case, the evidence supports mental illness as another example of the weak-organ theory. The reason one person is more susceptible to the damaging effects of stress than another may not be altogether clear, but evidence is mounting that one's perception or attitude plays a key role in the stress equation. A prime example demonstrating this relationship comes from the research that relates cardiovascular disease to stress. The realization that our attitude has such a significant impact on our health has led to a burgeoning new movement in psychology termed "positive psychology." Dr. Martin Segilman, professor of psychology at the University of Pennsylvania and father of the positive psychology movement, believes that optimism is a key factor in maintaining not only our mental health but our physical health as well. Dr. Segilman notes that while some people are naturally more optimistic than others, optimism can be learned.

One area in particular that appears to be influenced by the positive psychology movement is the area of stress management. Traditionally, stress management programs have focused on the elimination of stress but that is starting to change as new strategies approach stress as an essential component of life and a potential source of health. It is worth noting that this concept, of stress serving as a positive force in a person's life, was presented by Dr. Hans Selye in 1974 in his book *Stress without Distress*. Dr. Selye felt that there were three types of stress: negative stress (distress), normal stress, and positive stress (eustress). He maintained that positive stress not only increases a person's self-esteem but also serves to inoculate the person against the damaging effects of distress. Only time will tell if this change of focus, in the area of stress management, makes any real difference in patient outcome.

The causes of stress are many. Researchers have made significant strides in their understanding of the mechanisms that link emotional stress to physical ailments, but they are less clear on the mechanisms by which positive emotions bolster one's health. Although significant gains have been made in our understanding of the relationship between body and mind, much remains to be learned. What is known indicates that perception and one's attitude are the key elements in shaping our responses to stressors.

Article

Prepared by: Eileen Daniel, *SUNY College at Brockport*

Sound Mind, Sound Student Body

Challenges and Strategies for Managing the Growing Mental Health Crisis on College and University Campuses

KRISTEN DOMONELL

Learning Outcomes

After reading this article, you will be able to:

- Understand why there is an increased number of college students with mental illnesses.

- Describe why so many students with mental illness drop out before graduation.

- Explain ways in which colleges and universities can manage mental illness on their campuses.

B efore entering college, Nicole, a junior at a small liberal arts college in New England, had been getting treatment for anorexia for two years. Finding a college with adequate mental health services was one of her biggest concerns, so she was relieved when the director of counseling services at the college she selected promised her a full treatment, complete with a weekly dietician meeting and regular sessions with a psychiatrist and a therapist.

"I entered [college] full of hope, but was immediately disenchanted with the counselors," she says, noting that the dietician was in such high demand, she could only see her every three weeks. By the second semester of her freshman year, Nicole had relapsed.

"It was clear that there was no system in place," she says. "The physician did not find my symptoms serious enough, and the psychiatrist had found another job."

Nicole is now seeing a psychiatrist at school who she feels "makes a great effort to meet the medical needs of students on campus." Yet, she is still unsatisfied with the counseling services as a whole, specifically with graduate student interns working in the center who she feels are inexperienced and not equipped to diagnose complex disorders, let alone identify symptoms.

Nicole isn't alone in needing on-campus mental health services. One in four college-aged Americans has a diagnosable mental illness, and severe mental illness is more common among college students than it was a decade ago, according to the American Psychological Association. Meanwhile, state and local funding for higher education declined by 7 percent, to $81.2 billion, in 2012, and per-student funding dropped to the lowest level in 25 years, according to the State Higher Education Executive Officers Association.

With an increased demand for counseling services paired with budget restraints, experiences like Nicole's aren't uncommon.

Why the Increase?

Early intervention and a decreased stigma surrounding mental illness are two reasons campus counseling centers are seeing an increased demand.

After the shootings at **Virginia Tech** and **Northern Illinois University** in 2007 and 2008, most institutions began creating behavioral intervention teams—called early intervention teams, care teams, or threat assessment teams, depending on the campus.

"These intervention teams are keeping students from falling through the cracks—which is a good thing—but it increases the demands on counseling centers," explains Dan L. Jones, president of the Association for University and College Counseling Center Directors.

"It's kind of like a small town with four-lane highways coming into it. All the traffic is able to get into town, and then there's nowhere for it to go," explains Jones, who serves as director of the Counseling & Psychological Services Center at **Appalachian State University** (N.C.), as well.

A decrease in the stigma surrounding mental illness is also responsible for the increased services demand, as more students visit counseling centers from self-referrals.

"This generation of students seems more willing to seek counselling," says Jones. "There used to be more stigma to getting counseling, and since the stigma has diminished, that leads to more counseling."

Difficulty Meeting the Need

A 2012 survey by the American College Counseling Association found that more than one-third (37.4 percent) of college students seeking help have severe psychological problems, up from 16 percent in 2000. Of the 293 counseling centers surveyed, more than three-quarters reported more crises requiring immediate response than in the past five years.

Despite the increased need, tight budgets aren't allowing for many counseling staff hires to pick up the slack, with the number of counselors increasing only marginally over the past 20 or 30 years, shares Drew Walther, national chapter director for Active Minds, Inc., a mental health advocacy organization with more than 400 campus chapters dedicated to outreach.

Active Minds exists to help remove the stigma and start a larger conversation about the issues surrounding mental health. But it also helps fill a hole in the need for outreach. As counseling centers get busier, counselors who would normally be promoting available campus services wind up spending all their time fulfilling an increased need for therapy sessions, so outreach falls to the wayside.

Even with counselors working full throttle, students are still not able to receive as much help as they need. In non-emergency situations, it's common for students to have to sit on a waiting list for a month before getting their first therapy session, and about half of institutions use a short-term model, where students are only allowed 6 to 12 sessions per academic year, shares Jones.

Last February, before hiring a new staff member and taking on additional trainees to help with the client load, Appalachian State referred out 60 percent of the students who came in. Even after referrals, the center still had a waiting list 70 people long, shares Jones.

"Therapy works best in long chunks, and if you're only getting six sessions, how much progress can you be making?" points out Walther.

The most recent AUCCCD survey shows that more institutions are adding counseling positions, which could signal that administrators recognize the greater need for mental health services. But Jones points out that the trend is coming on the heels of the economic downturn when resources remained static, but demand was steadily growing.

"It's not like there's some huge trend of hiring lots of counseling center people. It's just better than the past few years," says Jones. "It's improving, but it's far from meeting the demands of university counseling services to see all the students that need to be seen in a timely manner."

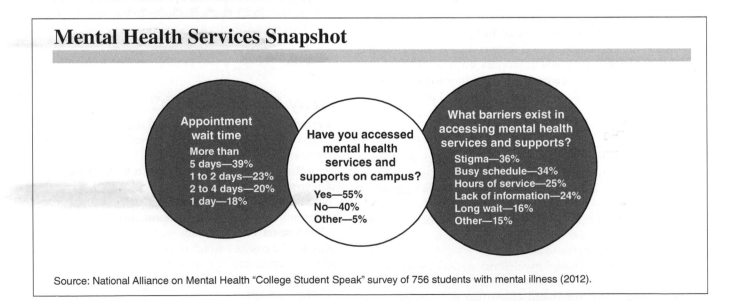

Mental Health Services Snapshot

Appointment wait time
More than
5 days—39%
1 to 2 days—23%
2 to 4 days—20%
1 day—18%

Have you accessed mental health services and supports on campus?
Yes—55%
No—40%
Other—5%

What barriers exist in accessing mental health services and supports?
Stigma—36%
Busy schedule—34%
Hours of service—25%
Lack of information—24%
Long wait—16%
Other—15%

Source: National Alliance on Mental Health "College Student Speak" survey of 756 students with mental illness (2012).

Consequences: Drop Outs, Violence, Litigation

A 2012 National Alliance on Mental Illness survey of 756 college students living with mental health conditions found that 64 percent of those who had stopped attending school within the past five years did so for a mental health-related reason. Half of those students didn't access mental health services and supports while they were attending.

In other words, at-risk students falling between the cracks and being unable to complete could harm a school's ability to retain students. In addition, without proper outreach and care, troubled students could harm themselves or others. Suicide is the second leading cause of death among college students (second to accidents), according to the Centers for Disease Control. Each year, 1,100 students die by suicide—figures that have remained steady in recent years.

There is also a risk for litigation. A noted 2002 wrongful-death lawsuit against MIT was a first in the higher education world. It implied that it's not only medical professionals who legally have a "special relationship" with their patients who could be held responsible for a death or other incident, but schools, administrators, and other employees could, as well.

In 2000, Elizabeth Shin, an MIT student, died from wounds inflicted by a fire in her dorm room. Shin had multiple suicide attempts and hospitalizations for mental illness in the past, although it was never proven whether her death was suicide or an accident.

In 2002, Shin's parents filed a $27 million wrongful death lawsuit against the institution, as well as administrators, campus police, and mental health employees, claiming their daughter did not receive enough mental health treatment and that the fire was not responded to properly. In 2006, the case was settled out of court for an undisclosed amount.

In the wake of a student suicide, the college or university, its administrators, and its other employees could be held financially responsible for the death—not just medical professionals who worked with the student.

"It was never clear what the results might have been, but it really shook up the university world," recalls Jones of AUCCCD.

A more recent example worth considering is the pending litigation over last year's movie theater shooting in Aurora, Colo.

against the **University of Colorado, Denver** and shooter James Holmes' psychiatrist Lynne Fenton.

Although Holmes left the institution a month before the tragedy, at least 20 tort claims have been filed saying that Fenton and the university's threat assessment team should have done more after it was brought to their attention that Holmes could have been dangerous.

Doing More with Less

While increasing resources is the best way to improve services, doing more with less is the option that's more realistic for many schools in the meantime. Here are some strategies that Jones has seen counseling centers across the country adopt to deal with the influx of students seeking services:

- Increased use of group therapy. "Outcome studies report equivalent results between group and individual therapy," says Jones. "Advocates for group therapy point out that it is cost-efficient and time-efficient since more people are served."
- Using trainees (such as field placement students or graduate assistants) to help serve clients with less severe illnesses, and interns or post-docs to help with the more severe clients. This requires adequate office space, which many centers are lacking, notes Jones.
- Increased use of technology and online services, including online and distance tele-counseling to help with excessive demands.
- Hiring part-time temporary contract therapists during peak usage times. Such staff often need advance notice to be available, and institutional administrators would likely need to complete time-consuming background checks before contract therapists can start working, points out Jones.

The Outlook

As with other big issues within higher education and the community at large, reaching agreement on how to improve mental health services won't come easily.

"There are so many decision makers, getting all of them on the same page and getting them all in line to be supportive of counseling centers—financially and resource wise—is difficult," Jones says.

But federal efforts could influence everyone, from state legislators to chancellors to boards of trustees.

The Garrett Lee Smith Memorial Reauthorization Act of 2013, a bill introduced in Congress earlier this year, may be one such step.

The bill would increase grant funding for colleges and universities from $5 million to $7 million for providing counseling services and training mental health providers, according to the office of Senator Jack Reed (D-R.I.), a sponsor of the bill. The original bill, enacted in 2004, provided funding for suicide prevention education and outreach, not for the delivery of services.

The act also funds the Suicide Prevention Resource Center and provides grants to states and tribes to support suicide prevention efforts.

"Over the past 10 years, we've been looking at what's been going on among children and young adults to see where improvements can be made and how schools, colleges, and universities are using their funding," according to the office of Senator Reed. The conclusion was that education institutions needed the flexibility to expand their use of the funds outside of outreach.

"When you think about kids going off to college and the services that universities offer, mental health is a critical component. If we don't have an infrastructure that's capable of providing treatment on those campuses, there are students who will go without."

Resources

Active Minds, Inc., www.activeminds.org
American College Counseling Association, www.collegecounseling.org
American Psychological Association, www.apa.org
Association of University and College Counseling Center Directors, www.aucccd.org
National Alliance on Mental Illness, www.nami.org

Critical Thinking

1. Why has the number of individuals with mental illnesses increased on college campuses?
2. What is the reason(s) why more students are willing to seek mental health counseling on college and university campuses?

Create Central

www.mhhe.com/createcentral

Internet References

American Psychological Association
    https://www.apa.org
National Alliance on Mental Illness
    http://www.nami.org/Content/NavigationMenu/Find_Support/NAMI_on_Campus1/Mental_Illness_Fact_Sheets/Mental_Health_Conditions_in_College_Students.htm
National Institutes of Mental Health
    http://www.nimh.nih.gov/index.shtml

Article   Prepared by: Eileen L. Daniel, *SUNY College at Brockport*

Anxiety Nation

Why are so many of us so ill at ease?

SOPHIE MCBAIN

Learning Outcomes

After reading this article, you will be able to:

- Understand the difference between psychological and socio-psychological explanations for anxiety.

- Understand the relationship between anxiety and depression.

- Be aware of the various drug therapies for anxiety.

For a condition that affects so many of us, there is very little agreement about what anxiety actually is. Is it a physiological condition, best treated with medication, or psychological—the product of repressed trauma, as a Freudian might suggest? Is it a cultural construct, a reaction to today's anomic society, or a more fundamental spiritual and philosophical reflection of what it means to be human? For most sufferers, the most pressing concern is whether drugs work, and if therapy is a good idea.

Our modern, medical definition of anxiety could be traced back to 1980 and the publication of the third edition of the *Diagnostic and Statistical Manual* (*DSM-III*), the doctor's and psychiatrist's bible for identifying mental illness. The authors of *DSM-III* suggested that, according to their new criteria, between 2 percent and 4 percent of the population would have an anxiety disorder. But three decades on, the *America's State of Mind Report* showed that one in every six people in the United States suffers from anxiety.

The most recent nationwide survey, which took place in 2007, found that three million people in the UK have an anxiety disorder. About 7 percent of UK adults are on antidepressants (often prescribed for anxiety, too) and one in seven will take benzodiazepines such as Xanax in any 1 year. Mental health charities warn that our anxiety levels are creeping even higher; they often blame our "switched-on" modern culture for this, or the financial crisis and the long recession that followed it.

And yet, it is difficult to quantify whether it is our feelings of anxiety that have changed, or whether it's just our perception of those feelings that is different: are we increasingly viewing ordinary human emotions as marks of mental illness? "In theory, it's possible that we've just watched too many Woody Allen films. That's a very difficult argument to definitively disprove," the clinical psychologist and author Oliver James told me.

If that seems like a slightly flippant way of framing the debate, that could be because James's books, including *The Selfish Capitalist and Britain on the Couch,* are premised on the idea that rates of depression and anxiety have reached record highs in the affluent consumer societies of the English-speaking world.

In January this year, Scott Stossel, who is the editor of the American magazine the *Atlantic,* published *My Age of Anxiety,* an account of his lifelong, debilitating battle with nerves. There has been a lot of interest in the book in both the United States and Europe. Stossel, who is 44, is a successful journalist and yet he is deeply insecure. He has been in therapy for three decades and has taken a cocktail of antidepressants, antipsychotic medications, and sedatives (not to mention more conventional cocktail ingredients such as gin, Scotch, and vodka) in an attempt to cope with any number of phobias, from the common (agoraphobia and fear of public speaking) to the more niche (turophobia: fear of cheese).

Stossel reveals in painful, intimate, and sometimes comical detail the humiliations of living with high anxious tension and very loose bowels. Despite the severity of his problems, he successfully concealed them from most of his friends and colleagues until the book was published. He told me when we spoke that in recent months co-workers have given him lots of hugs (which is sweet, but a little bit uncomfortable) and thousands of strangers have approached him because they so identify with the experiences he describes in the book.

"I was very nervous about coming out as anxious," Stossel says. "And now it's too late and I can't uncome out. It hasn't been a cure, but it has been something of a relief. I now feel there are practical things I can help with, like trying to reduce the stigma around anxiety."

He says we ought to view anxiety less as a "psychological problem" and more like a "medical condition, in the way gout or diabetes is. These are things that need to be managed and treated, and have an organic basis. It's not necessarily that you are weak, but that you have an illness."

Yet while we understand how our modern diet is making gout and diabetes more common, the causes of anxiety are more mysterious.

Anxiety has long been associated with depression, and often the two were subsumed under the notion of "melancholia": Robert Burton's great book *Anatomy of Melancholy* (1621) was as much about anxiety as sadness. But the *DSM-III* classified anxiety and depression as separate conditions: the former is related to feelings of worry, the latter to low mood, and loss of pleasure and interest. More often than not, however, the two occur together. The blurred lines between normality and illness, or depression and anxiety, make it very hard to grasp what it means to say that three million people in the UK suffer from anxiety.

If one in seven of us is taking pills to control or ward off anxiety, are we just medicalising an ordinary human emotion? Did the purveyors of the early antianxiety medicines such as Miltown—discovered in the 1940s, and the first in a line of blockbuster drugs including Prozac and Xanax—manage to create a new problem along with the solution they offered?

Stossel describes how in the 1950s a young psychiatrist called Donald Klein began randomly treating his patients with a new drug called imipramine. He noticed that patients on imipramine often remained very anxious but were less likely to suffer from acute paroxysms of anxiety. And so, having found a cure, he defined the problem—"panic attacks."

Until imipramine, panic attacks didn't "exist." This process of working backwards from new drugs to new illnesses is known as pharmacological dissection, and it is not uncommon. Yet even if modern drugs shaped our understanding of mental illness, that doesn't mean they made us sick.

As millions take pills, are we just medicalising an ordinary emotion?

Or maybe the UK's epidemic of anxiety isn't pathological at all but a product of historically unprecedented good health and affluence. Perhaps anxiety is a luxury that comes with wealth, freedom, and the privilege of having nothing fundamental to fear in our modern society.

This isn't an unpopular notion. A World Health Organization survey in 2002 found that, while 18.2 percent of Americans reported anxiety in any 1 year, south of the US border only 6.8 percent of Mexicans did. Of the 14 countries surveyed by WHO, Nigeria reported the lowest levels of anxiety, with only 3.3 percent of respondents experiencing anxiety in any year. Nigeria's per capita GDP is $2,690, about 6 percent that of the United States, and in 2010 84.5 percent of Nigerians were living on less than $2 a day, the international poverty line. Breaking out into a nervous sweat on the London Tube because you can't remember if you unplugged your hair straighteners is the kind of indulgence you can't afford if you're struggling to feed yourself, or so the argument goes.

However, it's not that simple. Again, it's very hard to tell whether feelings of anxiety vary internationally or if people label them differently. In countries with a large stigma against mental illness, people are less likely to report disorders, such as anxiety or depression. Yet the psychiatrist Vikram Patel, who recently featured on the BBC Radio 4 programme *The Life Scientific*, says his research in India and Zimbabwe has convinced him that rates of mental illness are the same all over the world.

The way we understand anxiety is cultural, says Beth Murphy, head of information at the mental health charity Mind. "If you're living on the breadline in a hand-to-mouth existence you might not recognise what you are feeling as anxiety, but it's quite probable that you're going to be pretty worried about where your next meal is coming from."

This raises another problem: if you are feeling anxious because it's very likely you could go hungry tomorrow, are you in any meaningful way unwell?

Just as sadness is natural but depression is an illness, most of the people I spoke to who suffered from anxiety instinctively drew a distinction between "good anxiety," the nervous adrenalin that helps you get stuff done and meet deadlines, and "bad anxiety," the destructive kind. Our common-sense interpretation of "bad anxiety" also suggests that the worries here should be disproportionate or irrational.

The *Diagnostic and Statistical Manual* used today identifies anxiety disorders according to how severe and persistent the feelings of worry are, and whether these feelings are accompanied by elements from a list of secondary symptoms, including sleep disturbance, muscle tension, poor concentration, and fatigue.

Although the anxiety should be "excessive," the focus is solely on the feelings, and not what caused them. This might go some way toward explaining the boom in prescriptions for mental illnesses; doctors sometimes prescribe antidepressants to someone who has suffered bereavement, something Oliver James described as "ludicrous." The counter-argument is: if a short course of drugs can make it easier to cope with the painful but completely healthy process of grieving, why not take them?

At its most extreme, anxiety is a debilitating, life-altering condition. I spoke to Jo, a volunteer at the charity Anxiety UK, and she told me that feelings of anxiety have "blighted" her life.

"It's stopped me from doing so many things that I would have liked to have been able to do and it's stopped me from living what I feel is a normal life, doing things like having relationships, perhaps getting married, having children, having a career. It's put paid to all that," she says bitterly.

Jo, who is in her fifties, has been overcome by anxiety since she was in her teens. She dropped out of school at 16, unable to cope with the pressure of exams, and when her anxiety peaks she is unable to work and is left isolated. Antianxiety drugs have helped ease the physical symptoms—such as headaches and irritable bowel syndrome—yet they've left her with "the same worries and fears."

What does anxiety feel like when it's at its worst? "It's an overwhelming feeling of being out of control, and overwhelmed by everything." Jo pauses, and then adds quietly, "It's not nice."

While researching this piece, I was struck by how many friends came forward with stories of anxiety-induced insomnia, phobias and stress, though mostly this didn't prevent them from working or socialising. I spent one strange dinner with a friend who is a lawyer. I noticed when we met that her hands were raw and bleeding slightly, and while we ate she repeatedly reached into her bag and disinfected them. Under stress from work, she had developed a huge fear of germs.

Another friend, a corporate lawyer, recently collapsed while out shopping after she suffered a panic attack. There's a recognisable stereotype of the neurotic, angst-filled high-flyer—and it has a historical precedent. In the 19th century, nervousness was seen as a mark of social standing because only the new leisured classes could afford such sensibility. But how closely related are these manifestations of unease and anxiety to those feelings experienced by people who are incapacitated by their nerves or phobias?

The triggers for people's nervous complaints can be idiosyncratic. I chatted about this to Andy Burrows, a musician and the former drummer of the indie band Razorlight. He says he has never felt overly anxious about performing to huge crowds at Wembley or the O$_2$ Arena in London—a prospect that might make most people break into a sweat—but he has suffered from anxiety since his teens and is so freaked out by lifts and tunnels that he can recite from memory the average time that a London overground train spends underground. It takes 16 seconds to travel through the tunnel from Hampstead Heath to Finchley Road and Frognal Station "at regular speed," he says—and sometimes he just has to get off the train and walk between the two.

Of course, phobias can seem funny to an outsider. I can laugh with friends about the time I leapt up from my chair, tipped over my coffee and ran out of a café because I suddenly couldn't cope with being in a confined space with a pigeon. And yet, for a brief few seconds, as someone with a fear of birds, I experienced a terror so profound that it overrode my usual instinct not to cause a scene.

In 2012, the National Health Service recorded 8,720 hospital admissions for acute anxiety. According to research for the Organisation for Economic Co-operation and Development, 40 percent of new claimants for disability benefits in the UK are suffering from mental illnesses, of which anxiety and depression are the most common. The effect of this is that Britain has a higher proportion of people claiming unemployment benefit for mental health conditions than any other developed nation. The estimated cost to the UK of mental illness is roughly 4.4 percent of GDP, through lost productivity and health-care costs.

What is going wrong? One problem is that we are not doing enough to support people with anxiety. The first port of call for most sufferers is their GP, and the response they get can vary. I know this because a few years ago, when I experienced a bereavement and a break-up in quick succession, I turned from a natural worrier into an unravelled bundle of nerves. I was unable to sleep, read, or concentrate.

Even sensitive GPs can be constrained in the solutions they can offer.

After a strange few months, spent mostly wandering aimlessly in London, as if somehow I might lose my panic down a backstreet, I burst into tears in front of my doctor. "Patient tearful but able to maintain eye contact," the GP typed on the large screen in front of us, leaving me feeling like some zoo exhibit. She advised me to book an appointment with someone who knew more about mental health.

In the end, I was lucky. The second doctor prescribed me a low dose of antidepressants (against his advice, I decided not to take these). Then, although the NHS waiting list for counselling was months long, my university counsellor could see me and within 2 months I felt almost normal again.

Even when they are very much aware of mental illness, GPs can often be constrained in the solutions they can offer. One in every 10 people in the UK has to wait more than a year for therapy and 54 percent have to wait for more than 3 months (people from black and ethnic-minority communities often wait the longest).

Anxiety is a broad, confusing label and is a condition with multiple causes. We are not the first generation to believe we live in an exceptionally anxious age, and yet in some ways, thanks to the development of drugs and talking therapies, anxiety is a peculiarly modern experience. Perhaps, at the very root of Britain's struggle with nerves—whether viewed in terms of its economic effects or from the perspective of plain, simple suffering, or whether one merely wonders why 3 million of us appear to be afflicted by a disorder we still can't quite define—is that we don't often talk about it.

In an odd way, it might be easier to admit in modern Britain that you're deeply sad than that you are anxious or scared. Collectively, we might be freaking out but most of us are suffering in silence.

Critical Thinking

1. Why is the rate of anxiety increasing in the developed world?
2. What is the relationship between anxiety and depression?
3. What is the role of drug therapy in the treatment of depression?

Internet References

Anxiety and Depression Association of America, ADAA
www.adaa.org/

Anxiety Helpguide
http://www.helpguide.org/home-pages/anxiety.htm

Listening to Xanax
http://nymag.com/news/features/xanax-2012-3/

Medline Plus
http://www.nlm.nih.gov/medlineplus/anxiety.html

National Institute of Mental Health
http://www.nimh.nih.gov/health/publications/anxiety-disorders/index.shtml

National Institutes of Mental Health
www.nimh.nih.gov/

Why Teenagers Act Crazy
http://www.nytimes.com/2014/06/29/opinion/sunday/why-teenagers-act-crazy.html?_r=0

SOPHIE MCBAIN is a staff writer for the New Statesman.

McBain, Sophie. "Anxiety Nation," *New Statesman*, 143(14), April 11, 2014, pp. 24–27.

Article   Prepared by: Eileen Daniel, *SUNY College at Brockport*

Go Forth in Anger

JOANN ELLISON RODGERS

Learning Outcomes

After reading this article, you will be able to:

- Explain why people should not work too hard to suppress their anger.

- Understand how and why anger evolved among humans.

- Describe the hormonal changes that occur in the body when we get angry.

Anger gets no respect. It's so yoked to "management" that we give it little consideration on its own. We aspire to the serene sangfroid in comedian John Cleese's description of the British as a people who rarely get more than "miffed" or "peeved," and haven't escalated to "a bit cross" since World War II when the Blitz cut tea supplies. Yoda framed the view well: "Anger leads to hate. Hate leads to suffering." Conclusion: The human race would be far better off without it altogether.

A growing cadre of social and evolutionary biologists, psychologists, and brain scientists begs to differ. With newly detailed neural maps of brain systems that underlie feelings and energize us to act on our goals, they have seriously dented the long-held view of anger as an all-time destructive and negative state worthy mostly of suppression. More to the point, they have uncovered its upside, and proposed a psychological model of anger framed as a positive, a force of nature that has likely fueled the ambitions and creativity of the famous and infamous.

Beethoven, for example, reportedly beat his students but still got the best from them. Mark Rothko's fury at pop art powered his own work and drove his towering mentorship of students. Marlon Brando was an angry young man whose anger later in life informed his bully pulpit for social justice. And Rosie O'Donnell built her career on a foundation of foul-mouthed feistiness—and later on efforts to control it.

Researchers are amassing evidence that anger is a potent form of social communication, a logical part of people's emotional tool kit, an appetitive force that not only moves us toward what we want but fuels optimism, creative brainstorming, and problem solving by focusing mind and mood in highly refined ways. Brainwise, it is the polar opposite of fear, sadness, disgust, and anxiety—feelings that prompt avoidance and cause us to move away from what we deem unpleasant. When the gall rises, it propels the irate toward challenges they otherwise would flee and actions to get others to do what they, the angry, wish.

"We need anger, and there are negative consequences for those without it," says Aaron Sell, a social psychologist at Australia's Griffith University, who, with pioneering evolutionary psychologists Lena Cosmides and John Tooby at the University of California Santa Barbara Center for Evolutionary Psychology, has helped lead the assault on old thinking about anger. It feels rewarding because it moves us closer to our goals. Wielded responsibly, scientists say, it even thwarts aggression.

GRRRR: the Neural Roots of Anger

The idea that anger is a positive feeling is not exactly new. Aristotle in 350 B.C. wrote that "the angry man is aiming at what he can attain, and the belief that you will attain your aim is pleasant." People resort to "mild to moderate" anger as often as several times a day and at least several times a week, finds James Averill, a professor of psychology at the University of Massachusetts. Such universality and frequency suggest that only our Stone Age forebears with the capacity to call forth anger pretty regularly, and get rewarded for it, survived to have descendants with the same makeup—us. "It's no surprise" that babies are born ready to express anger, notes Sell, because it's "the output of a cognitive mechanism engineered by natural

Hooray for Anger

Anger—the feeling—is one thing. Fury—its red-faced, fist-first expression—is another. Fury is hardly a useful modality, but anger has positive value in our emotional lives. Here's what that means for most of us:

Anger Offers a Sense of Control

If the true function of anger is to impose costs or withhold benefits from others to increase our Welfare Tradeoff Ratio, it should follow that people who have enhanced abilities to inflict costs are more likely to prevail in conflicts, consider themselves entitled to better treatment, think better of themselves, and be prone to anger. In other words, they control their destinies more than less angry people do.

Psychologist Aaron Sell and coworkers found that strong men report more success resolving interpersonal conflicts in their favor than weak men and are, by their own account, more prone to anger. They endorse personal aggression and are likely to approve the use of military force in global conflicts. The more a woman considers herself attractive—a counterpart to masculine might—the more she is prone to anger, feelings of entitlement, and success in getting her way.

Anger May Promote Cooperation

The association between attractiveness in women or strength among men and "entitlement anger" also suggests that anger enables cooperative relationships by means of getting two parties to "yes" before hostilities break out.

Harvard's Jennifer Lerner examined Americans' reactions to the terrorist attacks of 9/11 and found that feelings of anger evoked a sense of certainty and control on a mass scale, helping to minimize paralyzing fear and allowing people to come together for common cause. Those who became angry were less likely to anticipate future attacks, while those who were fearful expected more attacks.

Anger preserves a sense of control and the desire to defend what's yours, but only insofar as it leaves both parties more or less OK, because you may need the hungry oaf who stole your dinner to help you hunt down the next meal.

Anger Fuels Optimism

Boston College psychologist Brett Ford has found that anxiety drives people to be extremely vigilant about threats, while a state of excitement makes them hyperaware of rewards within their reach. Anger increases visual attention to rewarding information. It helps people home in on what they hope things can be, rather than on an injury. Fearful people not only have "strikingly different" assessments of the level of risk in the environment compared to angry people, their fear leads to higher perceptions of risk.

Anger Enables Leadership

Dutch psychologist Gerben van Kleef has found that anger deployed by a leader gets underlings to perform well, but only if the underlings are high in their motivation to read the leader. Cheerfulness in a leader is more effective among teams with low interest in reading emotional tea leaves.

Beware of becoming a volcanic Steve Jobs, however. Eventually, the strategy of using either consistent or intermittent explosive anger becomes obvious and may be ignored or resisted. Jobs was notoriously and chronically angry, and he used that emotion to exact extraordinary performance from his most creative employees. But finally, his anger lost its impact and became so dangerous to his effectiveness that he was forced out of the company he had founded.

"If you get a bang for the buck for anger and you don't ever get punished for it and it gets you what you want, you can lose control of the benefit and still keep at it when it's self-destructive," says Michael Cataldo, a psychologist at Johns Hopkins.

Anger Boosts Focus on the Practical

Approach motivation toward anger-related objects occurs only when people perceive they can actually get a reward, finds psychologist Henk Arts of Utrecht University in the Netherlands. In the absence of such a reward context, avoidance motivation prevails. The findings suggest that our anger system is pretty fine-tuned to go after the gettable, not the impossible.

Anger Abets Creativity and Ambition

After establishing that anger often accompanies brainstorming, in which people throw conflicting ideas out for debate, a team of Dutch researchers elicited anger, sadness, or a neutral state from subjects, and then had them brainstorm about ways to protect the environment. Those in the anger group had lots more ideas and more creative ideas than sad or neutral participants—although, over time, things evened out.

Consider the work of superior talents who were famously angry at the world: Francis Bacon's screaming faces. David Mamet's masterful plays, Adrienne Rich's feminist poem, "Diving Into the Wreck," and anything by Virginia Woolf.

It's likely that anger stirs energizing hormones and focuses attention, all while disinhibiting social interactions, creating less "politically correct" behavior.

Anger Is Emotionally Intelligent

People who prefer to feel useful emotions (such as anger) even when they are unpleasant to experience—when confronting others, for example—"tend to be higher in emotional intelligence" than people who prefer to feel happiness, Brett Ford and Maya Tamir report. "Wanting to feel bad may be good at times and vice versa."

Anger Aids Understanding of Others

In advance of an Israeli-Palestinian summit conference convened by President George W. Bush in 2007, a team of Israeli and American psychologists set out to see whether anger would have constructive effects. Experimentally inducing anger in Israelis toward Palestinians several weeks before the summit increased support for making compromises among those with low levels of hatred. Even when anger was evoked just days before the summit, it led to increased support for compromise in the same low-hatred group.

Anger makes people more willing to accept risks, a major feature of leadership.

—JER

selection." Nature favored and preserved anger for the same reasons it conserved love, sex, fear, sadness, and anxiety: survival and advantage.

Biologically, when people are aroused to some degree of anger and let off steam, their heart rate, blood pressure, and testosterone levels all increase. This might suggest that anger freaks us out and harms us. But in fact, levels of the stress hormone cortisol drop, suggesting that anger helps people calm down and get ready to address a problem—not run from it. In studies in which she and her colleagues induced indignation among volunteer subjects, Jennifer Lerner, a psychologist at Harvard, found that anger diminished the effects of cortisol on heart reactivity.

Although anger has long been considered a fully negative emotion, recent neuroscience has overturned that view. Scientists know that two basic motivational forces underlie all behavior—the impulse to approach, or move toward something desired, and the impulse to withdraw, or move away from unpleasantness. Hardwired in the brain, these behaviors are headquartered in the frontal cortex, which acts as the executive branch of the emotions. Brain imaging and electrical studies of the brain consistently show that the left frontal lobe is crucial to establishing approach behaviors that push us to pursue desired goals and rewards in rational, logical, systematic, and ordered ways and that activation of the right frontal cortex is tied to the more negative, withdrawal motivational system, marked by inhibition, timidity, and avoidance of punishment and threat.

Brain scans show that anger significantly activates the left anterior cortex, associated with positive approach behaviors. Anger, moreover, appears to be downright rewarding, even pleasurable, in studies showing predominant left-brain activation when angry subjects perceive they can make things better.

"Expecting to be able to act to resolve the [angering] event should yield greater approach motivational intensity," contend social psychologists Charles Carver of the University of Miami and Eddie Harmon-Jones of the University of New South Wales, long-time collaborators in anger scholarship. In a variety of studies, Harmon-Jones has found that subjects who score high on a scale that measures a tendency to anger display a characteristic asymmetry in the prefrontal cortex—they exhibit higher levels of left anterior (frontal) EEG activity and lower levels of right anterior activation. Randomly insulting subjects, compared with treating them neutrally in verbal communications, stimulates greater relative left frontal activity.

Spurred by the findings on anger, neuroscientists have begun to move away from thinking of any emotion as either negative or positive, preferring instead to characterize emotions by "motivational direction"—whether they stimulate approach behaviors or avoidance/withdrawal behaviors. Viewed within this framework, they explain, it's not strange that anger produces happiness. "The case of anger," reports a team of Spanish scientists led by Neus Herrero, "is different because although it is considered or experienced as negative, based on findings of increased left brain activity it produces a motivation of closeness, or approach." When we get mad, in other words, we "show a natural tendency to get closer to what made us angry to try to eliminate it."

Herrero looked at psychological and biological measures—heart rate (increase), testosterone levels (increase), cortisol levels (decrease), and brain activation (asymmetric left activation)—at the same time he induced anger. The findings support the notion that nature intends us to respond to anger in ways that increase motivation to approach what is sending heart rate up and cortisol down and left brains into thinking up creative ways to make it go away. In short, venting calms us enough to think straight.

Harmon-Jones's studies add detail. "When individuals believed there was nothing they could do to rectify an angering situation, they still reported being angry," he reports, "but they did not show increased left frontal activity compared to right frontal activity." Overall, he adds, it's most accurate to say that anger is associated with left frontal activity only when the anger is associated with approach inclinations, the perception that there is an opportunity to fix the situation, at the least cost to oneself.

Director of the University of Wisconsin's influential Laboratory for Affective Neuroscience, Richard Davidson has studied the neural origins of emotions for 40 years. His pioneering investigations of the asymmetric brain response to anger show that the emotion is "intrinsically rewarding, with a positive quality that mobilizes resources, increases vigilance, and facilitates the removal of obstacles in the way of our goal pursuits, particularly if the anger can be divorced from the propensity to harm or destroy."

The Real Function of Anger

Nature wired us over time to get angry when others insult or exploit us or, in the jargon of evolutionary psychologists, impose too high a cost on us (in our opinion) to get an unjustifiably (again in our opinion) small benefit for themselves. So states the Recalibration Theory of Anger put forth by Cosmides, Tooby, and Sell. Moreover, they contend, anger was designed by natural selection to nonconsciously regulate our response to personal conflicts of interest in ways that help us bargain to our advantage. In other words, anger prods the aggrieved to behave in ways that increase the weight the wrongdoer puts on her value and welfare. If the angry person is successful, it not only produces benefits ("I win!") but also pleasure—enough to reinforce deploying anger this way repeatedly.

Using studies that probe people's true emotions by gauging reactions to hypothetical scenarios, along with argument analysis, computerized measures of facial expressions, and voice analysis, Sell finds that anger erupts naturally when someone puts a "too low value, or weight, on your welfare relative to their own when making decisions or taking actions that affect both of you." Sell and his colleagues call this index the Welfare Tradeoff Ratio or WTR. And the purpose of the anger is to recalibrate that ratio.

Anger is likely the primary way people have of addressing conflicts of interest and other "resource conflicts," says Sell. Anger allows us to detect our own value in any conflicting interaction, then motivates us to get others to rethink our positions, to pay a lot more attention to what it will cost us to get what we want—and whether it's worth the cost.

Sell proposes that anger essentially makes the target of the anger "less willing to impose costs and more willing to tolerate costs." Studies conducted with Cosmides and Tooby show that anger, by WTR measure, is more prevalent in physically strong men, who would be perceived as able to get away with anger as a bargaining tactic. The trio has also found when two parties both want exclusive access to, or the lion's share of, something, arguments seasoned with anger work well in divvying up the spoils in ways that allow for winners without destroying the losers.

Recalibration theory explains a lot of everyday human behavior in which anger serves a positive purpose as a social value indicator and regulator and ironically, perhaps, as a check on aggression. "My classmate uses my sleeve to wipe ketchup off his chin in order to keep his shirt clean," Sell offers as an example. Such behavior arouses anger not because he is really harmed by it (no one dies of a ketchup stain), but because it's an indication his classmate has little respect for his worth. The ketchup wipee might respond with a laugh if the wiper is a buddy, but if not, showing anger gets the afflicted to behave in ways that increase the value the wrongdoer puts on him by escalating the social cost of misbehaving.

Standing up for your shirtsleeve is standing up for yourself. You don't need to throw a punch; an angry frown or a loud "Hey!" will probably recalibrate. Anger, then, can be a way of increasing the likelihood of evening out respectful relationships, even among friends—in essence, encouraging cooperation. Without anger, Sell adds, there would be no emotional environment in which to persuade, negotiate, and progress in a relatively safe way without overt war and mayhem at every frustration.

"I keep finding that anger, across different settings, can have positive consequences," says Gerben van Kleef, professor of social psychology at the University of Amsterdam. He has found that negotiators led to believe that their counterparts are angry are more likely to make concessions, a nice edge for those especially good at reading and calculating WTRs. Our innate anger system guides the angered person to do things that encourage an offender to treat the angry person better by some combination of conferring benefits or lowering costs.

If there's a take-home message to all the good news about anger, Davidson says it might be that while anger can be healthy or toxic depending on the situation at hand, people should not work too hard to suppress it. "In general, it's better to let emotions unfold than to externally suppress them," he says.

"Ultimately," insists Harvard's Lerner, "research will provide evidence for the view that the most adaptive and resilient individuals have highly flexible emotional response systems. They are neither chronically angry nor chronically calm." Anger, she adds, is good for you, "as long as you keep the flame low."

Critical Thinking

1. Is it physically and emotionally better to try to suppress anger or let our emotions unfold?

2. How does the recalibration theory explain the positive purpose of anger?

3. Why is anger considered to be a form of social communication?

Create Central

www.mhhe.com/createcentral

Internet References

American Psychological Association
   http://apa.org/topics/anger/index.aspx
Psychology Today
   http://www.psychologytoday.com/basics/anger

JOANN ELLISON RODGERS is a writer based in Baltimore.

Article

Prepared by: Eileen L. Daniel, *SUNY College at Brockport*

Stress: Its Surprising Implications for Health

HONOR WHITEMAN

Learning Outcomes

After reading this article, you will be able to:

- Describe the health risks associated with exposure to stress.

- Discuss how one can protect against stress-induced health problems.

Whether it is down to work pressure, money worries or relationship troubles, most of us experience stress at some point in our lives. In fact, around 75% of us report experiencing moderate to high levels of stress over the past month. It is well known that stress can cause sleep problems, headache, and raise the risk of depression. But in this Spotlight, we look at some of the more surprising ways in which stress may harm our health.

The National Institute of Mental Health (NIMH) defines stress as the "brain's response to any demand." In other words, it is how the brain reacts to certain situations or events.

It is important to note that not all stress is negative. Many of us who have been in a pressurized situation may have found that stress has pushed us to perform better. This is down to a "fight-or-flight" response, whereby the brain identifies a real threat and quickly releases hormones that encourage us to protect ourselves from perceived harm.

It is when this fight-or-flight response overreacts that problems arise, and this usually happens when we find ourselves exposed to constant threats.

"Stress is caused by the loss or threat of loss of the personal, social and material resources that are primary to us. So, threat to self, threat to self-esteem, threat to income, threat to employment and threat to our family or our health," Stevan Hobfoll, PhD, the Judd and Marjorie Weinberg Presidential Professor

and Chair at Rush University Medical Center in Chicago, IL, and member of the American Psychological Association (APA), told *Medical News Today*.

Stress Levels "Too High" in Americans

Earlier this month, the APA released their annual "Stress in America" Survey, which assesses the attitudes and perceptions of stress and identifies its primary causes among the general public.

The survey, completed by 3,068 adults in the US during August 2014, revealed that the primary cause of stress among Americans is money, with 72% of respondents reporting feeling stressed about finances at some point over the past month. Of these, 22% said they had felt "extreme stress" in the past month as a result of money worries.

The second most common cause of stress among Americans was found to be work, followed by the economy, family responsibilities, and personal health concerns.

On a positive note, average stress levels among Americans have decreased since 2007. On a 10-point scale, respondents rated their stress levels as 4.9 last year, compared with 6.2 in 2007. However, the APA say such levels remain significantly higher than the 3.7 stress rating we consider to be healthy.

"This year's survey continues to reinforce the idea that we are living with a level of stress that we consider too high," says Norman B. Anderson, CEO and executive vice president of the APA, adding:

"All Americans, and particularly those groups that are most affected by stress—which include women, younger adults and those with lower incomes—need to address this issue sooner than later in order to better their health and well-being."

The Surprising Health Implications of Stress

"Stress is significantly associated with virtually all the major areas of disease," Prof. Hobfoll told *MNT*. "Stress is seldom the root cause of disease, but rather interacts with our genetics and our state of our bodies in ways that accelerate disease."

Some of the more well-known implications of stress that many of you may have experienced include sleep deprivation, headache, anxiety, and depression. But increasingly, researchers are uncovering more and more ways in which stress can harm our health.

Heart Health

According to the American Heart Association (AHA), stress can influence behaviors that have negative implications for heart health.

Have you ever arrived home after a stressful day at work and reached for that bottle of wine? Many of us have. Last month, *MNT* reported on a study that found working long hours was associated with risky alcohol use, which the study researchers say is partly down to the belief that "alcohol use alleviates stress that is caused by work pressure and working conditions."

Some of us may smoke in response to stress, while others may "comfort eat," which can lead to obesity. All of these are factors that can contribute to poor heart health by raising blood pressure and causing damage to the walls of the arteries.

According to a study reported by *MNT* in November 2014, stress may also reduce blood flow to the heart—particularly for women. The study researchers found that in patients with coronary heart disease, stressed women had a three times greater reduction in blood flow than stressed men.

Stress has also been associated with increased risk of heart attack. In 2012, a study published in *The Lancet* found that work stress may raise the risk of heart attack by 23%. And earlier this week, *MNT* reported on a study by researchers from the University of Sydney in Australia, which found periods of intense anger or anxiety may raise heart attack risk by more than nine times.

Even after a heart attack, stress may continue to affect health. A study published in the journal *Circulation* earlier this month found women were more likely to experience higher levels of mental stress following a heart attack, which results in poorer recovery.

Diabetes

You may be surprised to learn that stress has been associated with increased risk of diabetes. Last month, a study published in *JAMA Psychiatry* found that women with symptoms of post-traumatic stress disorder (PTSD)—a condition triggered by very distressing events—were more likely to develop the condition than those without PTSD.

Periods of stress increase production of the hormone cortisol, which can increase the amount of glucose in the blood—a potential explanation for why stress has been linked to higher risk of diabetes.

For people who already have diabetes, stress can lead to poorer management of the condition. As well as interfering with stress hormones and increasing blood glucose levels, the American Diabetes Association note that stressed patients with diabetes may be less likely to take care of themselves.

"They may drink more alcohol or exercise less. They may forget, or not have time, to check their glucose levels or plan good meals," notes the organization.

Alzheimer's disease

Alzheimer's disease affects more than 5 million people in the US and is the sixth leading cause of death in the country.

While the exact causes of the condition are unclear, past studies have suggested that stress may contribute to its development.

In March 2013, *MNT* reported on a study by researchers from the University of Gothenburg in Sweden, which found that high levels of stress hormones in the brains of mice were associated with larger amounts of beta-amyloid plaques—proteins believed to play a role in Alzheimer's.

Another study published in 2010 by Finnish researchers found that women who had either high blood pressure or higher cortisol levels—both symptoms of stress—were more than three times as likely to develop Alzheimer's, compared with patients who did not have these symptoms.

Most recently, a study published in *The American Journal of Geriatric Psychiatry* found that for seniors with mild cognitive impairment, anxiety could speed up progression toward Alzheimer's.

In 2012, the UK's Alzheimer's Society revealed that they are embarking on a 3-year project to find out more about the association between stress and Alzheimer's disease.

"All of us go through stressful events. We are looking to understand how these may become a risk factor for the development of Alzheimer's," said lead investigator of the project Prof. Clive Holmes, of the University of Southampton in the UK.

Fertility

Approximately 1 in 8 couples in the US have problems getting pregnant or sustaining a pregnancy. Increasingly, researchers are suggesting stress may be a contributing factor.

In May 2014, we reported on a study published in the journal *Fertility and Sterility* that found stress in men can lead to reduced sperm and semen quality, which may negatively affect fertility.

The researchers behind that study, including first author Teresa Janevic, PhD, an assistant professor at Rutgers School of Public Health in Piscataway, NJ, hypothesize that stress could trigger the release of glucocorticoids—steroid hormones that affect the metabolism of carbohydrates, fats and proteins. This could lower testosterone levels and sperm production in men.

"Stress has long been identified as having an influence on health," says Janevic. "Our research suggests that men's reproductive health may also be affected by their social environment."

And women may not be free from the effects of stress on fertility. In 2014, a study led by researchers from Ohio State University found that women with high levels of a stress-related enzyme in their saliva—alpha-amylase—were 29% less likely to become pregnant than women with low levels of this enzyme. What is more, these women were also more than twice as likely to be infertile.

How Can You Protect against Stress-induced Health Problems?

Of course, the best way to reduce the risk of stress-related health implications is to tackle the stress itself.

In order to do this, you first need to recognize the symptoms of stress. Though these vary in each individual, they commonly include difficulty sleeping, fatigue, overeating or undereating and feelings of depression, anger or irritability. You may also be smoking or drinking more in an attempt to manage stress, and some people many even engage in drug abuse.

According to the NIMH, one of the best ways to tackle stress is to seek support from others, be it friends, family or religious organizations. If an individual feels unable to cope with stress,

is having suicidal thoughts or has engaged in drug or alcohol use to try and manage stress, the organization recommends seeking help from a qualified mental health provider.

Exercise can also be an effective aid for stress. The Mayo Clinic explain that physical activity increases production of "feel-good" neurotransmitters in the brain, called endorphins. Exercise has also been associated with reduced symptoms of depression, as well as improved sleep quality.

The AHA provide some other ways to help deal with stress:

- **Positive self-talk:** turn negative thoughts into positive ones. Instead of saying "I can't do this," say "I'll do the best I can." Negative self-talk increases stress levels
- **Emergency stress stoppers:** if you start to feel stressed, count to 10 before you talk, take a few deep breaths or go for a walk
- **Finding pleasure:** engaging in activities you enjoy is a great way to stave off stress. Take up a hobby, watch a movie or have a meal with friends
- **Daily relaxation:** engage in some relaxation techniques. Meditation, yoga and tai chi have all been shown to reduce stress levels.

Critical Thinking

1. Why are stress levels so high among Americans?
2. What are techniques to relieve stress?
3. How does stress exposure increase the risk of diabetes?

Internet References

American Institute of Stress
www.stress.org
American Psychological Association-Stress
http://www.apa.org/topics/stress/
National Institutes of Mental Health
http://www.nimh.nih.gov

Unit 3

UNIT

Prepared by: Eileen L. Daniel, *SUNY College at Brockport*

Nutritional Health

For years, the majority of Americans paid little attention to nutrition other than to eat three meals a day and, perhaps, take a vitamin supplement. While this dietary style was generally adequate for the prevention of major nutritional deficiencies, medical evidence began to accumulate linking the American diet to a variety of chronic illnesses. In an effort to guide Americans in their dietary choices, the U.S. Dept. of Agriculture and the U.S. Public Health Service review and publish Dietary Guidelines every five years. The recent Dietary Guidelines recommendations are no longer limited to food choices; they include advice on the importance of maintaining a healthy weight and engaging in daily exercise. In addition to the Dietary Guidelines, the Department of Agriculture developed the *MyPlate* to show the relative importance of food groups.

Despite an apparent ever-changing array of dietary recommendations from the scientific community, five recommendations remain constant: (1) eat a diet low in sugar, (2) eat whole grain foods, (3) drink plenty of fresh water daily, (4) limit your daily intake of salt, and (5) eat a diet rich in fruits and vegetables. These recommendations, while general in nature, are seldom heeded and in fact many Americans don't eat enough fruits and vegetables and eat too much sugar and unhealthy fats.

Of all the nutritional findings, the link between transfat and coronary heart disease remains the most consistent throughout the literature. Current recommendations suggest that the types of fats consumed may play a much greater role in disease processes than the total amount of fat consumed. As it currently stands, most experts agree that it is prudent to limit our intake of trans fat that appears to raise LDLs (the bad cholesterol) and lower HDLs (the good cholesterol) and thus increases the risk of heart disease. There's also evidence that trans fats increase the risk of diabetes.

While the basic advice on eating healthy remains fairly constant, many Americans are still confused over exactly what to eat. Should their diet be low carbohydrate, high protein, or low fat? When people turn to standards such as MyPlate, even here there is some confusion. MyPlate was originally called the Food Pyramid and was designed by the Department of Agriculture over 20 years ago. It recommended a diet based on grains, fruits, and vegetables with several servings of meats and dairy products. It also restricts the consumption of fats, oils, and sweets. While MyPlate offers guidelines as to food groups, individual nutrients are not emphasized. One nutrient, vitamin D, has been in the news recently. New research on the "sunshine" vitamin suggests current recommendations may not be adequate, especially for senior citizens. The data also indicate that vitamin D may help lower the incidence of cancers, type 1 diabetes, and multiple sclerosis.

Of all the topic areas in health, food and nutrition is certainly one of the most interesting, if for no other reason than the rate at which dietary recommendations change. One recommendation that hasn't changed is the adage that a good breakfast is the best way to start the day. There is a definite link between better grades and breakfast among schoolchildren. Despite all the controversy and conflict, the one message that seems to remain constant is the importance of balance and moderation in everything we eat.

Article   Prepared by: Eileen L. Daniel, *SUNY College at Brockport*

The Truth about Gluten

The biggest trend in the food world shows no signs of slowing down. But will going gluten-free really make you healthier? Here are the six realities behind the labels.

Learning Outcomes

After reading this article, you will be able to:

- Describe the potential risks from consuming a gluten-free diet.
- Understand who needs to avoid gluten.
- Identify what foods contain gluten.

Eighteen months ago, Ahmed Year wood decided to go gluten-free. "A few years earlier, I'd given up processed foods and felt great," the 41-year-old business owner recalls. "I figured cutting out gluten would make me feel even better. Everyone told me I'd have more energy and lose weight." He lasted less than a month. "Everything was rice this and rice that—it was way too restrictive," he says. "And I didn't feel any different healthwise than I did before." Yearwood reverted to his former eating habits. "Some of the grains I eat have gluten, but I still feel amazing."

Just as fat was vilified in the 1990s and carbs have been scorned more recently, gluten—a protein found in wheat, barley, and rye—has become the latest dietary villain, blamed for everything from forgetfulness to joint pain to weight gain. Some people must avoid it because they have celiac disease—an autoimmune condition in which gluten causes potentially life-threatening intestinal damage—or gluten sensitivity. But less than 7 percent of Americans have those conditions.

According to a recent survey of more than 1,000 Americans by the Consumer Reports National Research Center, 63 percent thought that following a gluten-free diet would improve physical or mental health. About a third said they buy gluten-free products or try to avoid gluten. Among the top benefits they cited were better digestion and gastrointestinal function, healthy weight loss, increased energy, lower cholesterol, and a stronger immune system.

Yet there's very limited research to substantiate any of those beliefs, notes Alessio Fasano, M.D., director of the Center for Celiac Research at Massachusetts General Hospital in Boston. Unless you have celiac disease or a true gluten sensitivity, there's no clear medical reason to eliminate it, Fasano says. In fact, you might be doing your health a disservice. "When you cut out gluten completely, you can cut out foods that have valuable nutrients," he says, "and you may end up adding more calories and fat into your diet." Before you decide to ride the wave of this dietary trend, consider why it might not be a good idea.

1 Gluten-Free Isn't More Nutritious (And May Be Less So)

A quarter of the people in our survey thought gluten-free foods have more vitamins and minerals than other foods. But a recent Consumer Reports review of 81 products free of gluten across 12 categories revealed that they're a mixed bag in terms of nutrition. "If you go completely gluten-free without the guidance of a nutritionist, you can develop deficiencies pretty quickly," warns Laura Moore, R.D., a dietitian at the University of Texas Health Science Center at Houston. Many gluten-free foods aren't enriched or fortified with nutrients such as folic acid and iron; the products that contain wheat flours are.

And it may come as a surprise to learn that ditching gluten often means adding sugar and fat. "Gluten adds oomph to foods—wheat, rye, and barley all have strong textures and flavors," says Angela Lemond, a registered dietitian nutritionist in Dallas and a spokeswoman for the Academy of Nutrition and Dietetics. Take it out of food that usually contains it and you might find that extra fat, sugar, or sodium have been used to compensate for the lack of taste. For example, the Walmart regular blueberry muffins we looked at had 340 calories, 17 grams of fat, and 24 grams of sugars. Gluten-free blueberry muffins from Whole Foods had 370 calories, 13 grams of fat, and 31 grams of sugars. Thomas' plain bagels had 270 calories and 2 grams of fat; Udi's plain gluten-free bagels had 290 calories and 9 fat grams. We found similar differences in all 12 food categories. It may not seem like much, but a few grams here and there can add up. A gluten-free bagel for breakfast and two slices of gluten-free bread at lunch means 10 to 15 additional grams of fat.

Gluten may actually be good for you. There's some evidence that the protein has beneficial effects on triglycerides and may help blood pressure. The fructan starches in wheat also support healthy bacteria in your digestive system, which in turn may reduce inflammation and promote health in other ways. One small study found that healthy people who follow a gluten-free diet for a month have significantly lower levels of healthy bacteria.

2 You'll Probably Increase Your Exposure to Arsenic

About half of the gluten-free products Consumer Reports purchased contained rice flour or rice in another form. In 2012 we reported on our tests of more than 60 rices and packaged foods with rice (such as pasta, crackers, and infant cereal). We found measurable levels of arsenic in almost every product tested. Many of them contained worrisome levels of inorganic arsenic, a carcinogen. We've done more testing to see whether there are some types of rice we can recommend as lower in arsenic than others, and whether other grains (gluten-free ones like quinoa as well as bulgur and barley) contain significant levels of arsenic. We've also done additional analyses of data from the Food and Drug Administration to determine arsenic levels in packaged foods that have rice.

A 2009-10 study from the Environmental Protection Agency estimates that 17 percent of an average person's dietary exposure to inorganic arsenic comes from rice. That may be an underestimate, especially for people on a gluten-free diet. It's getting easier to find gluten-free packaged foods that don't contain rice (see "Gluten-Free Foods [With No Rice!] That Passed Our Taste Test"), but the majority of them do. "If you don't have to give up gluten, the likelihood that you'll consume a significant amount of arsenic following a typical gluten-free

How Foods Stack Up

Gluten-free doesn't necessarily mean healthier

Walmart Blueberry Muffin	VS.	Whole Foods Gluten-Free Blueberry Muffin	Bob's Red Mill Old Country Style Muesli	VS.	Bob's Red Mill Gluten-Free Muesli
3½ oz.	SERVING	3½ oz.	¼ cup	SERVING	¼ cup
340	CALORIES	370	110	CALORIES	110
17	FAT(g)	13	3	FAT (g)	3
340	SODIUM (mg)	390	0	SODIUM (mg)	0
1	FIBER (g)	1	4	FIBER (g)	2
24	SUGARS (g)	31	5	SUGARS (g)	5
$1	PRICE*	$2	$0.25	PRICE*	$0.31

Thomas' Plain Bagel	VS.	Glutino Original New York Style Bagel	Nabisco Multigrain Wheat Thins	VS.	Nabisco Gluten-Free Rice Thins
3½ oz.	SERVING	4 oz.	14 crackers	SERVING	13 crackers
270	CALORIES	340	130	CALORIES	120
2	FAT (g)	7	4	FAT (g)	2
460	SODIUM (mg)	660	190	SODIUM (mg)	115
2	FIBER (g)	1	3	FIBER (g)	2
7	SUGARS (g)	14	3	SUGARS (g)	<1
$0.78	PRICE*	$1.36	$0.31	PRICE*	$0.57

* Per serving.

diet should give you pause," says Michael Crupain, M.D., M.P.H., associate director of Consumer Safety and Sustainability at Consumer Reports. In a 2014 Spanish study, researchers estimated the arsenic intake of adults with celiac disease. They devised a daily menu that assumed someone would eat rice or a rice product high in arsenic at every meal and snack. A 128-pound woman following such a diet would get 192 micrograms of inorganic arsenic per week from rice and rice foods alone. For a man weighing 165 pounds, it would be 247 micrograms. "These levels are close to 10 times the amount of inorganic arsenic we think consumers should get in their diets on a weekly basis," Crupain says.

3 You Might Gain Weight

More than a third of Americans think that going gluten-free will help them slim down, according to our survey. But there's no evidence that doing so is a good weightloss strategy; in fact, the opposite is often true. In a review of studies on nutrition and celiac disease published in the *Journal of Medicinal Food,* researchers said that a gluten-free diet "seems to increase the risk of overweight or obesity." The authors attributed that to the tendency for gluten-free foods to have more calories, sugars, and fat than their regular counterparts.

People who have celiac disease often gain weight when they go gluten-free, Fasano notes. That's because the damage gluten does to their small intestine prevents them from digesting food properly. Their digestive system heals after they have given up gluten and they're able to absorb key vitamins and nutrients from the foods they eat, including calories. In a study of 369 people with celiac disease, 42 percent of those who were overweight or obese lost weight after almost three years on a gluten-free diet, but 27 percent of them gained weight. In another study, 82 percent of those who were overweight at the start of it gained weight.

What about those who say they got rid of their belly when they ditched the wheat? There's no evidence that it was due to cutting gluten. "If people lose weight on a gluten-free diet, it might be because they're cutting calories, eating less processed food or sweets, or cutting portions of starchy foods like pasta and bread," says Samantha Heller, R.D., senior clinical nutritionist at NYU Langone Medical Center. "Instead of a cookie, they're eating an apple. Instead of pasta, they're eating a high-fiber, gluten-free whole grain like quinoa. Eating more fiber helps satiety and may aid in weight loss."

4 You'll Pay More

Our research found that in every category except ready-to-eat cereal, the gluten-free versions were more expensive than their regular counterparts, about double the cost, and in some cases considerably more. For example, brownies made from the

Duncan Hines regular mix cost about 8 cents per serving; Betty Crocker's gluten-free mix cost 28 cents per serving. The per-serving cost of Nabisco's Multigrain Wheat Thins is 31 cents; it's 57 cents for the company's gluten-free Sea Salt & Pepper Rice Thins. DiGiorno's Pizzeria Four Cheese frozen pizza is $1.38 per serving; Freschetta's Gluten Free Thin & Crispy Four Cheese frozen pizza is $2.50 per serving.

Why are foods without gluten more expensive? "One factor in the price differential may be attributed to the added costs incurred by the manufacturer to meet certification and labeling regulations," explains Andrea Levario, executive director of the American Celiac Disease Alliance, a nonprofit group.

5 You Might Miss a Serious Health Condition

If you're convinced that you have a problem with gluten, see a specialist to get a blood test to check for certain antibodies associated with celiac disease. You need to be eating gluten when the test is done to get a proper diagnosis, notes Peter Green, M.D., director of the Celiac Disease Center at Columbia University's medical school. If it's positive, then you should have an endoscopic biopsy of your small intestine to check for damage.

Your symptoms may also be a reaction to something other than gluten in your diet. "We commonly see patients who go on a gluten-free diet and feel better for a week or two," explains Joseph Murray, M.D., a gastroenterologist at the Mayo Clinic. "It may be the placebo effect or simply because they're eating less. For some, their symptoms come back, so they decide to drop another food group, and then a few weeks later, when they're still not feeling any better, they make an even more drastic change, like going completely vegan. By the time they enter my office, they're on a severely restricted diet and still have symptoms." The reason? It often turns out their condition wasn't celiac disease or even gluten sensitivity at all, but another condition, such as irritable bowel syndrome.

Some people may benefit from something called the low-FODMAPs diet. The acronym stands for fermentable oligodi-monosaccharides and polyols. They're the carbohydrates fructose (found in fruit and honey); lactose (in dairy); fructans (in wheat, garlic, and onions); galactans (in legumes) and polyols (sugar-free sweeteners); and stone fruit like apricots, cherries, and nectarines. The diet is complicated, however, and you might need to work with a GI specialist or nutritionist to help you figure out which foods to eat.

6 You Might Still Be Eating Gluten, Anyway

A recent study in the *European Journal of Clinical Nutrition* looked at 158 food products labeled gluten-free over three years.

It found that about 5 percent—including some that were certified gluten-free—didn't meet the FDA's limit of less than 20 parts per million of gluten. The products were tested before the FDA's rule went into effect last summer. Still, that standard doesn't stipulate that manufacturers must test their products before making a gluten-free claim. "Cross-contamination can occur," Levario explains. "Gluten-free products may be manufactured on the same equipment used for wheat or other gluten-containing products." That can also happen when wheat is grown next to other grains. For example, oats are often grown in or near fields where wheat has been grown. As a result, wheat finds its way into the oat harvest and contaminates its subsequent products.

There's no way to completely protect yourself, but you can call manufacturers. "They should be transparent about what tests they use to determine whether a product is gluten-free," says the study's author, Tricia Thompson, M.S., R.D., founder of Gluten Free Watchdog. "If they insist that it's proprietary information, that should set off an alarm."

Another concern is that some products, particularly chips and energy bars, that carry a no-gluten claim contain malt, malt extract, or malt syrup, which are usually made from barley. As the study notes, "some manufactures mistakenly believe that the only criterion for labeling a food gluten-free is that it tests less than 20 ppm gluten." The FDA also stipulates that the food can't contain an ingredient derived from a gluten grain that has not been processed to remove the gluten. For people with celiac disease, inaccurate claims can be damaging. As always, it's best to read the ingredients list.

Gluten-Free: The Common-Sense Version

If you must cut out gluten, be sure to do it the healthy way

Get your grains. Whether you're on a gluten-free diet or not, eating a variety of grains is healthy, so don't cut out whole grains. Replace wheat with amaranth, corn, millet, quinoa, teff, and the occasional serving of rice.

Shop the grocery store perimeter. Stick with naturally gluten-free whole foods: fruit, vegetables, lean meat and poultry, fish, most dairy, legumes, some grains, and nuts.

Read the label! Minimize your intake of packaged foods made with refined rice or potato flours; choose those with no-gluten, non-rice whole grains instead. Whenever you buy processed foods, keep an eye on the sugar, fat, and sodium content of the product.

The Meteoric Rise of Gluten-Free Marketing

Since 2012 sales of "gluten-free" products have risen 63 percent, with 4,599 products introduced last year. For marketers, it's a gold mine. The label can lead to increased sales and premium pricing, says Richard George, a food marketing expert. "Perception is reality, and if consumers believe gluten-free products are better, then logic no longer matters." Here, some gluten-free items:

Potato Chips The no. 1 no-gluten snack. (They're naturally free of gluten.) Sales of products with the label have soared 456 percent since 2012.

Not Just for People Last year almost twice as many gluten-free pet foods were launched than breakfast cereals.

Or for Eating Beauty and hair products, and even household cleaners, carry the label.

Source: Mintel Group

Gluten-Free Foods (With No Rice!) That Passed Our Taste Test

Our professional tasters gave these a thumbs-up. Still, be mindful of nutrition.

Flax 4 Life Wild Blueberry Muffin

Moist, dense, and dark brown. Flavorful and fairly complex, with oats, apple, cinnamon, and nutmeg. Denser and less cakelike than you might expect of a blueberry muffin; more like an apple-cinnamon muffin than a blueberry one.

Nutritional info

(1 muffin): 300 calories, 14 g fat, 420 mg sodium, 10 g fiber, 22 g sugars.

Absolutely Gluten-Free Original Crackers

With nicely browned edges, this product looks and tastes like a typical water cracker. Toasted grain notes and moderate saltiness are well-balanced in this crispy and crunchy snack.

Nutritional info

(9 crackers): 60 calories, 2 g fat, 50 mg sodium, <1 g fiber, 0 g sugars.

(continued)

Maninis Papa's Pane Rustic Multigrain Bread Mix

We had to add ¼ tsp. sugar to the yeast to get good results with this mix. Moist, tender, and nutty with a flavorful crust. Better toasted.

Nutritional info

(¼ loaf): 120 calories, 4.5 g fat, 160 mg sodium, 2 g fiber, 1 g sugars.

General Mills Corn Chex, Gluten Free

Crispy-crunchy woven squares taste of toasted corn. Straightforward taste, mild and clean.

Nutritional info

(1 cup): 120 calories, 0.5 g fat, 220 mg sodium, 2 g fiber, 3 g sugars.

Lucy's Gluten-Free Chocolate Chip Cookies

Toasted oatmeal flavors give them more of an oatmeal-cookie taste. On the salty side, with slight-moderate sweetness; very light and crispy texture. Sodium is a bit high.

Nutritional info

(3 cookies): 130 calories, 5 g fat, 170 mg sodium, 2 g fiber, 12 g sugars.

Bob's Red Mill Gluten-Free Pancake Mix

More browned-looking than a regular pancake. Mixed nonspecific grain flavors with toasted notes and slight sweetness. Overall, the flavor is better than the texture. Sodium was significantly higher than in similar mixes.

Nutritional info

(2 4-inch pancakes): 210 calories, 6 g fat, 700 mg sodium, 2 g fiber, 5 g sugars.

Smart Flour Classic Cheese Pizza

Browned mozzarella cheese on a toasted, thin, crispy crust and a slightly sweet tomato sauce. Flavors are well-balanced overall. High in sodium.

Nutritional info

(½ pizza): 340 calories, 14 g fat, 830 mg sodium, 3 g fiber, 5 g sugars.

XO Baking Company Fudge Brownie Gourmet Mix

Dense, moist; makes a fudgy rather than cakelike brownie. Calories and fat are similar to a regular mix.

Nutritional info

(1 brownie): 170 calories, 8 g fat, 95 mg sodium, 2 g fiber, 19 g sugars.

Mission White Corn Tortillas

Light tan with brown flecks, they have a rubbery feel in the hand, but that doesn't translate to the palate. A basic corn tortilla.

Nutritional Info

(2 tortillas): 100 calories, 2 g fat, 10 mg sodium, 3 g fiber, 2 g sugars.

Live G Free Gluten-Free Penne Rigate 100% Corn Pasta (Aldi)

Mild corn flavor makes it a good substitute for regular pasta flavorwise, but it has a chalky texture. Adding sauce helped.

Nutritional info

(2 oz., dry): 190 calories, 0.5 g fat, 0 mg sodium, 2 g fiber, 1 g sugars.

Against the Grain Gourmet Original Rolls

Slight eggy flavor; mild overall. Toasting improves texture and flavor. Relatively high in fat and sodium.

Nutritional Info

(1 roll): 223 calories, 11 g fat, 272 mg sodium, 0 g fiber, 0 g sugars.

Kind Plus Peanut Butter Dark Chocolate + Protein Bar

Lots of big pieces of nuts, with a dark-chocolate coating on the bottom and chocolate drizzle on top. Moderately sweet; a firm and chewy bar with some crunchiness from the nuts.

Nutritional Info

(1 bar): 200 calories, 13 g fat, 40 mg sodium, 2.5 g fiber, 9 g sugars.

Other Products Worth Trying

1. XO Baking Company Gluten-Free Pancake & Waffle Gourmet Mix
2. Glutino Original New York Style Bagels
3. Against the Grain Sesame Bagels
4. Maninis Classic Peasant Bread Mix Miracolo Pane
5. Kashi Organic Promise Indigo Morning breakfast cereal
6. Flax 4 Life Mini Flax Muffins, Chocolate Brownie
7. Bob's Red Mill Gluten-Free Brownie Mix
8. Mediterranean Snacks Lentil Crackers, Sea Salt
9. Against the Grain Gourmet
10. Three Cheese frozen pizza
11. Sam Mills Pasta d'Oro 100% Corn Pasta Penne Rigate
12. Lärabar Peanut Butter Chocolate Chip snack bar
13. Nature Valley Roasted Nut Crunch Peanut Crunch snack bar

Critical Thinking

1. Why do so many consumers choose a gluten-free diet even if it's not medically necessary?
2. What are the risks from a gluten-free diet?

Internet References

Academy of Nutrition and Dietetics
www.eatright.org/

Celiac Disease Foundation
www.celiac.org

Society for Nutrition Education and Behavior
www.sneb.org

Article   Prepared by: Eileen L. Daniel, *SUNY College at Brockport*

Food Myths

What Science Knows (and Does Not Know) about Diet and Nutrition

HARRIET HALL

Learning Outcomes

After reading this article, you will be able to:

- Explain the relationship between diet and cancer prevention.

- Understand the basics of the Paleolithic diet.

- Describe the impact of genetically modified food on health.

Koalas have it easy. What to eat? No worries: they eat eucalyptus leaves, period. We humans have it tougher. Ever since Eve and the apple, we have had to make decisions about what to eat. Today we are constantly bombarded with conflicting advice about food. "Eat fish because it's a great source of omega-3S." "Don't eat fish because it contains toxic mercury." (Actually both of those statements are true, so we need to quantify the actual content in specific varieties of fish and carefully consider the risk/benefit ratio.)

Fad diets and "miracle" diet supplements promise to help us lose weight effortlessly. Different diet gurus offer a bewildering array of diets that promise to keep us healthy and make us live longer: vegan, Paleo, Mediterranean, low fat, low carb, raw food, gluten-free. . . the list goes on. Obviously, they can't all be right. Food myths abound, often supported by the strongest of convictions and emotions. What are we to believe?

We live in the Information Age. Unfortunately, bad information comes mixed with the good. The only reliable guide to reality is science, but when it comes to food, there's a problem. It's hard to do a gold standard double-blinded randomized controlled study on diet. We could learn a lot if we could divide infants into two groups, insert feeding tubes, pour competing diets directly into their stomachs throughout their lifetimes, and see which group lived longer and had fewer illnesses. But that just isn't feasible. So we have to rely on less conclusive forms of evidence. We can compare two groups who eat different diets (such as vegans v. meat-eaters, or Mediterraneans v. Americans), but those groups almost always differ in other ways that affect results, ways that we didn't think to control for. We can ask people what they eat, but we can't trust their answers to be accurate; people tend to misremember, to misestimate portion sizes, and to misreport what they eat in the direction they think the researcher will approve of. We can tell people what to eat for a study, or even provide the food we want them to eat; but compliance is a problem, and studies are time-limited.

It's not hopeless, because we can combine less ideal types of research and reach a reasonable conclusion if the evidence from all the avenues of inquiry converges. We didn't need lifelong blinded trials to learn that smoking causes cancer: the evidence from animal studies, analysis of tobacco for carcinogens, various kinds of studies comparing smokers to nonsmokers, etc., all pointed in the same direction. If the evidence from diet studies were as coherent, as consistent, and as strong as the evidence from tobacco studies, science would have reached a consensus by now, and we would know which diet is optimal. Unfortunately, the evidence for different diets is inconsistent or lacking. If anyone claims to *know* how you should eat, you can pretty much guarantee they are wrong. We have hints, but we don't have a definitive answer about which diet is best, and we have pretty good evidence that some of the pronouncements on diet are just plain wrong.

What We Know Is True

Science has given us a lot of reliable information about nutrition. It took a while to realize that "our daily bread" alone wouldn't keep us healthy. As late as the 19th century we had no explanation for scurvy, beriberi, kwashiorkor, and other nutritional deficiency diseases. Vitamins were not discovered until the 1920s. Today we know that we need six categories of nutrients: proteins, fats, carbohydrates, vitamins, minerals, and water. We know that some nutrients like vitamin K are stored in body fat for future use while excess amounts of others, like vitamin C, are excreted in the urine and must be replenished more frequently. We can measure blood levels and body stores of various nutrients. We know that there are 14 essential vitamins and 17 essential minerals plus a few ultra-trace minerals that the body requires in only the tiniest amounts. We have identified the nine amino acids in protein that are "essential" in diet—the ones that the body can't synthesize: phenylalanine, valine, threonine, tryptophan, methionine, leucine, isoleucine, lysine, and histidine. (Serendipity led early Mexicans to a diet based on corn and beams, which together provide all the essential amino acids.) We know that there are two components of fat that are essential fatty acids for humans; omega-3s like alpha-linolenic acid, DHA and EPA, and omega-6s like linoleic acid and arachidonic acid. We know the approximate daily requirements of every nutrient, and they are provided on package labels as Recommended Daily Allowances (RDAs). Dietitians can analyze the nutrient content of a person's diet and can prescribe appropriate diets for various health conditions like diabetes. We understand nutritional requirements well enough that we are able to provide total parenteral nutrition intravenously to patients whose gastrointestinal tract is unable to function for some reason.

We know that the gastrointestinal tract digests what you eat and breaks it down into its component nutrients. The original source of the nutrients is relatively unimportant. Eskimos get most of their nutrients from raw meat and blubber; the Maasai eat raw meat, raw milk, and raw blood from their cattle; vegans eat no animal products of any kind. Throughout human history, people have eaten a wide variety of diets, some rich in plant foods, some poor in plant foods and rich in animal foods. People can thrive on a wide variety of diets; they can even live on raw meat alone. It has all the nutrients we need, even vitamin C, which is not present in cooked meat because it is destroyed by heat. (Not that I would recommend a raw meat diet!) Those are things that we know are true.

What We Know Is Not True

There are other things people think they know about diet that simply aren't true. Some people claim that a proper diet will prevent all cancer and even cure existing cancers. The scientific evidence does not support that claim. The American Cancer Association estimates that a healthy diet could prevent only around a third of all cancers. There's no way diet could prevent the 5–10% of cancers that are genetic, the 25–30% that are caused by tobacco, the 15–20% that are caused by infection, or the 10–15% that are caused by other environmental factors such as sun exposure, radiation, and environmental carcinogens. Some foods reduce the risk of cancer, others increase it. Foods that have shown the strongest correlation with reduced risk of cancer include broccoli, berries, tomatoes, and garlic. The dietary factors that are most strongly associated with cancer include overeating (obesity), alcohol, high intake of red meat and processed meats, and low intake of fruits and vegetables.

Since the days of Hippocrates, people have thought of food as medicine. Recently, one naturopath called it the "most powerful drug," and some have claimed that all disease could be prevented and/or cured by just eating right. Wouldn't that be nice! Too bad it's only wishful thinking. A nutritious diet is essential to health, but food is not medicine except when it is used to correct a dietary deficiency, like citrus fruits for scurvy to correct a lack of vitamin C.

The changing advice about cholesterol and heart disease has confused the public and engendered distrust of science. At first, consumers were told to avoid eggs and other sources of dietary cholesterol; product labels trumpeted "contains no cholesterol." Then further research showed that cholesterol in the diet had little effect on blood cholesterol levels and on the incidence of heart attacks, and recommendations evolved to become more precise as we learned more. We were advised to worry less about dietary cholesterol and worry more about total fat intake, then to avoid saturated fat, and finally to avoid trans fats and not worry so much about the other fats. While it can be frustrating to see science change its mind like this, we should appreciate that science follows the best currently available evidence, in contrast to diet myths that were never based on any credible evidence and never change in response to new evidence.

Opinions about the healthiest diet for humans often rely on arguments from evolution: we should eat what our ancestors evolved to eat. There are some serious pitfalls in that reasoning. There was not one Paleolithic diet: there were many. Our ancestors ate whatever they could get. If they lived near water, they ate fish and shellfish. If they were good hunters in an area with plentiful game, they ate meat. If hunting was not very productive, they relied on gathering food from plants. If fruit was in season, they picked fruit. If nothing was ripe, they dug roots. If there was a plague of locusts, they ate the locusts. Like my smart-aleck brother, they were on a "seefood" diet: "When I see food, I eat it." Studies of traditional diets from around the world have shown a wide variation in macronutrient content, from 30 to 78% carbohydrate, 7 to 40% fat, and 15 to 50% protein. Archaeological evidence indicates that different human groups thrived on a great variety of diets. Our ancestors would not have been able to migrate to new continents or to survive Ice Age climate changes if they had not been able to readily adapt their diets to what was available.

Our homeostatic mechanisms can maintain an equilibrium across a wide range of nutritional inputs. If we eat more vitamin C than we need, we pee out the excess; if we don't eat enough cholesterol, our body manufactures the rest of what it needs. There are hints that exercise may be able to compensate for some of the harmful effects of nutritional deficiencies by activating antioxidant defenses.[1]

The Paleo Diet: What Is "Natural"?

Paleolithic diet proponents argue that eating grain is not "natural," but there is archaeological and other evidence indicating that humans were already eating grains well back in Paleolithic times, long before the development of agriculture. In reality, most of the foods that our Paleolithic ancestors ate no longer exist. Instead of big cars of corn, they gathered tiny teosinte ears. Ancient avocados had only a few millimeters of edible flesh surrounding a huge pit. Ancient chickens were tough and scrawny, and their eggs were small. We have modified essentially all of our foods by selective breeding. Our ancestors gladly traded their "natural" diet for a better, "unnatural" one. Paleo is not healthier. It consists of 50% meat, and studies have shown that increased meat intake increases the rate of death.[2] It recommends avoidance of dairy foods, but a 2010 review found that eating more dairy products was associated with a *lower* risk of heart disease, stroke, diabetes and death.[3] And heavy consumption of whole grain is associated with a *lower* death rate.[4] The Paleo folks explain away all that scientific evidence by accusing researchers of being controlled by the food industry. I don't think industry is powerful enough to corrupt all the scientists studying nutrition.

If evolution teaches us anything, it's that humans are remarkably adaptable and that we have continued to evolve since the Paleolithic. Our early ancestors were all lactose intolerant as adults; babies produce lactase so they can digest breast milk, but adults lose that ability. Now a substantial part of the population continues to produce the lactase enzyme throughout their lifetime. Part of the human population has evolved to take advantage of a new source of nutrition: the milk from dairy cows. After the introduction of dairy farming in northern Europe, the prevalence of lactase-persistence genes rose to over 80% of the population, while in other parts of the world where dairy farming was not practiced it remained essentially zero.[5] Similarly, populations with high-starch diets have more copies of the gene for amylase (needed to digest starch) than those with low-starch diets.[6] These are examples of evolution in action; we have evolved beyond the Paleo days, so it is not logical to revert to Paleo eating habits.

Travellers commonly develop GI upsets as they encounter new foods and new microbes; with prolonged residence in a new area, they adapt through changes in their intestinal flora and through other mechanisms. In diet studies, Dr. Antonis Kafatis found that when Cretans and British subjects were fed olive-oil-based meals, the Cretans had faster clearance of blood lipids, but after 3–4 weeks the British subjects' clearance became equal to that of the Cretans.[7] People have a fixed set of genes, but the expression of those genes can change when they change their diet. When African Bushmen were switched to a high-starch European diet, the amylase levels in their saliva increased fourfold.[8] Epigenetics turns genes on and off and can sometimes transmit those changes in gene expression to the next generation or two.

We evolved to become exceptionally skilled omnivores with the intelligence and inventiveness to create technology that increases food production and creates new food sources. One of those technological advances was cooking. Advocates of the raw food diet have an underlying vitalistic philosophy; they believe that there is some kind of life force energy in raw foods (although they don't go quite as far as the "live food" advocates). They try to justify their ideology with science. They argue that fire was a late discovery and cooking is not "natural." They argue that cooking destroys nutrients and destroys the natural enzymes in foods, but we know that digestion disassembles those enzymes so they don't act in the human body. And cooking actually increases the availability of many nutrients. They argue that cooking produces toxins, and there is some truth to that, especially for fried foods, but the amounts are small. There is no evidence that a raw food diet is healthier. In fact, cooking was a discovery that allowed humans to take advantage of foods that would otherwise have been indigestible, to spend less energy chewing, and to extract more nutrients from some foods. And cooking has been around for longer than they think, with current estimates going back as far as a million years or more.[9] It has even been suggested that cooking provided the increased energy to facilitate the evolution of larger brains. It could be argued that we "should" do whatever evolution has insured that we "could" do, such as agriculture, cooking, selective breeding, and food processing.

Cooking is a form of food processing. Processed foods are typically demonized, but they can be either good or bad. According to the IFIC (the International Food Information Council), "processed foods" encompass four categories: (1) foods that are processed to preserve freshness (like canned salmon and frozen fruits and vegetables); (2) foods combined with sweeteners, colors, spices, or preservatives (like rice, cake mix, salad dressing, and pasta sauce); (3) "ready-to-eat" foods (like breakfast cereal, yogurt, rotisserie chicken, granola bars, cookies, crackers, and sodas); and (4) prepared foods (like deli foods, frozen meals, and pizzas). The IFIC further identifies a "minimally processed" food category, which includes washed and packaged fruits and vegetables, bagged salads, and ground nuts.[10]

We humans have always processed our foods. We seldom just grab an animal or plant and devour it without any preparation. Most of the food we eat is processed in one way or another, by washing, chopping, grinding, cooking, canning, freezing, drying, skinning, smoking, adding preservatives so foods will stay edible longer, etc. Food processing is not inherently evil. It should be considered on a case-by-case basis; processing that adds sugar or toxins or removes nutrients is not healthy, but other kinds of processing increase food availability and nutritional value.

Dietary Morals and Weight Loss Myths

There is a moral aspect to dietary recommendations. In his book *Diet Cults,*[11] Matt Fitzgerald argues that a propensity to make moral judgments based on others' food choices began as a practical way to encode trial and error knowledge about safe foods and later became hardwired into human behavior because of the survival advantage of group cohesion. Our tribe vilifies those other tribes who "don't eat right." Taboo foods that are perfectly healthy have been encoded into religious rules like halal and kosher because taboos serve to strengthen group identity. Today's environmentalists and animal rights activists are almost religious in their zeal to condemn those who eat in ways that they consider bad for the environment or for animal welfare.

Peer pressure is powerful but is not necessarily in line with truths about diet. Even without explicit rules, we tend to eat like our parents or our social groups. Who is attracted to the Paleo diet? Mostly men (the virile caveman image?). On the other hand, 60% of vegetarians are women (appeal to compassion?). Both are attractive as a form of rebellion and rejection of artificial modern life. People believe that they have chosen a diet rationally, but they really choose for social and emotional reasons and then try to justify their choice with post hoc reasoning.

One of the major reasons people adopt diets is to lose weight. Pretty much all weight-loss diets succeed in the short term but fail to keep the weight off permanently. Studies have shown that people who lost weight and kept it off did so by using all kinds of different methods; no one diet was more effective than another. Motivation was the key. Common factors for those who kept the weight off included keeping a food diary, self-weighing, exercise, and consistency (not varying eating habits on weekends and special occasions).

All diets are essentially ways to trick yourself into tolerating a lower calorie intake. Different tricks work better for different people. Satiety is important; bulky, low calorie density foods provide satiety with fewer calories. A low fat diet helps some people control calories because fat contains nine calories per gram while protein and carbs provide only four calories per gram. If you eat fewer calories than you burn, you will necessarily lose weight. A reduction of 500 calories a day equates to the loss of a pound a week. It's simple physics in principle, but it can be diabolically difficult in practice. Some people argue that calorie counting won't work because not all calories sire equal. It's true that there are differences in absorption, satiety, metabolism, and effect on hormones, but in practice those differences are too small to matter very much.

Low carb diets have been recommended both for weight loss and for health. High carb intake has been blamed for the obesity epidemic, but studies have found that, if anything, people who eat more carbs are less likely to be overweight.[12] Comparison of weight loss diets shows that it is the calorie restriction that matters, not the macronutrient content.[13] In some studies, people have lost weight more rapidly with low carb, but the long-term results are no different. Low carb cam be a convenient way to reduce calorie intake; but the initial enthusiasm for diets like the Atkins diet and the South Beach diet is waning, and some people prefer other diets that work just as well. Some athletes bought into the fad and tried to reduce their dependence on carbohydrates, but the diet of the world's best endurance athletes (from Africa) is 75% carbohydrate. Gary Taubes, in his impressive 640-page tome *Good Calories, Bad Calories,*[14] argues that the official low fat diet recommendations for heart disease prevention were not based on good science and had the unintended effect of making people eat more carbohydrates, so low fat diets indirectly caused the obesity epidemic. He advocates low carb not just for weight loss but for prevention of the so-called diseases of civilization (obesity, heart disease, diabetes, cancer, Alzheimer's, etc.). He marshals an impressive mass of data about insulin resistance, fat storage, the metabolic syndrome, inflammation, and other factors to support his thesis. He doesn't say much about other research that contradicts his thesis, and he admits that his ideas haven't yet been properly tested against competing ideas; but he urges readers to adopt his diet recommendations without waiting for the testing to be done. So in essence, he is doing exactly what he vilified the low fat advocates for doing, advising population-wide dietary changes based on inadequate evidence. Chris Voight (executive director of the Washington State Potato Commission) did an informal test. He went on a potatoes-only diet for 60 days; according to low carb theories he should have gained weight and raised his blood sugar, but instead he lost 21 pounds and lowered his blood sugar.[15] His cholesterol and triglyceride levels dropped too. He felt well and had plenty of energy, although he got awfully tired of eating 20 potatoes a day.

I would love to see Gary Taubes in a debate with Colin Campbell, a man who believes just the opposite and thinks he has just as good evidence. Campbell wrote *The China Study,*[16] subtitled *The Most Comprehensive Study of Nutrition Ever Conducted And the Startling Implications for Diet, Weight Loss, And Long-term Health.* For him, carbs are not the enemy, animal protein and dairy products are. He relies on epidemiologic studies from villages in China and arguments based on laboratory research. He claims that heart disease can be prevented and even reversed by a healthy diet, but the evidence he provides is inadequate to support that claim. He advocates a vegetarian diet devoid of all animal protein and dairy products. Like Taubes, he marshals an impressive mass of data but fails to include other data that tend to discredit his thesis. Obviously, he and Taubes can't possibly both be right; but they could both be wrong, or even wrong in some aspects and right in others.

Good and Bad Foods

Some foods have more of certain nutrients than others, but the idea of "superfoods" is a myth. No food is a perfect source of all nutrients. Yes, spirulina has an impressive array of nutrients; but spinach has even more. Superfood lists disagree with each other and can include as many as 200 foods. If these were all superfoods, almost all foods would be superfoods, making the concept meaningless. So many healthy foods are left off the lists that you could eat a healthy diet while avoiding everything on the list. There's no advantage to eating special, expensive, or exotic foods high in certain nutrients if you can easily get the same nutrients from other foods that are cheaper and easier to find.

No foods are perfectly good, and no foods are perfectly bad. Several supposedly healthy diets prohibit coffee, but the bulk of current evidence indicates that coffee is healthy. A 2012 study in the *New England Journal of Medicine* found that regular coffee drinkers were 10% less likely to die over the next 13 years.[17] The caffeine in coffee is a stimulant, but coffee (whether caffeinated or decaffeinated) is also the number one source of antioxidants in the American diet.[18] Coffee drinkers are less likely to develop certain diseases.

Sugar has been demonized—even called "addicting"—but there's no reason it can't be part of a healthy, nutritious, calorie-controlled diet. Fructose has been demonized, too, especially in the form of high-fructose corn syrup. Table sugar is a combination of one molecule of fructose and one of glucose. So it is 50% fructose. High-fructose corn syrup is not much higher, it's 55% fructose, and its increased sweetness allows using fewer calories for the same effect. And it's cheaper. Apples and peaches have higher percentages of fructose than high-fructose corn syrup.

Even alcohol, despite the harm it does, can be part of a healthy diet when used in moderation; moderate alcohol intake is more effective at reducing the risk of heart attacks and strokes than other interventions like diet and blood pressure control. It is the second-best way to reduce cardiovascular risk after smoking cessation.[19] The benefits of red wine have been attributed to resveratrol, which has been put into pills and hyped way beyond the scientific evidence. Of course, alcohol can't be generally recommended for health because of the dangers of intoxication and addiction.

Water is essential to life, but too much is as bad as too little: people can die of water intoxication. It is important for athletes to replenish lost fluids, but overhydration has killed marathon runners. There are many myths about dehydration, from the myth that we need to drink 8-10 glasses of water a day to Dr. Batmanghelid's "Water Cure" and his claim that dehydration is the main cause of disease.[20] It isn't. It doesn't cause all those diseases, and it doesn't cause most of the symptoms people attribute to it. For most people, in most situations, it is sufficient to drink when you feel thirsty, and the source of the water is not important. You can even get it from coffee and from solid foods that have a high water content.

Organic v. GMO

People worry about the sources of their food. They commonly believe that organic is healthy and GMO is unhealthy. The evidence doesn't support those beliefs. A recent systematic review[21] of 240 published studies concluded that "The published literature lacks strong evidence that organic foods are significantly more nutritious than conventional foods." It suggested that consumption of organic foods may reduce exposure to pesticide residues and antibiotic-resistant bacteria, but it didn't show that this reduction had any significant implications for human health. The amounts are tiny, organic farming also uses pesticides, and simply washing produce removes most residues. People also argue that organic tastes better, but blinded taste tests don't bear that out, and taste probably depends more on freshness than on methods of cultivation. Much of the hype about organic food is based on the "natural is better" fallacy rather than on any actual evidence. Organic food tends to be higher priced, which makes it harder for consumers to buy sufficient nutritious food.

Demonization of GMOs is based on the natural fallacy, on scientific illiteracy, on distrust of large corporations with financial motivations, and on the myth of the evil Frankenstein who tries to play God. As Neil deGrasse Tyson recently tweeted, "Most who fear genetically altered food are unaware that nearly all food has been genetically altered via artificial selection." No one rejects seedless watermelons or wants to trade their corn on the cob for teosinte. Modern science doesn't do anything unique or fundamentally different, it only allows us to speed up the process of genetic modification and improve food for human benefit. Genetic modification has been used to increase a plant's resistance to disease, improve herbicide and insecticide tolerance so less can be used, and increase agricultural yields to feed more people. Golden rice was modified to provide vitamin A to third world children with nutritional deficiencies; it has prevented untold cases of blindness and death. GM foods have been extensively studied and no adverse effects on human health have been found. The highly publicized Seralini study that allegedly showed harmful effects in rats was so flawed that it has now been retracted. As with any technology, genetic modification has the potential for harm, either deliberate or through unforeseen consequences. Continued testing and monitoring is warranted; blanket rejection is not.

Fad Diets

Fad diets and diet cults appeal to emotion, not to evidence-based reasoning. They give their followers a sense of belonging, a sense of control over their health, and a virtuous feeling of doing something that is difficult but good for them. Decisions come first, rationalizations come later. True believers can always find a few cherry-picked scientific studies that tend to support their beliefs. Confirmation bias allows them to notice any feelings of improvement and give diet the credit.

Those magazines at the grocery checkout stands can be relied on to keep you up to date on the latest fad diets that your favorite celebrities are trying. The variety is astounding; the proof is nonexistent; and the premises are often mindbogglingly silly. An article in the *Huffington Post* recently listed the "14 worst fad diets you should absolutely never try":[22]

1. **The Raw Food Diet.** It prohibits any food that is cooked or processed in any way, ignoring the fact that cooking can improve access to nutrients. Raw food preparation is onerous, requiring hours of juicing, germinating, sprouting, dehydrating and rehydrating, blending, cutting, chopping, etc. And while it does put a healthy emphasis on fruits and vegetables, most people find the diet unpalatable, inconvenient, and hard to stick to long-term.

2. **Alkaline Diets.** They prohibit meat, dairy, and a lot of other healthy foods, based on the concept that acidic foods are bad for you. The underlying rationale is pseudoscientific and the diet has never been demonstrated to improve health. Misguided devotees monitor their urine pH, failing to understand that nothing in their diet can change their blood pH, which is maintained in a narrow range by homeostatic mechanisms. Changes in urine pH only show that the kidneys are doing their job.

3. **The Blood Type Diet.** Popularized by naturopath Peter D'Adamo, it postulates that people with different blood types need to avoid certain foods. There isn't a

shred of credible evidence either for the rationale or the effectiveness of the recommendations, and the diet restricts a lot of perfectly healthy foods.

4. **The Werewolf Diet.** This requires fasting during full moon or new moon, and eating differently for each phase. (Why? Because werewolves do it? Because of the tides? This may serve as a reminder that the origin of the word "lunacy" derives from moon.) Fasting can produce temporary loss of a few pounds, but the weight will come right back. The myth of the moon's effect on human physiology is as silly as astrology. And speaking of astrology, there's also a Zodiac diet.

5. **The Cookie Diet.** 500–600 calories a day of special high-protein, high-fiber cookies plus a normal dinner. A gimmick to limit calorie intake, unnecessarily restrictive and the deprivation during the day may lead to binging at dinner.

6. **The Five-Bite Diet.** You can eat whatever you want, but you must skip breakfast and eat 5 bites of food for lunch and dinner. Unless you take improbably huge bites, your calorie intake will be limited to unhealthy levels and nutrition will suffer.

7. **The Master Cleanse/Lemonade Diet.** This one buys into the detoxification myth. For several days, dieters subsist on lemon juice, cayenne pepper, and maple syrup mixed with water. This is a starvation diet that will indeed drop pounds but that will cause unpleasant side effects (fatigue, nausea, dizziness, etc.). And you lose muscle instead of losing fat. *Skeptic* publisher Michael Shermer tried this diet for a week during his cycling days and bonked horribly during long rides. When he returned to a normal diet he got sick from that as well since his body wasn't used to processing food.

8. **The Baby Food Diet.** This allows up to 14 jars of baby food a day, each containing 20–100 calories, followed by a low calorie dinner. Just another gimmick to decrease total calorie intake, and an embarrassment when others see you carrying around jars of baby food.

9. **The Cabbage Soup Diet.** You prepare a fat-free cabbage soup and eat it three times a day along with a few other low calorie foods. That much cabbage produces bloating and gas, and the diet is deficient in protein and other nutrients.

10. **The Grapefruit Diet.** This one has been around for 80 years and is based on the myth that grapefruit produces fat-busting enzymes. We know that enzymes in food are destroyed in the stomach and don't survive to act as enzymes in our bodies. How it really works is that people get so tired of monotonously eating one food item that they eat less. This diet is very low in calories but is not healthy.

11. **The Sleeping Beauty Diet.** If you're sleeping, you're not eating. Sedatives will put you to sleep. I don't think I need to explain why this is not a good idea.

12. **The HCG Diet.** The hormone human chorionic gonadotropin allegedly acts as an appetite suppressant. It must be injected and accompanied by a 500-calorie diet. It has been tested and proven not to work: people lose weight just as well on 500 calories without the injections. To compound the silliness, there is a homeopathic HCG diet using drops that have all the HCG diluted out of them.

13. **The Tapeworm Diet.** Dieters deliberately consume tapeworm eggs so the adult worms will take up residence in their intestines and eat some of the partially digested food, thereby limiting the amount available for humans to absorb, so they tend to lose weight. Tapeworm infections can cause a variety of unpleasant symptoms and can lead to serious complications when masses of them block the intestine or when they migrate to other parts of the body like the liver, heart, eyes, and brain. The yuck factor alone ought to be sufficient to deter most people from following this diet.

14. **The Cotton Ball Diet.** Fiber, anyone? They have to soak the cotton balls in orange juice to get them down. This is dangerous, deprives the body of nutrients, and can lead to intestinal blockages.

This list is incomplete. There are so many more! The "ycast connection" blames a lot of nonspecific symptoms on an alleged overgrowth of yeast in the body that can't be diagnosed with medical tests, and prescribes avoidance of foods that are falsely believed to encourage the growth of yeast. The Maker's Diet restricts dieters to foods that are mentioned in the Bible. Pastor Rick Warren has developed The Daniel Plan based on a story in the book of Daniel about captive Israelites in Babylon. Nebuchadnezzar allowed Daniel and three other captive Israelites to try a diet of vegetables and water, and at the end of 10 days they appeared healthier than those who dined at the king's table. Weight loss was not even mentioned, and this is hardly the kind of experimental evidence we can trust. Even if the story is true, the Bible has lower scientific standards than *The New England Journal of Medicine* and no peer review.

The Gluten Free Fad

One of the biggest fads today is the gluten-free craze. Celiac disease is a serious autoimmune disease; patients must scrupulously avoid gluten or risk severe symptoms and permanent damage to the cells lining the small bowel. People who have not been diagnosed with celiac disease by a doctor and do not meet the criteria

for the disease often believe that they must avoid gluten because they are "gluten sensitive" and get symptoms from eating it. A randomized controlled trial showed evidence for the existence of non-celiac gluten sensitivity. But then a better trial showed that it was not gluten these patients were sensitive to, but FODMAPS (fermentable oligo-di-monosaccharides and polyols).[23] Examples of FODMAPS are fructans in foods like wheat, garlic, and artichokes; fructose (found in fruits and other foods); lactose in dairy products; and galactans found in some legumes. A low-FODMAP diet has been developed and has been successful in treating irritable bowel syndrome (IBS).

People who have no idea what gluten or celiac mean have jumped on the gluten-free bandwagon because some celebrity is on it and they have the mistaken idea that it will produce weight loss and is a healthier way to eat in general. A cardiologist named William Davis has contributed to the mythology by inventing the Wheat Belly Diet, claiming that the traditional foods relied on by billions of people through the ages, including wheat, rice, corn, and potatoes are unhealthy, cause a big belly, and damage the brain. This is just another low carb diet that ignores the bulk of the scientific evidence, makes false associations, and exaggerates grains (pun intended) of truth into delusional mountains.

Variations of Vegetarianism

Fruitarians limit themselves to a diet of at least 75% fruits. Some eat only fallen fruit. They are under the illusion that humans evolved to eat only fruit, that we are frugivores rather than carnivores or omnivores. Of course, that is demonstrably untrue. Some of them argue that the human body is unable to digest meat, also demonstrably untrue. A fruit-only diet doesn't make sense and it leads to nutritional deficiencies, especially in children. Fruitarians can develop protein-energy malnutrition, anemia, and low levels of iron, calcium, essential fatty acids, vitamins, and minerals.

Then there are vegetarians and vegans: 10% of Italians and Swedes, 13% of Americans, and 20–42% of Indians self-identify as vegetarians. Vegans avoid animal products entirely, lacto-ovo-vegetarians allow eggs and milk, and some consider themselves vegetarians but occasionally eat small amounts of fish or even meat. Some vegetarians are more concerned about the environment or about animal cruelty than about health, but there is evidence that a vegetarian diet is a healthy one, and it is certainly healthier than the standard American diet. Seventh-Day Adventists are vegetarians; studies show that they live longer and are healthier than non-Adventists but that could be due to other aspects of their healthy lifestyle. And other studies have suggested that any advantages accruing to vegetarians are likely due to the ample amounts of vegetables in their diet rather than to avoidance of animal products.[24]

Dietary Restriction, Detoxification, and Fasting

The one thing that has been proven to increase longevity in animals is severe calorie restriction (to 40% of the usual intake). Studies in roundworms, flies, fish, mice, and other animals are encouraging; but no human studies have demonstrated increased longevity, and primate studies have had mixed results. Some researchers think that genetics and dietary composition may be more important for longevity than calorie restriction. It is hard to maintain good nutrition with severe calorie restriction, and it is not a diet most people are able to stick to over the long term. In the Minnesota Starvation Experiment,[25] a semi-starvation diet led to serious physical and psychological problems.

What about intermittent fasting? It has a long tradition in religions, where it has instrumental in triggering visions and ecstatic states, and where it has been endowed with meanings for self-control, purification, sacrifice, and group cohesion. Intermittent fasting works well to reduce overall calorie intake, as long as dieters don't compensate by eating more once the fast is over. The daytime fasting/nighttime feasting of Ramadan often results in weight gain.[26]

Fasting is sometimes associated in the modern mind with "detoxification," as in the pseudo-religious juice cleanse purification rituals. The need for detoxification is a myth; the kidneys and liver do the job quite well, and there is no evidence that colon irrigation, detoxification footbaths, or any other detoxification methods actually remove any toxins or improve health in any way.

There are hints that fasting might benefit certain diseases, but it might also lead to inadequate nutrition and compromise the immune system.

Some cancer patients have given up sugar because of the misguided idea that cancers feed on sugar. This myth is based on a misunderstanding of Otto Warburg's 1924 study of cancer metabolism; restricting sugar in the diet has no effect on cancer outcomes.

Some diet advisers not only want to tell you what to eat, but how to eat. Certain foods shouldn't be mixed, they claim; food should be eaten in a certain order; you should avoid drinking liquids with meals. Advocates of Fletcherizing even want to tell you how to chew. Fletcher said each mouthful of food must be chewed 32 times. His slogan was "Nature will castigate those who don't masticate."

Dietary Supplements

The diet supplement industry is big business that capitalizes on irrational fears. Some people argue that the nutritional content of our produce is diminishing over time. There may be a grain of truth to the claim, but as Steven Novella says, "It's complicated" and the practical importance is negligible.[27] People take multivitamins as psychotherapy, to assuage worries that they are not eating a good enough diet.

Although some people need dietary supplements for medical reasons (for instance folic acid to prevent birth defects or iron supplements for iron deficiency anemia), recent research has questioned the wisdom of vitamin supplementation for the general population. Every vitamin can be toxic in large amounts, and studies have found harmful effects from antioxidant supplements and even for the time-honored daily multivitamin. More and more studies are finding a link between both individual vitamins and daily multivitamins and adverse health effects. Vitamin E supplements and high levels of omega-3 are associated with an increased risk of prostate cancer; multivitamins, iron, and copper are associated with a higher rate of death in postmenopausal women; antioxidants like vitamin A, E, and beta-carotene may increase mortality;[28] a large study in Sweden found that vitamin supplements did not improve mortality;[29] smokers who take beta carotene are more likely to die of lung cancer; etc. The body processes vitamins differently depending on whether they are ingested alone in large amounts or combined with other nutrients in food. It makes far more sense to eat a more nutritious diet than to continue with an inadequate diet and try to compensate with supplement pills.

Bodybuilders and other athletes tend to overdo the supplements and protein shakes because they have been misled about their protein requirements. Science tells us there is no advantage to eating more than the 1.2 g per kg of body weight that the typical American diet provides.[30] Once the muscles have become developed, protein requirements drop, and overdoing the protein counteracts natural adaption so that a body builder might tend to lose muscle weight if he stops chugging the protein shakes that he didn't really need in the first place.

What Should We Eat?

The typical American diet is not a very healthy one. It includes too much meat, too many processed foods, too many calories, too few fruits and vegetables, too many empty calories from sugar and high fructose corn syrup that have no other nutritional value, and too much fast food. Much has been written about the evils of big corporations and mass production. Our crops are becoming monocultures and losing genetic variety. The practice of feeding antibiotics to livestock promotes the development of antibiotic resistant strains of bacteria. Feedlots and battery cages are cruel to cows and chickens. Industry has been blamed for manipulating the food choices of the whole population in an unhealthy direction for its own profit. Restaurants are blamed for excess salt, large portion sizes, and a paucity of healthier, low calorie options. Fast food is blamed for its corrupting influences. There are certainly downsides to industrialized food, but we mustn't lose sight of the many benefits. Mass production has made more food, safer food, and food of more consistent quality available to more people at lower prices. We can look for ways to correct the bad practices of big corporations without throwing out the baby with the bath water.

People have tried to blame all our modern health problems on poor eating habits. Gluten, yeast, acid foods, and other components of a healthy diet have served as handy scapegoats. There's a plethora of diets but a paucity of proof. People who follow fad diets are convinced that they work. They are satisfied that they are getting the results they want, but they don't stop to wonder whether other diets might work just as well to get those same results. Since humans can thrive on a variety of diets, it's easy to become convinced that whatever you are eating is the healthiest choice.

In the future, science-based nutritionists maybe able to provide individual diet advice tailored to each person's specific genetic makeup, but we're not there yet. Several companies offer direct-to-consumer genome tests; some of them advise customers about the best diet for their genes and conveniently sell them dietary supplements. They promise more than they can deliver; they are not much better than the "individualized" diets based on ABO blood groups or horoscopes. Individual differences are likely to be small; basic nutrition depends on physiology and is the same for every member of the species.

So what's the answer to the question of what we should eat? The answer is that there is no answer. As Matt Fitzgerald says,[31]

Science has not identified the healthiest way to eat. In fact, it has come as close as possible (because you can't prove a negative) to confirming that there is no such thing as the healthiest diet. To the contrary, science has established quite definitively that humans are able to thrive equally well on a variety of diets. Adaptability is the hallmark of man as eater. For us, many diets are good while none is perfect.

Until better evidence is available, I think the best plan is to adopt the diet advice that most nutrition experts are able to agree on and that is epitomized by Michael Pollan's pithy "Eat food. Not too much. Mostly plants." More fruits and vegetables, less red meat, less processed food, more variety, limit the calories, control your weight.

In his book Diet Cults,[32] Matt Fitzgerald lists a hierarchy of 10 food categories from more healthy to less healthy:

- Vegetables
- Fruits
- Nuts, seeds and healthy oils
- High quality meat and seafood
- Whole grains
- Dairy
- Refined grains
- Low quality meat and seafood
- Sweets
- Fried foods

He recommends eating foods in amounts that correspond to their place on the hierarchy with the major emphasis on vegetables and fruits. Foods that are lower on the list need not be avoided, but the amounts should decrease as you go down the list. One could argue with his list, and it hasn't been established that his plan will keep people healthier or make them live longer, but it is as good a place as any to start, and it is consistent with the limited evidence that we do have about nutrition.

Finally, remember that health and longevity are not the only reasons we eat. Think about eating to make you happy, not just eating to make you healthy. Eating is one of the great pleasures of life. Is it worth gambling on uncertain diet advice if it means you have to forgo the pleasures of your favorite foods and of shared dining experiences? There's an old joke where a doctor tells an elderly patient he will live longer if he stops smoking, drinking, eating unhealthy foods, and having sex; the old guy replies, "You call that living?!"

References

1. *http://bit.ly/YAxkkE*
2. http://1.usa.gov/1p006Ar
3. http://1.usa.gov/1rmJv1B
4. http://bit.ly/VFZx7z
5. http://1.usa.gov/1z26TiY
6. http://1.usa.gov/1sVdwVO
7. http://bit.ly/1pLA3BW
8. http://bit.ly/YAy5KH
9. http://bit.ly/1mmGOka
10. http://bit.ly/1tmrjmh
11. Fitzgerald, Matt. 2014. *Diet Cults: The Surprising Fallacy at the Core of Nutrition Fads and a Guide to Healthy Eating for the Rest of Us. Pegasus* Books.
12. http://1.usa.gov/1naTKhW
13. http://1.usa.gov/VFZKb4
14. Taubes, Gary. 2008. *Good Calories, Bad Calories*. Anchor.
15. http://bit.ly/1w9L05h
16. Campbell, T. Colin, and Thomas M. Campbell. 2006. *The China Study: The Most Comprehensive Study of Nutrition Ever Conducted And the Startling Implications for Diet, Weight Loss, and Long-term Health.* BenBella Books.
17. http://1.usa.gov/1q0WMc9
18. http://bit.ly/1viwkwk
19. http://bit.ly/1z27zoC
20. http://bit.ly/1mmGjve
21. http://bit.ly/1oecTiG
22. http://huff.to/1AnvzGd

23. http://1.usa.gov/1i5bl79
24. http://1.usa.gov/1uXzYP4
25. http://bit.ly/1do4lzZ
26. http://latimesblogs.latimes.com/world_now/2012/07/cairo
    -the-sun-slips-beyond-the-nile-and-the-fast-is-broken-as-they
    -have-done-for-centuries-during-the-holy-month-of-ramad.html
27. http://theness.com/neurologicablog/index.php/
    nutritional-content-of-produce/
28. http://www.ncbi.nlm.nih.gov/pubmed/24241129
29. http://www.ncbi.nlm.nih.gov/pubmed/17764599
30. http://faculty.washington.edu/crowther/Misc/RBC/protein.shtml
31. Fitzgerald, op cit., 10
32. Fitzgerald, op cit, 260-61.

Critical Thinking

1. What is the best diet to prevent cancer?
2. Is there benefit to eating a Paleolithic diet?
3. What are the moral aspects regarding dietary recommendations?

Internet References

Academy of Nutrition and Dietetics
www.eatright.org/

Society for Nutrition Education and Behavior
www.sneb.org

Article   Prepared by: Eileen L. Daniel, *SUNY Brockport*

Fat Facts and Fat Fiction

New research can help you make the best choices for your health.

CONSUMER REPORTS ON HEALTH

Learning Outcomes

After reading this article, you will be able to:

- Explain the difference between healthy and less healthy fats.

- Understand why consumers believe they should try to eliminate most fats from their diets.

- Understand the role of healthy fats in the diet.

If you're confused about fats these days, you're in good company. With research coming in at breakneck speed in recent years, even experts have a hard time agreeing about which fats we should consume, and in what exact proportions, to improve our health and prevent chronic disease. Here we review what the strongest evidence says about healthy choices to make at the grocery store and in your kitchen.

Are Saturated Fats Still "Bad"?

Yes, the best available evidence suggests that saturated fat found in such food as meat, full-fat cheese, ice cream, and cake is still worse for you than the unsaturated fat in vegetable oils, nuts, and avocados. According to a recent report from the United Nations, there is convincing evidence that replacing saturated fat with polyunsaturated fat reduces the risk of heart disease. And a 2012 review of studies by the independent Cochrane Collaboration found that replacing saturated fat with unsaturated fat lowered the risk of cardiovascular events, such as heart attacks and strokes. The authors reported that for every 1,000 people in the studies, there were 77 such events for people on a regular diet compared with 66 for those on a reduced saturated-fat diet.

There's an important caveat, which can make the message here somewhat confusing: When cutting saturated fats, substitute with healthful alternatives, not refined carbohydrates (which are found in such items as white bread, pizza, and snack foods). Otherwise, you probably won't reduce your risk of heart disease and may well increase it, according to the U.N. report. As Penny Kris-Etherton, Ph.D., distinguished professor of nutrition at Penn State University, puts it: "It's not that saturated fats aren't bad anymore. It's that saturated fats and refined carbohydrates are equally bad."

Which Are Better: Mono- or Polyunsaturated Oils?

Nutritionists can't agree about this one, though they do agree that unsaturated fats are better than saturated ones. On the one hand, there is plenty of evidence to support the health benefits of the Mediterranean diet, which calls for generous amounts of olive oil, a mostly mono-unsaturated fat. But when researchers make direct comparisons of mono- and polyunsaturated fats, they generally find stronger evidence of a cardio-protective effect for polyunsaturated fat, found abundantly in safflower, soybean, and sunflower oils.

The American Heart Association recommends minimum dietary intake levels for certain polyunsaturated fats that the body has trouble synthesizing on its own. For example, it suggests getting at least 5 percent to 10 percent of fat calories from omega-6 polyunsaturated fats, and eating at least two servings a week of fish rich in omega-3 polyunsaturated fats. But it makes no specific minimum recommendation for mono-unsaturated fat.

Choosing a variety of plant-based oils, plus low-mercury fish such as salmon twice a week, will help you meet the recommended intake levels and get plenty of all the "good" fats.

Should I Consider the Omega-6 to Omega-3 Ratio?

Omega-6 and omega-3 are two types of polyunsaturated fat—a "good" fat. Many studies suggest that diets rich in two omega-3 fats—eicosapentaenoic acid (EPA) and docosahexaenoic acid (DHA), found in high levels in fish—are linked to lower rates of cardiovascular disease.

To maximize those heart benefits, some experts recommend limiting omega-6 fat found in sources such as corn oil and soybean oil, which have become common in the human diet only in the past 100 years or so, and getting more omega-3s from traditional sources such as fish.

According to some experts, getting too much omega-6 fat might be harmful because it could promote inflammation—which can lead to cardiovascular and other problems—and block the beneficial anti-inflammatory effects of omega-3s. While the jury is still out, recent evidence suggests that omega-6 fats may not in fact increase inflammation.

Can you get enough omega-3 from oils without consuming fish or taking supplements? Probably not. Only a small amount of the alpha-linoleic acid (ALA) found in such oils as canola, flaxseed, and soybean is converted in the body to the more-beneficial omega-3s—EPA and DHA.

The American Heart Association's current position is that both omega-3 and omega-6 fats are beneficial. They say it is more important to meet the minimum recommended intakes for both fats than to try to achieve any specific consumption ratio. Still, there are important gaps and limitations in the research, and conclusions may change as more evidence surfaces.

Can Fats Affect Cancer Risk?

It's your body fat—not the fat in your food—that you should be worrying about most when it comes to cancer risk. According

---

Shopper's guide to fats and oils

Oils with the lowest amount of saturated fat are listed first in each category. Solid fats, such as stick margarine and shortening, are likely to contain trans fats, which should be avoided. Unrefined oils will have a stronger, more distinctive taste than refined oils.

Type of fat/oil	Fatty acids %[1]			Taste	Cost[2]	Best uses
	Mono	Poly	Sat			
Everyday oils						
Safflower	14	75	6	Neutral	$$	Good all-purpose oils for salads and cooking, including pan-frying and deep-frying. Suitable for some baked items (brownies, muffins).
Canola	63	28	7	Neutral	$	
Sunflower	20	66	10	Neutral	$$	
Grapeseed	16	70	10	Neutral	$$	
Corn	28	55	13	Neutral	$	
Olive	73	11	14	Distinctive fruitiness in better virgin oils	$$ to $$$	Extra-virgin is good for salads and light sautéeing. Use lower-grade oils for higher-heat cooking.
Soybean	23	58	16	Neutral	$	Good all-purpose oil; sometimes labeled "vegetable oil."
Peanut	46	32	17	Neutral to mild nutty flavor	$$	Good for all-around use. Unrefined oil adds flavor to Asian dishes.
Tub margarine (vegetable-oil base)	32	46	21	Mild	$	Good substitute for butter for most uses.
Specialty oils (use occasionally)						
Almond	70	17	8	Distinctive	$$$	Unrefined oils are good for dipping, in salads, or drizzled on food. Toasted oils pack extra flavor.
Flaxseed	18	68	9	Distinctive	$$$	
Walnut	23	63	9	Distinctive	$$$	
Sesame	40	42	14	Distinctive	$$$	
Solid fats (use sparingly)						
Stick margarine	39	24	15	Mild	$	Solid fats are best for some baked goods (flaky piecrusts, pastries) or when used judiciously to impart richness (in buttery sauces, for example). Shortening and stick margarine can contain trans fats, which should be avoided.
Shortening	45	26	25	Neutral to mild	$	
Lard (pork fat)	45	11	39	Mild, savory	$	
Palm	37	9	49	Mild	$$	
Butter	21	3	51	Mild	$	
Coconut	6	2	87	Mild	$$ to $$$	

[1] Percentages calculated per 100 grams. Percentages do not add up to 100 because we did not include some minor constituents. "High-oleic" versions of some oils have higher monounsaturated and lower polyunsaturated fat content. [2] Cost calculations based on an Informal shopper survey.

to a comprehensive 2007 review of studies by the World Cancer Research Fund and the American Institute for Cancer Research, there is no strong, convincing evidence that eating more or less total fat, or any individual type of fat, has any significant effect on cancer.

Since obesity is one of the few diet-related factors that is strongly and consistently linked to a risk of cancer, the best diet for cancer prevention may be one that can help you maintain a healthy weight.

Are Coconut and Palm Oil Good for You or Not?

The consensus is that those oils are loaded with cholesterol-raising saturated fat. But dissenters say there is emerging evidence that tropical oils, especially coconut oil, behave differently in the body than animal-derived saturated fats, and might have under-appreciated health benefits.

Philip Calder, Ph.D., professor of nutritional immunology at the University of Southampton in England and editor-in-chief of the *British Journal of Nutrition,* notes that while more research is needed, for now, "There's not that much evidence that coconut oil offers an advantage over other types of oil, and it's likely to raise your cholesterol."

What to do? Your best bet for the time being is to limit consumption of those oils but keep an open mind.

How Does Processing Affect the Benefits and Risks of Oil?

Oils may be processed using mechanical pressing or heat and chemicals, a method that can affect its flavor and potentially its health benefits. Olive oil, for example, is prized for the complex flavors that are strongest when the oil is fresh from the fruit. That's why higher grades (extra virgin and virgin) are given only to mechanically pressed oil that hasn't been treated with heat or chemicals. Those premium oils contain higher quantities of antioxidants, which are eliminated or reduced from lesser oils during processing.

Processed or refined oils do have some pluses, though. They are less expensive, last longer, and can hold up to high-heat uses like frying without smoking and breaking down into potentially toxic compounds. On the minus side, refined oils may have been extracted with hexane, an industrial solvent. A form of hexane is classified as an air pollutant by the Environmental Protection Agency and as a neurotoxin by the Centers for Disease Control and Prevention, and environmental groups have raised concerns about residues that might be left behind in the oil.

Testing by an organic advocacy group found trace amounts of hexane residue (less than 10 parts per million) in a sample of soybean oil. However, almost all of the research on hexane toxicity has involved factory workers breathing in high concentrations of air-borne hexanes.

At very low exposure levels through food, there is no reason to think it should be a health problem, says toxicologist John L. O'Donoghue, Ph.D., of the University of Rochester School of Medicine and Dentistry.

If you're concerned about hexane in oil, look for labels that say it was "expeller pressed." Oils that carry the "USDA Organic" label are also produced without hexane.

Bottom line. According to the 2010 U.S. Dietary Guidelines, 20 to 35 percent of the calories in a healthful diet should come from fats. Most of that total should consist of plant oils such as canola, olive, and soybean oil (usually labeled simply as vegetable oil). Coconut and palm oils are an exception.

Overall, limit your intake of saturated fats to less than 10 percent of your daily calories. That's about 4 teaspoons for someone eating a typical 2,000-calorie-a-day diet. To achieve that, eat less animal-based food (full-fat cheese, processed meats, and dairy desserts like ice cream) and highly processed snack food (cakes and cookies). In addition, reduce saturated fat by filling most of your plate with fruit and vegetables.

Critical Thinking

1. What is the difference between healthy and unhealthy fat in the diet?
2. What type of foods will increase healthy fats in the diet?

Create Central

www.mhhe.com/createcentral

Internet References

The American Dietetic Association
   www.eatright.org
Center for Science in the Public Interest (CSPI)
   www.cspinet.org

Article   Prepared by: Eileen L. Daniel, *SUNY Brockport*

Yes, Healthful Fast Food Is Possible. But Edible?

A tofu taco from Lyfe Kitchen, Buffalo "wings" with ranch dressing from Veggie Grill and Veggie Grill's "cheeseburger" on kale.

Mark Bittman

Learning Outcomes

After reading this article, you will be able to:

- Explain what has driven the market for healthy fast food.
- Describe what consumers are seeking besides nutrition when they opt for healthy fast food.
- Understand why so many fast food companies are investing in healthier options.

When my daughter was a teenager, about a dozen years ago, she went through a vegetarian phase. Back then, the payoff for orthodontist visits was a trip to Taco Bell, where the only thing we could eat were bean burritos and tacos. It wasn't my favorite meal, but the mushy beans in that soft tortilla or crisp shell were kind of soothing, and the sweet "hot" sauce made the experience decent enough. I usually polished off two or three.

I was thinking of those Taco Bell stops during a recent week of travel. I had determined, as a way of avoiding the pitfalls of airport food, to be vegan for the length of the trip. This isn't easy. By the time I got to Terminal C at Dallas/Fort Worth, I couldn't bear another Veggie Delite from Subway, a bad chopped salad on lousy bread. So I wandered up to the Taco Bell Express opposite Gate 14 and optimistically asked the cashier if I could get a bean burrito without cheese or sour cream. He pointed out a corner on the overhead display where the "fresco" menu offered pico de gallo in place of dairy, then upsold me on a multilayered "fresco" bean burrito for about 3 bucks. As he was talking, the customers to my right and left, both fit, suit-wearing people bearing expressions of hunger and resignation, perked up. They weren't aware of the fresco menu, either. One was trying to "eat healthy on the road"; the other copped to "having vegan kids." Like me, they were intrigued by a fast-food burrito with about 350 calories, or less than half as many as a Fiesta Taco Salad bowl. It wasn't bad, either.

Twelve years after the publication of "Fast Food Nation" and nearly as long since Morgan Spurlock almost ate himself to death, our relationship with fast food has changed. We've gone from the whistle-blowing stage to the higher-expectations stage, and some of those expectations are being met. Various states have passed measures to limit the confinement of farm animals. In-N-Out Burger has demonstrated that you don't have to underpay your employees to be profitable. There are dozens of plant-based alternatives to meat, with more on the way; increasingly, they're pretty good.

The fulfillment of these expectations has led to higher ones. My experience at the airport only confirmed what I'd been hearing for years from analysts in the fast-food industry. After the success of companies like Whole Foods, and healthful (or theoretically healthful) brands like Annie's and Kashi, there's now a market for a fast-food chain that's not only healthful itself, but vegetarian-friendly, sustainable and even humane. And, this being fast food: cheap. "It is significant, and I do believe it is coming from consumer desire to have choices and more balance," says Andy Barish, a restaurant analyst at Jefferies LLC, the investment bank. "And it's not just the coasts anymore."

I'm not talking about token gestures, like McDonald's fruit-and-yogurt parfait, whose calories are more than 50 percent sugar. And I don't expect the prices to match those of Taco Bell or McDonald's, where economies of scale and inexpensive ingredients make meals dirt cheap. What I'd like is a place that serves only good options, where you don't have to resist the junk food to order well, and where the food is real—by which I mean dishes that generally contain few ingredients and are recognizable to everyone, not just food technologists. It's a place where something like a black-bean burger piled with vegetables and baked sweet potato fries—and, hell, maybe even a vegan shake—is less than 10 bucks and 800 calories (and way fewer without the shake). If I could order and eat that in 15 minutes, I'd be happy, and I think a lot of others would be, too. You can try my recipes for a fast, low-calorie burger, fries and shake.

In recent years, the fast-food industry has started to heed these new demands. Billions of dollars have been invested in more healthful fast-food options, and the financial incentives justify these expenditures. About half of all the money spent on food in the United States is for meals eaten outside the home. And last year McDonald's earned $5.5 billion in profits on $88 billion in sales. If a competitor offered a more healthful option that was able to capture just a single percent of that market share, it would make $55 million. Chipotle, the best newcomer of the last generation, has beaten that 1 percent handily. Last year, sales approached $3 billion. In the fourth quarter, they grew by 17 percent over the same period in the previous year.

Numbers are tricky to pin down for more healthful options because the fast food industry doesn't yet have a category for "healthful." The industry refers to McDonald's and Burger King as "quick-serve restaurants"; Chipotle is "fast casual"; and restaurants where you order at the counter and the food is brought to you are sometimes called "premium fast casual." Restaurants from these various sectors often deny these distinctions, but QSR, an industry trade magazine—"Limited-Service, Unlimited Possibilities"—spends a good deal of space dissecting them.

However, after decades of eating the stuff, I have my own. First, there are those places that serve junk, no matter what kind of veneer they present. Subway, Taco Bell (I may be partial to them, but really. . .), McDonald's and their ilk make up the Junk Food sector. One step up are places with better ambience and perhaps better ingredients—Shake Shack, Five Guys, Starbucks, Pret a Manger—that also peddle unhealthful food but succeed in making diners feel better about eating it, either because it tastes better, is surrounded by some healthful options, the setting is groovier or they use some organic or sustainable ingredients. This is the Nouveau Junk sector.

Chipotle combines the best aspects of Nouveau Junk to create a new category that we might call Improved Fast Food. At Chipotle, the food is fresher and tastes much better than traditional fast food. The sourcing, production and cooking is generally of a higher level; and the overall experience is more pleasant. The guacamole really is made on premises, and the chicken (however tasteless) is cooked before your eyes. It's fairly easy to eat vegan there, but those burritos can pack on the calories. As a competitor told me, "Several brands had a head start on [the Chipotle founder Steve] Ells, but he kicked their [expletive] with culture and quality. It's not shabby for assembly-line steam-table Mexican food. It might be worth $10 billion right now." (It is.)

Chipotle no longer stands alone in the Improved Fast Food world: Chop't, Maoz, Freshii, Zoës Kitchen and several others all have their strong points. And—like Chipotle—they all have their limitations, starting with calories and fat. By offering fried chicken and fried onions in addition to organic tofu, Chop't, a salad chain in New York and Washington, tempts customers to turn what might have been a healthful meal into a calorie bomb (to say nothing of the tasteless dressing), and often raises the price to $12 or more. The Netherlands-based Maoz isn't bad, but it's not as good as the mom-and-pop falafel trucks and shops that are all over Manhattan. There are barely any choices, nothing is cooked to order, the pita is a sponge and there is a messy serve-yourself setup that makes a $10 meal seem like a bit of a rip-off.

Despite its flaws, Improved Fast Food is the transitional step to a new category of fast-food restaurant whose practices should be even closer to sustainable and whose meals should be reasonably healthful and good-tasting and inexpensive. (Maybe not McDonald's-inexpensive, but under $10.) This new category is, or will be, Good Fast Food, and there are already a few emerging contenders.

Veggie Grill is a six-year-old Los Angeles–based chain with 18 locations. Technically, it falls into the "premium fast casual" category. The restaurants are pleasantly designed and nicely lighted and offer limited service. The food is strictly vegan, though you might not know it at first.

Kevin Boylan and T. K. Pillan, the chain's founders, are vegans themselves. They frequently refer to their food as "familiar" and "American," but that's debatable. The "chickin" in the "Santa Fe Crispy Chickin" sandwich is Gardein, a soy-based product that has become the default for fast-food operators looking for meat substitutes. Although there are better products in the pipeline, Gardein, especially when fried, tastes more or less like a McNugget (which isn't entirely "real" chicken itself). The "cheese" is Daiya, which is tapioca-based and similar in taste to a pasteurized processed American cheese. The "steak," "carne asada," "crab cake" (my favorite) and "burger" are also soy, in combination with wheat and pea protein. In terms of animal welfare, environmental damage and resource usage, these products are huge steps in the right direction. They save animals, water, energy and land.

Boylan wanted to make clear to me that his chain isn't about haute cuisine. "We're not doing sautéed tempeh with a peach reduction da-da-da," he said. "That may be a great menu item, but most people don't know what it is. When we say 'cheeseburger'—or 'fried chickin' with mashed potatoes with gravy and steamed kale—everyone knows what we're talking about." He's probably right, and the vegetables are pretty good, too. The mashed potatoes are cut with 40 percent cauliflower; the gravy is made from porcini mushrooms and you can get your entree on a bed of kale instead of a bun.

When I first entered a Veggie Grill, I expected a room full of skinny vegans talking about their vegan-ness. Instead, at locations in Hollywood, El Segundo and Westwood, the lines could have been anywhere, even an airport Taco Bell. The diners appeared mixed by class and weight, and sure looked like omnivores, which they mostly are. The company's research shows that about 70 percent of its customers eat meat or fish, a fact that seems both reflected in its menu and its instant success. Veggie Grill won best American restaurant in the 2012 Los Angeles Times readers' poll, and sales are up 16 percent in existing stores compared with last year. The plan is to double those 18 locations every 18 months for the foreseeable future—"fast enough to stay ahead of competitors, but not so fast as to lose our cultural DNA," Boylan said. In 2011, the founders brought in a new C.E.O., Greg Dollarhyde, who helped Baja Fresh become a national chain before its sale to Wendy's for nearly $300 million.

Veggie Grill is being underwritten partly by Brentwood Associates, a small private-equity firm that's invested in various consumer businesses, including Zoës Kitchen, a chain that offers kebabs, braised beans and roasted vegetables. "For a firm like us to get involved with a concept like Veggie Grill, we have to believe it's a profitable business model, and we do," Brentwood's managing director, Rahul Aggarwal, told me. "Ten years ago I would've said no vegan restaurant would be successful, but people are looking for different ways to eat and this is a great concept."

I admire Veggie Grill, but while making "chickin" from soy is no crime, it's still far from real food. I have a long-running argument with committed vegan friends, who say that Americans aren't ready for rice and beans, or chickpea-and-spinach stew, and that places like Veggie Grill offer a transition to animal-and-environment-friendlier food. On one level, I agree. Why feed the grain to tortured animals to produce lousy meat when you can process the grain and produce it into "meat"? On another level, the goal should be fast food that's real food, too.

Much of what I ate at Veggie Grill was fried and dense, and even when I didn't overeat, I felt as heavy afterward as I do after eating at a Junk Food chain. And while that Santa Fe Crispy Chickin sandwich with lettuce, tomato, red onion, avocado and vegan mayo comes in at 550 calories, 200 fewer than Burger King's Tendercrisp chicken sandwich, the "chickin" sandwich costs $9. The Tendercrisp costs $5, and that's in Midtown Manhattan.

Future growth should allow Veggie Grill to lower prices, but it may never be possible to spend less than 10 dollars on a meal there. Part of that cost is service: at Veggie Grill, you order, get a number to put on your table and wait for a server. It's a luxury compared with most chains, and a pleasant one, but the combination of the food's being not quite real and the price's being still too high means Veggie Grill hasn't made the leap to Good Fast Food.

During my time in Los Angeles, I also ate at Native Foods Café, a vegan chain similar to Veggie Grill, where you can get a pretty good "meatball" sub (made of seitan, a form of wheat gluten), and at Tender Greens, which, though it is cafeteria-style (think Chipotle with a large Euro-Californian menu), flirts with the $20 mark for a meal. It can't really be considered fast food, but it's quite terrific and I'd love to see it put Applebee's and Olive Garden out of business.

In Culver City, I visited Lyfe Kitchen (that's "Love Your Food Everyday"; I know, but please keep reading). Lyfe has the pedigree, menu, financing, plan and ambition to take on the major chains. The company is trying to build 250 locations in the next five years, and QSR has already wondered whether it will become the "Whole Foods of fast food."

At Lyfe, the cookies are dairy-free; the beef comes from grass-fed, humanely raised cows; nothing weighs in at more than 600 calories; and there's no butter, cream, white sugar, white flour, high-fructose corn syrup or trans fats. The concept was the brainchild of the former Gardein executive and investment banker Stephen Sidwell, who quickly enlisted Mike Roberts, the former global president of McDonald's, and Mike Donahue, McDonald's U.S.A.'s chief of corporate communications. These three teamed up with Art Smith, Oprah's former chef, and Tal Ronnen, who I believe to be among the most ambitious and talented vegan chefs in the country.

According to Roberts, Lyfe currently has more than 250 angel investors who "represent a group of people that are saying, 'We've been waiting for something like this.' " The Culver City operation opened earlier this year, and two more California locations are scheduled to open before the year is out. New York locations are being actively scouted, and a Chicago franchise is in the works.

When I visited the Culver City operation, shortly before its official opening, I sampled across the menu and came away impressed. There are four small, creative flatbread pizzas under $10; one is vegan, two are vegetarian and one was done with chicken. I tasted terrific salads, like a beet-and-farro one ($9) that could easily pass for a starter at a good restaurant, and breakfast selections, like steel-cut oatmeal with yogurt and real maple syrup ($5) and a tofu wrap ($6.50), were actually delicious.

Lyfe, not unlike life, isn't cheap. The owners claim that an average check is "around $15" but one entree (roast salmon, bok choy, shiitake mushrooms, miso, etc.) costs exactly $15. An "ancient grain" bowl with Gardein "beef tips" costs $12, which seems too much. Still, the salmon is good and the bowl is delicious, as is a squash risotto made with farro that costs $9— or the price of a "chickin" sandwich at Veggie Grill or a couple of Tendercrisp sandwiches at Burger King.

How in the world, I asked Roberts and Donahue, can they expect to run 250 franchises serving that salmon dish or the risotto or their signature roasted brussels sprouts, which they hope to make into the French fries of the 21st century? Donahue acknowledged that it was going to be a challenge, but nothing that technology couldn't solve. Lyfe will rely on digital order-taking, G.P.S. customer location—a coaster will tell your server where you're sitting—online ordering and mobile apps. Programmable, state-of-the-art combination ovens store recipes, cook with moist or dry heat and really do take the guesswork out of cooking. An order-tracking system tells cooks when to start preparing various parts of dishes and requires their input only at the end of each order. Almost all activity is tracked in real time, which helps the managers run things smoothly.

Lyfe isn't vegan, so much as protein-agnostic. You can get a Gardein burger or a grass-fed beef burger, "unfried" chicken or Gardein "chickin." You can also get wine (biodynamic), beer (organic) or a better-than-it-sounds banana-kale smoothie. However, I fear that Lyfe's ambition, and its diverse menu, will drive up equipment and labor costs, and that those costs are going to keep the chain from appealing to less-affluent Americans. You can get a lot done in a franchise system, but its main virtues are locating the most popular dishes, focusing on their preparation and streamlining the process. My hope is that Lyfe will evolve, as all businesses do, by a process of trial and error, and be successful enough that they have a real impact on the way we think of fast food.

Veggie Grill, Lyfe Kitchen, Tender Greens and others have solved the challenge of bringing formerly upscale, plant-based foods to more of a mass audience. But the industry seems to be focused on a niche group that you might call the health-aware sector of the population. (If you're reading this article, you're probably in it.) Whole Foods has proved that you can build a publicly traded business, with $16 billion in market capitalization, by appealing to this niche. But fast food is, at its core, a class issue. Many people rely on that Tendercrisp because they need to, and our country's fast-food problem won't be solved—no matter how much innovation in vegan options or high-tech ovens—until the prices come down and this niche sector is no longer niche.

It was this idea that led me, a few years ago, to try to start a fast-food chain of my own, modeled after Chipotle. I wanted to focus on Mediterranean food, largely on plant-based options like falafel, hummus, chopped salad, grilled vegetables and maybe a tagine or ratatouille. I wanted to prioritize sustainability, minimize meat and eliminate soda, and I'd treat and pay workers fairly. But after chatting with a few fast-food veterans, I soon recognized just how quixotic my ideas seemed. Anyone with industry experience would want to add more meat, sell Coke and take advantage of both workers and customers to maximize profits. I lost my stomach for the project before I even really began, but recent trends suggest that there may have been hope had I stuck to my guns. Soda consumption is down; meat consumption is down; sales of organic foods are up; more people are expressing concern about G.M.O.s, additives, pesticides and animal welfare. The lines out the door—first at Chipotle and now at Maoz, Chop't, Tender Greens and Veggie Grill—don't lie. According to a report in Advertising Age, McDonald's no longer ranks in the top 10 favorite restaurants of Millennials, a group that comprises as many as 80 million people. Vegans looking for a quick fix after the orthodontist have plenty of choices.

Good Fast Food doesn't need to be vegan or even vegetarian; it just ought to be real, whole food. The best word to describe a wise contemporary diet is flexitarian, which is nothing more than intelligent omnivorism. There are probably millions of people who now eat this way, including me. My own style, which has worked for me for six years, is to eat a vegan diet before 6 p.m. and then allow myself pretty much whatever I want for dinner. This flexibility avoids junk and emphasizes plants, and

Lyfe Kitchen, which offers both "chickin" and chicken—plus beans, vegetables and grains in their whole forms (all for under 600 calories per dish)—comes closest to this ideal. But the menu offers too much, the service raises prices too high and speed is going to be an issue. My advice would be to skip the service and the wine, make a limited menu with big flavors and a few treats and keep it as cheap as you can. Of course, there are huge players who could do this almost instantaneously. But the best thing they seem able to come up with is the McWrap or the fresco menu.

In the meantime, I'm throwing out a few recipes to the entire fast-food world to help build a case that it's possible to use real ingredients to create relatively inexpensive, low-calorie, meat-free, protein-dense, inexpensive fast food. If anyone with the desire can produce this stuff in a home kitchen, then industry veterans financed by private equity firms should be able to produce it at scale in a fraction of the time and at a fraction of the price. You think people won't eat it? There's a lot of evidence that suggests otherwise.

Critical Thinking

1. What are consumers looking for in fast food besides good nutrition?
2. Why are so many fast food companies investing in healthier menu options?

Create Central

www.mhhe.com/createcentral

Internet References

The American Dietetic Association
www.eatright.org
Center for Science in the Public Interest (CSPI)
www.cspinet.org

MARK BITTMAN *is a food writer for the magazine.*

Unit 4

UNIT

Prepared by: Eileen Daniel, *SUNY College at Brockport*

Exercise and Weight Management

Recently, a new set of guidelines, dubbed "Exercise Lite," has been issued by the U.S. Centers for Disease Control and Prevention in conjunction with the American College of Sports Medicine. These guidelines call for 30 minutes of exercise, 5 days a week, which can be spread over the course of a day. The primary focus of this approach to exercise is improving health, not athletic performance. Examples of activities that qualify under the new guidelines are walking your dog, playing tag with your kids, scrubbing floors, washing your car, mowing the lawn, weeding your garden, and having sex. From a practical standpoint, this approach to fitness will likely motivate many more people to become active and stay active. Remember, because the benefits of exercise can take weeks or even months before they become apparent, it is very important to choose an exercise program that you enjoy so that you will stick with it.

While a good diet cannot compensate for the lack of exercise, exercise can compensate for a less than optimal diet. Exercise not only makes people physically healthier, it also keeps their brains healthy. While the connection hasn't been proven, there is evidence that regular workouts may cause the brain to better process and store information, which results in a smarter brain.

Although exercise and a nutritious diet can keep people fit and healthy, many Americans are not heeding this advice. For the first time in our history, the average American is now overweight when judged according to the standard height/weight tables. In addition, more than 25 percent of Americans are clinically obese, and the number appears to be growing. Why is this happening, given the prevailing attitude that Americans have toward fat? One theory that is currently gaining support suggests that while Americans have cut back on their consumption of fatty snacks and desserts, they have actually increased their total caloric intake by failing to limit their consumption of carbohydrates. The underlying philosophy goes something like this: Fat calories make you fat, but you can eat as many carbohydrates as you want and not gain weight. The truth is that all calories count when it comes to weight gain, and if cutting back on fat calories prevents you from feeling satiated, you will naturally eat more to achieve that feeling. While this position seems

reasonable enough, some groups, most notably supporters of the Atkins diet, have suggested that eating a high-fat diet will actually help people lose weight because of fat's high satiety value in conjunction with the formation of ketones (which suppress appetite). Whether people limit fat or carbohydrates, they will not lose weight unless their total caloric intake is less than their energy expenditure.

America's preoccupation with body weight has given rise to a billion-dollar industry. When asked why people go on diets, the predominant answer is for social reasons such as appearance and group acceptance, rather than concerns regarding health. Why do diets and diet aids fail? One of the major reasons lies in the mindset of the dieter. Many dieters do not fully understand the biological and behavioral aspects of weight loss, and consequently they have unrealistic expectations regarding the process. While many people reasonably need to lose weight, many college women strive and compete with each other for the thinnest and most perfect body. This practice has led to an increase in the number of young women suffering from eating disorders.

Being overweight not only causes health problems; it also carries with it a social stigma. Overweight people are often thought of as weak-willed individuals with little or no self-respect. The notion that weight control problems are the result of personality defects is being challenged by new research findings. Evidence is mounting that suggests that physiological and hereditary factors may play as great a role in obesity as do behavioral and environmental factors. Researchers now believe that genetics dictate the base number of fat cells an individual will have, as well as the location and distribution of these cells within the body.

The study of fat metabolism has provided additional clues as to why weight control is so difficult. These metabolic studies have found that the body seems to have a "setpoint," or desired weight, and it will defend this weight through alterations in basal metabolic rate and fat-cell activities. While this process is thought to be an adaptive throwback to primitive times when food supplies were uncertain, today, with our abundant food supply, this mechanism only contributes to the problem of weight control.

It should be apparent by now that weight control is both an attitudinal and a lifestyle issue. Fortunately, a new, more rational approach to the problem of weight control is emerging. This approach is based on the premise that you can be perfectly healthy and good looking without being pencil-thin. The primary focus of this approach to weight management is the attainment of your body's "natural ideal weight" and not some idealized, fanciful notion of what you would like to weigh. The concept of achieving your natural ideal body weight suggests that we need to take a more realistic approach to both fitness and weight control and also serves to remind us that a healthy lifestyle is based on the concepts of balance and moderation.

Article Prepared by: Eileen L. Daniel, *SUNY College at Brockport*

The Trouble with Diet Pills

Prescription weight-loss drugs and supplements promise a lot. But the dangers may outweigh the benefits.

Learning Outcomes

After reading this article, you will be able to:

- Explain the risks associated with prescription diet pills.
- Identify the benefits of low fat and low carbohydrate diets.
- Describe the risks and benefits of bariatric surgery.

As everyone on the planet probably knows, Americans have a weight problem. In fact, 69 percent of adults are overweight and 35 percent qualify as obese. (A body mass index, or BMI, of more than 25 puts you in the overweight category; if it's over 30, you're obese. To calculate yours, go to *ConsumerReportsHealth.org/bmi.*)

Consumers spend billions annually in a desperate search for a solution, whether in the form of supplements, over-the-counter and prescription drugs, or even weight-loss surgery. The problem with all of those would-be magic bullets is that with weight loss—as with most health problems—there *is* no magic bullet. And each of those approaches carries well-documented and potentially serious health risks.

As yet another prescription diet pill, *Contrave,* has just come onto the market, we thought it was a good moment to survey the field of weight-loss aids so that we could share our findings.

Weight-Loss Supplements: Billions Spent on Snake Oil

Dietary supplements that manufacturers promise will help you lose weight—including the green coffee bean extract once touted by Dr. Oz—are among the most consumed. About one in four Americans has used weight-loss supplements, and half of supplement consumers have taken them in the past year, according to a new Consumer Reports survey of almost 3,000 adults. Twenty-eight percent said that they thought supplements

worked better than other weight-loss methods. About half of those users reported at least one side effect, most often a faster heart rate, jitters, digestive problems, or dry mouth.

But unlike drugs, which must be proved safe and effective before being marketed, supplements are assumed to be safe unless proved otherwise. "Supplements are legally promoted as if they're safe and effective for weight loss," says Pieter Cohen, M.D., a physician at Harvard Medical School. In fact, he says, they are neither. "There's no 'natural' herb in legitimate supplements that leads to weight loss. And because natural ingredients don't work, unethical manufacturers are putting drugs into supplements."

Indeed, the Food and Drug Administration has recalled hundreds of weight-loss supplements that contained drugs that were rarely listed on labels. In 2013, 97 cases of severe hepatitis and liver failure (including one that led to death) were linked to OxyElite Pro, a weight-loss supplement containing the little-known substance aegeline. The stimulant 1,3-dimethylbutylamine (DMBA), which has never been studied in humans, was recently detected in the widely sold weight-loss supplements MD2 Meltdown and OxyTherm Pro, among others. The health risks of DMBA aren't fully known, but it's chemically related to DMAA, a stimulant that the FDA has barred supplement makers from using because it can lead to elevated blood pressure and cardiovascular problems. And last year the drug lorcaserin (available by prescription only under the brand name *Belviq*) was found in the supplement Lose Quickly, according to a study in the *Journal of Pharmaceutical and Biomedical Analysis.* Other weight-loss supplements contain FDA-banned drugs such as sibutramine, which can increase the risk of heart attack and stroke, and the laxative phenolphthalein, which animal studies linked to an increased risk of certain cancers. (Despite their recall, at press time many of the supplements containing banned drugs were still being sold.)

"Some supplement manufacturers are willing to put consumers in the line of fire," Cohen says, "even when the FDA has made clear that those ingredients are dangerous."

The word "natural" on a label is no guarantee of safety, although about one-third of the supplement users in our survey thought that it meant the product was safer than prescription medication. For example, yohimbe extract, which is derived from the bark of an African tree and marketed as a weight-loss supplement, may cause elevated blood pressure and panic attacks.

CR's take: Don't take weight-loss supplements. They're mostly unregulated, they don't work, and they could harm you.

Prescription Diet Pills: A checkered past

Between 1997 and 2010, three weight-loss drugs—*Fen-Phen* (a combination of fenfluramine and phentermine), *Acomplia* (rimonabant), and *Meridia* (sibutramine)—either failed to get FDA approval or were taken off the market because of dangerous side effects, including an increased risk of heart attack and stroke. Now there are four weight-loss medications available to consumers. But they're only for people with a BMI of 30 or greater, or those with a BMI of 27 and a weight-related health condition. Here's a rundown:

Alli/Xenical (orlistat): In both of its forms—over the counter (*Alli*) and prescription (*Xenical*)—orlistat works by blocking the enzyme that allows you to digest and absorb dietary fat. After a voluntary recall last March (the manufacturer suspected tampering after consumers reported bottles containing tablets in various shapes and colors), *Alli* is expected to return to stores in the first half of 2015. In clinical trials, after a year of treatment with orlistat, severely overweight patients on a reduced-calorie diet lost 7 pounds more than those who took a placebo. Orlistat has been linked, on rare occasions, to severe liver damage, liver failure (resulting in a transplant), and even death. Last summer the manufacturer added a new warning to the label, noting that the drug might interfere with the absorption of antiseizure and other medications. Orlistat may decrease the absorption of vitamins A, D, E, and K. Other side effects include gas and involuntary discharge of stool.

Belviq (lorcaserin): This medication promotes weight loss by activating brain receptors for serotonin, a neurotransmitter that triggers feelings of fullness. After a year, those taking it lost only 6 pounds more than those who took a placebo. After another year, participants gained back about a quarter of the weight they had lost. They also had trouble staying on the drug; side effects include headaches, dizziness, fatigue, nausea, constipation, memory and attention problems, and (rarely) a leaky heart valve. As a result, the FDA has mandated studies to rule out heart problems. Like many prescriptions, *Belviq* can also interact dangerously with other drugs. If you take it with antidepressants or a migraine medication, for example, you can develop serotonin syndrome, which is characterized by agitation, diarrhea, a fast heart rate, and hallucinations.

The Best Way to Lose Weight

Despite the dizzying array of diets out there, losing weight is actually pretty simple. In a 2014 analysis of 48 diets published in *The Journal of the American Medical Association*, participants achieved significant weight loss by following *any* low-fat or low-carbohydrate diet. Here are a few tips:

- Pick a reasonable goal. Studies and surveys have found that an initial weight-loss goal of 5 percent is realistic and offers important health benefits, including reduced blood cholesterol and glucose levels, and a lowering of blood pressure, to name just a few.
- Portion control is key. Aim to consume fewer than 2,000 calories per day—ideally around 1,200 to 1,500 per day for women and 1,500 to 1,800 for men.
- Cook and eat at home, where you have more control over calories you take in.
- Eat more fruit and vegetables, choose whole over refined grains, and select lean meats and seafood.
- Eat a protein-rich breakfast.
- Reduce your sugar intake to 10 percent (or less) of your total daily calories.

Qsymia (phentermine/topiramate): This drug is a combination of two prescription medications—the stimulant phentermine, which suppresses appetite, and the antiseizure drug topiramate, which sometimes causes weight loss as a side effect. *Qsymia* leads to more weight loss than the other medications. After a year of taking it, patients who lost 10 percent of their body weight outnumbered those who took a placebo by 7 percent. But it increases heart rate and may lead to memory, attention, or speech problems, anxiety, insomnia, and depression (including suicidal thoughts). About 40 percent of clinical trial participants stopped taking it. To ensure that it doesn't cause cardiovascular problems, the FDA has requested a postmarket study.

Contrave (naltrexone/bupropion): This combination of naltrexone (an addiction medicine) and bupropion (an antidepressant) may reduce appetite and curb cravings. After a year on the drug, nondiabetic patients in a clinical trial lost 4.1 percent more weight than those who took a placebo. Nausea, constipation, headache, vomiting, dizziness, insomnia, dry mouth, and diarrhea are the most common side effects. More troubling, the drug may cause seizures. And because it contains the antidepressant bupropion, it must carry a boxed warning saying that it might increase suicidal thoughts and behavior. The FDA is concerned about the medication's effect on the heart and is requiring more studies.

CR's take: Skip those drugs and stick with calorie reduction and exercise to drop pounds. (See "The Best Way to Lose Weight".)

Is Bariatric Surgery Right for You?

About 113,000 weight-loss surgeries are performed on morbidly obese people per year (those with a BMI of 40 or above or those with a BMI above 35 who also have a serious health condition such as type 2 diabetes, severe joint pain, or sleep apnea). About 80 to 90 percent of patients who undergo the two most common procedures—gastric bypass and sleeve gastrectomy—experience long-term weight loss, according to John Birkmeyer, M.D., chief academic officer of the Dartmouth-Hitchcock Health System in New Hampshire. The procedures have also been shown to improve or resolve type 2 diabetes as well as high blood pressure and cholesterol abnormalities. But anyone with a blood-clotting disorder or a history of heart attack, stroke, or kidney failure may not qualify.

- **Roux-en-Y gastric bypass** The surgeon divides the upper part of the stomach to make an egg-sized pouch, then connects it to the lower half of the small intestine. Because your stomach is so small, you feel full soon after eating. This procedure, the most effective of all weight-loss surgeries (patients usually lose 62 to 68 percent of their excess weight in the first year), also has the greatest number of adverse incidents.

About 10 percent of patients develop diarrhea, cramps, and facial flushing after eating; 3 to 4 percent develop a stomach ulcer or bowel obstruction.

- **Laparoscopic sleeve gastrectomy** Doctors remove about 85 percent of your stomach, leaving a banana-shaped pouch. That restricts food intake and affects the appetite-related stomach hormone, leaving you feeling less hungry. Within a year, patients lose an average of 33 percent of excess weight.
- **Laparoscopic adjustable gastric banding (Lap-Band)** An adjustable band placed around the upper part of the stomach limits the amount of food it can hold. The band can be tightened or loosened periodically. After two years, weight loss ranges from 45 to 75 percent of excess body weight. This surgery, unlike the previous two, is reversible.
- **Endoscopic sleeve gastroplasty** In this new (and reversible) procedure, doctors place a flexible tube with a suturing device into your stomach. Using stitches, they "sew" your stomach so that it shrinks to a narrow bananalike tube, rendering you unable to eat much. Patients can expect to lose up to 30 pounds in the first six months. Most regain some weight but largely sustain the loss after a year.

Critical Thinking

1. What are the financial costs associated with dieting and weight loss?
2. What are the risks associated with the use of weight loss supplements and prescription diet pills?

Internet References

American Board of Obesity Medicine
abom.org/

Academy of Nutrition and Dietetics
www.eatright.org/

Society for Nutrition Education and Behavior
www.sneb.org

Article Prepared by: Eileen L. Daniel, *SUNY Brockport*

Dieting on a Budget

Plus the secrets of thin people, based on our survey of 21,000 readers.

Learning Outcomes

After reading this article, you will be able to:

- Explain how it's possible to lose weight on a limited budget.
- Describe a diet plan of low-cost, low-calorie foods.
- Explain the components of a healthy weight loss program.

With jobs being cut and retirement accounts seemingly shrinking by the day, it's too bad our waistlines aren't dwindling, too. We can't rectify that cosmic injustice, but in this issue we aim to help you figure out the most effective, least expensive ways to stay trim and fit.

Though most Americans find themselves overweight by middle age, an enviable minority stay slim throughout their lives. Are those people just genetically gifted? Or do they, too, have to work at keeping down their weight?

To find out, the Consumer Reports National Research Center asked subscribers to *Consumer Reports* about their lifetime weight history and their eating, dieting, and exercising habits. And now we have our answer:

People who have never become overweight aren't sitting in recliners with a bowl of corn chips in their laps. In our group of always-slim respondents, a mere 3 percent reported that they never exercised and that they ate whatever they pleased. The eating and exercise habits of the vast majority of the always-slim group look surprisingly like those of people who have successfully lost weight and kept it off.

Both groups eat healthful foods such as fruits, vegetables, and whole grains and eschew excessive dietary fat; practice portion control; and exercise vigorously and regularly. The only advantage the always-slim have over the successful dieters is that those habits seem to come a bit more naturally to them.

"When we've compared people maintaining a weight loss with controls who've always had a normal weight, we've found that both groups are working hard at it; the maintainers are just working a little harder," says Suzanne Phelan, Ph.D., an assistant professor of kinesiology at California Polytechnic State University and co-investigator of the National Weight Control Registry, which tracks people who have successfully maintained a weight loss over time. For our respondents, that meant exercising a little more and eating with a bit more restraint than

Price vs. Nutrition: Making Smart Choices

Although healthful foods often cost more than high-calorie junk such as cookies and soda, we unearthed some encouraging exceptions. As illustrated below, two rich sources of nutrients, black beans and eggs, cost mere pennies per serving—and less than plain noodles, which supply fewer nutrients. And for the same price as a doughnut, packed with empty calories, you can buy a serving of broccoli.

- **Cooked black beans**
  - Serving size 1/2 cup
  - Calories per serving 114
  - Cost per serving 74¢
- **Hard-boiled egg**
  - Serving size one medium
  - Calories per serving 78
  - Cost per serving 94¢
- **Cooked noodles**
  - Serving size 3/4 cup
  - Calories per serving 166
  - Cost per serving 134¢
- **Glazed doughnut**
  - Serving size 1 medium
  - Calories per serving 239
  - Cost per serving 324¢
- **Cooked broccoli**
  - Serving size 1/2 cup chopped
  - Calories per serving 27
  - Cost per serving 334¢
- **Chicken breast**
  - Serving size 4 oz.
  - Calories per serving 142
  - Cost per serving 364¢

Sources: Adam Drewnowski, Ph.D., director of the Center for Public Health Nutrition, University of Washington: USDA Nutrient Database for Standard Reference.

an always-thin person—plus using more monitoring strategies such as weighing themselves or keeping a food diary.

A total of 21,632 readers completed the 2007 survey. The always thin, who had never been overweight, comprised 16 percent

Stay-Thin Strategies

Successful losers and the always thin do a lot of the same things—and they do them more frequently than failed dieters do. For the dietary strategies below, numbers reflect those who said they are that way at least five days a week, a key tipping point, our analysis found. (Differences of less than 4 percentage points are not statistically meaningful.)

Lifetime Weight History

Failed dieters: overweight and have tried to lose, but still close to highest weight. **Always thin:** never overweight. **Successful losers:** once overweight but now at least 10 percent lighter and have kept pounds off for at least three years.

Strength Train at Least Once a Week

Always thin   31%
Successful loser 32%
Failed dieter   23%

Do Vigorous Exercise at Least Four Days a Week

Always thin   35%
Successful loser 41%
Failed dieter   27%

Eat Fruit and Vegetables at Least Five Times a Day

Always thin   49%
Successful loser 49%
Failed dieter   38%

Eat Whole Grains, Not Refined

Always thin   56%
Successful loser 61%
Failed dieter   49%

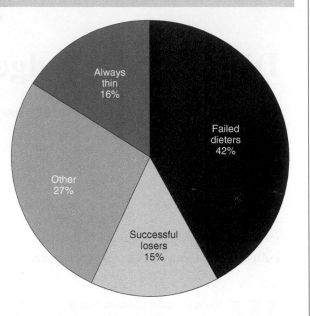

Eat Less Than 1/3 Calories from Fat

Always thin   47%
Successful loser 53%
Failed dieter   35%

Observe Portion Control at Every Meal

Always thin   57%
Successful loser 62%
Failed dieter   42%

Count Calories

Always thin   9%
Successful loser 47%
Failed dieter   9%

of our sample. Successful losers made up an additional 15 percent. We defined that group as people who, at the time of the survey, weighed at least 10 percent less than they did at their heaviest, and had been at that lower weight for at least three years. Failed dieters, who said they would like to slim down yet still weighed at or near their lifetime high, were, sad to say, the largest group: 42 percent. (The remaining 27 percent of respondents, such as people who had lost weight more recently, didn't fit into any of the categories.)

An encouraging note: More than half of our successful losers reported shedding the weight themselves, without aid of a commercial diet program, a medical treatment, a book, or diet pills. That confirms what we found in our last large diet survey, in 2002, in which 83 percent of "superlosers"—people who'd lost at least 10 percent of their starting weight and kept it off for five years or more—had done it entirely on their own.

6 Secrets of the Slim

Through statistical analyses, we were able to identify six key behaviors that correlated the most strongly with having a healthy body mass index (BMI), a measure of weight that takes height into account. Always thin people were only slightly less likely than successful losers to embrace each of the behaviors—and significantly more likely to do so than failed dieters. By following the behaviors, you can, quite literally, live like a thin person.

Watch portions. Of all the eating behaviors we asked about, carefully controlling portion size at each meal correlated most strongly with having a lower BMI. Successful losers—even those who were still overweight—were especially likely (62 percent) to report practicing portion control at least five days per week. So did 57 percent of the always thin, but only 42 percent of failed dieters.

Portion control is strongly linked to a lower BMI.

Limit fat. Specifically, that means restricting fat to less than one-third of daily calorie intake. Fifty-three percent of successful losers and 47 percent of the always thin said they did that five or more days a week, compared with just 35 percent of failed dieters.

Eat fruits and vegetables. The more days that respondents ate five or more servings of fruits or vegetables, the lower their average BMI score. Forty-nine percent of successful losers and the always thin said they ate that way at least five days a week, while 38 percent of failed dieters did so.

Choose whole grains over refined. People with lower body weights consistently opted for whole-wheat breads, cereals, and other grains over refined (white) grains.

Eat at home. As the number of days per week respondents ate restaurant or takeout meals for dinner increased, so did their weight. Eating at home can save a lot of money, too.

Exercise, exercise, exercise. Regular vigorous exercise—the type that increases breathing and heart rate for 30 minutes or longer—was strongly linked to a lower BMI. Although only about one quarter of respondents said they did strength training at least once a week, that practice was significantly more prevalent among successful losers (32 percent) and always thin respondents (31 percent) than it was among failed dieters (23 percent).

What Didn't Matter

One weight-loss strategy is conspicuously absent from the list: going low-carb. Of course we asked about it, and it turned out that limiting carbohydrates was linked to higher BMIs in our survey. That doesn't necessarily mean low-carb plans such as the Atkins or South Beach diets don't work. "If you go to the hospital and everyone there is sick, that doesn't mean the hospital made them sick," says Eric C. Westman, M.D., associate professor of medicine and director of the Lifestyle Medicine Clinic at Duke University Medical School. "Just as people go to hospitals because they're ill, people may go to carb restriction because they have a higher BMI, not the other way around." At the same time, the findings do suggest that cutting carbs alone, without other healthful behaviors such as exercise and portion control, might not lead to great results.

Are You Overweight?

A body mass index under 25 is considered normal weight: from 25 to 29, overweight; and 30 or above, obese. To calculate your BMI, multiply your weight in pounds by 703, then divide by your height squared in inches.

Eating many small meals, or never eating between meals, didn't seem to make much difference one way or another. Including lean protein with most meals also didn't by itself predict a healthier weight.

Realistic Expectations

Sixty-six percent of our respondents, all subscribers to *Consumer Reports,* were overweight as assessed by their body mass index; that's the same percentage as the population as a whole. One third of the overweight group, or 22 percent of the overall sample, qualified as obese.

Although that might seem discouraging, the survey actually contains good news for would-be dieters. Our respondents did much better at losing weight than published clinical studies would predict. Though such studies are deemed successful if participants are 5 percent lighter after a year, our successful losers had managed to shed an average of 16 percent of their peak weight, an average of almost 34 pounds. They had an impressive average BMI of 25.7, meaning they were just barely overweight.

One key to weight loss success is having realistic goals and our subscribers' responses proved encouraging. A staggering 70 percent of them said they currently wanted to lose weight. But when we asked how many pounds they hoped to take off, we found that their goals were modest: The vast majority reported wanting to lose 15 percent or less of their overall body weight; 65 percent sought to lose between 1 and 10 percent. Keeping expectations in check might help dieters from becoming discouraged when they don't achieve, say, a 70-pound weight loss or drop from a size 20 to a size 6—a common problem in behavioral weight loss studies.

Realistic goals are one key to weight loss.

What You Can Do

Weight loss is a highly individual process, and what matters most is finding the combination of habits that work for you. But our findings suggest that there are key behaviors common to people who have successfully lost weight and to those who have never gained it in the first place. By embracing some or all of those behaviors, you can probably increase your chances of weight-loss success, and live a healthier life in the process. In addition to following the steps above, consider these tips:

Don't get discouraged. Studies show that prospective dieters often have unrealistic ideas about how much weight they can lose. A 10 percent loss might not sound like much, but it significantly improves overall health and reduces risk of disease.

Ask for support. Though only a small minority of respondents overall reported that a spouse or family member interfered with their healthful eating efforts, that problem was much more likely among failed dieters, 31 percent of whom reported some form of spousal sabotage in the month prior to the survey. Ask housemates to help you stay on track by, for example, not pestering you to eat foods you're trying to avoid, or not eating those foods in front of you.

Get up and move. While regular vigorous exercise correlated most strongly with healthy body weight, our findings suggest that any physical activity is helpful, including activities you might not even consider exercise. Everyday activities such as housework, yard work, and playing with kids were modestly tied to lower weight. By contrast, hours spent sitting each day, whether at an office desk or at home watching television, correlated with higher weight.

Critical Thinking

1. What does a healthy weight loss diet consist of?
2. How can one lose weight without spending a fortune on "diet" foods?

Create Central

www.mhhe.com/createcentral

Internet References

The American Dietetic Association
 www.eatright.org
Cyberdiet
 www.cyberdiet.com

Article   Prepared by: Eileen L. Daniel, *SUNY College at Brockport*

Can Government Regulate Portion Sizes?

JENNIFER L. POMERANZ AND KELLY D. BROWNELL

Learning Outcomes

After reading this article, you will be able to:

- Understand why larger portions encourage greater intake of food.

- Describe how external cues can influence eating behaviors.

External cues can have powerful effects on people's eating habits. One thoroughly studied environmental trigger is portion size: studies show that larger portions encourage greater consumption of a range of foods and beverages.[1] This effect is especially problematic when it comes to sugar-sweetened beverages, which are associated with obesity and diabetes and are being sold in ever-increasing portion sizes. The original Coca-Cola bottle was 6.5 oz (190 ml); many bottles intended for individual consumption are now triple that size.

There are no government restrictions on portion sizes for food prepared and consumed outside the home, which accounts for more than 43% of Americans' food expenditures.[2] A regulation enacted by the New York City Board of Health that limited portion sizes of sugar-sweetened beverages was struck down in 2014.[3] Although this case applies only in New York State, the precedent it set may help address fundamental questions about whether restricting food and beverage portion sizes is defensible on public health and legal grounds in other U.S. jurisdictions.

The New York City Board of Health adopted the portion-cap rule in 2012, limiting the size of sugar-sweetened beverages sold in food-service establishments—which are licensed by the city—to 16 oz (470 ml).[4] Grocers and convenience stores are regulated by New York State and hence were not subject to the rule. The ordinance applied to calorically sweetened beverages with more than 25 calories per 8 oz (235 ml) and excluded drinks containing more than 50% milk or milk substitute.[4] Consumers were free to purchase multiple drinks, and sellers could offer free refills. State

and national nonprofit and labor organizations representing food-service establishments and the beverage industry sued the city to prevent enforcement of the law. The state's highest court, the New York Court of Appeals, ultimately struck down the ordinance.[3]

The first industry complaint in the litigation was that the Board of Health exceeded the authority granted to it by the City Charter and thus improperly acted in a legislative capacity—an argument based on the separation of powers. The Board of Health is part of an administrative agency in the executive branch of the government, and therefore it can act only within the parameters set forth by the legislative body. According to the court's majority opinion, the Board exceeded this authority because the regulation interfered with activities preferred by large numbers of people and required "complex value judgments" concerning public health, personal autonomy, and economics.[3] The court found that the Board of Health made difficult choices among "broad policy goals" and engaged in a form of "policy-making," an activity reserved for legislatures, rather than standard agency "rule-making," which consists of "subsidiary policy choices" based on an enabling legislation's requirements.[3]

The second industry argument was that the ordinance was "arbitrary and capricious" and hence not rational. States—and to the extent permitted, local governments—possess the authority to enact laws to protect, preserve, and promote the health, safety, and welfare of their citizens (known as the "police power"), as long as such regulation has a rational basis. The Court of Appeals did not address this argument because it struck down the law on the basis of the separation-of-powers issue. According to the dissenting opinion, however, "the Rule easily passes this test."[3] Neither lower court had found that regulating portion sizes of sugar-sweetened beverages was irrational (although both courts similarly struck down the law). The trial court found that the exceptions in the rule, outlined above, were arbitrary, and the appellate division did not address this issue but noted that the "deleterious effects (e.g., obesity) associated with excessive soda consumption are well-known."[5]

Legally, the rule remains viable because there is a valid argument that regulating portion sizes of a known public health threat such as sugar-sweetened beverages is rational. The binding outcome of the case is that administrative agencies in New York State cannot pass a serving-size regulation without a legislative mandate. The state legislature or the New York City Council could still pass a similar measure, as could any state or local legislature in the United States. Regulatory agencies can enact portion-cap rules if they have broad authority or are granted express authority by their legislatures; otherwise, they, too, risk a court finding that they encroached on policymaking activities reserved for the legislative branch.

State and local governments have not yet attempted to regulate portion sizes for public health reasons, but they have successfully done so for other purposes deemed rational by the Supreme Court. In several cases from the early 20th century, the Court upheld states' ability to enact laws related to the weight, measure, and ingredients of foods, calling such regulation a valid and common exercise of the police power. For example, in 1913, the Court upheld a Chicago ordinance prescribing the standard size of bread loaves, and in 1916, it upheld a North Dakota statute restricting the weight of lard containers, in both cases in order to prevent fraud and despite consumer demand for products of different sizes and businesses' willingness to supply them. In a precedent with implications for the argument that New York City was "singling out" sugar-sweetened beverages, in 1981, the Supreme Court upheld a Minnesota law that banned plastic—but not cardboard—milk containers as a way of addressing environmental concerns regarding plastic. Although these ordinances were enacted for different reasons, the public health rationale, which supports a serving-size restriction for sugar-sweetened beverages, is also well established as valid under the police power.

Jurisdictions seeking to address portion size can learn from New York City. Although opposition groups argued that the ordinance was a slippery slope that could lead to portion-size restrictions on other foods, the targeting of another type of food or beverage without robust public health data would most likely not be deemed rational by a court. In addition, legislatures need not limit portion-size restrictions to food-service establishments. Retailers that sell large fountain beverages (such as 7-Eleven) could be similarly covered under such laws to avoid challenges based on claims of irrationality. Conversely, governments may not wish to prevent grocery sales of multiple-liter bottles of sugar-sweetened beverages, which may be consumed at home, by families, or over time, because such a ban would not be supported by the same rationale behind addressing large portion sizes consumed in one sitting away from home.

Jurisdictions could also independently determine whether 16 oz is the appropriate size to target by conducting studies and surveys and engaging with local businesses. Finally, methods of enforcing portion-cap rules could be integrated into current inspection procedures to minimize administrative burdens. Jurisdictions could license retailers and require compliance with the law as a condition of maintaining the license, with licensing fees covering enforcement, inspection, and paperwork costs.

Political obstacles are important, as the dissent in the New York City case argued: the law was simply "unpopular."[3] Beverage manufacturers contributed to this sentiment with a major public-relations campaign. In the future, advocacy groups and grassroots movements could conduct surveys to ascertain the most promising way to frame the messages conveyed about such a policy to gain the support of the public and elected officials. Other nutrition-related policies, including revised school-meal standards, menu labeling, and taxes on sugar-sweetened beverages, were initially met with skepticism and industry opposition, but government actions have led to their greater acceptance. It is quite possible that the history of portion-size limits will follow the same course. Limiting portion sizes is a promising frontier in nutrition policy, with legally viable options available to support public health.

1. Cohen DA, Story M. Mitigating the health risks of dining out: the need for standardized portion sizes in restaurants. *Am J Public Health* 2014;104:586–90.
2. U.S. Department of Agriculture, Economic Research Service. Food consumption and demand: food away from home (http://www.ers.usda.gov/topics/food-choices-health/food-consumption-demand/food-away-from-home.aspx#.VBcdRaP4ei0).
3. *In the matter of New York Statewide Coalition of Hispanic Chambers of Commerce v. the New York City Department of Health and Mental Hygiene,* No. 134 New York Court of Appeals (2014).
4. New York City Department of Health and Mental Hygiene, Board of Health Notice of Adoption of an Amendment (§81.53) to Article 81 of the New York City Health Code.
5. *New York Statewide Coalition of Hispanic Chambers of Commerce v. New York City Dept. of Health & Mental Hygiene,* 110 A.D.3d 1 (NY App. 1st Dept 2013).

Critical Thinking

1. Why do larger portions encourage overeating?
2. Should portion sizes be regulated?

Internet References

Academy of Nutrition and Dietetics
www.eatright.org/

American Board of Obesity Medicine
abom.org/

Society for Nutrition Education and Behavior
www.sneb.org

Pomeranz, Jennifer L. and Brownell, Kelly D. "Can Government Regulate Portion Sizes?" *New England Journal of Medicine,* November 20, 2014. Copyright © 2014 by Massachusetts Medical Society. Reprinted by permission.

Unit 5

UNIT

Prepared by: Eileen Daniel, *SUNY College at Brockport*

Drugs and Health

As a culture, Americans have come to rely on drugs not only as a treatment for disease but also as an aid for living normal, productive lives. This view of drugs has fostered a casual attitude regarding their use and resulted in a tremendous drug abuse problem. Drug use and abuse has become so widespread that there is no way to describe the typical drug abuser. There is no simple explanation for why America has become a drug-taking culture, but there certainly is evidence to suggest some of the factors that have contributed to this development.

From the time that we are children, we are constantly bombarded by advertisements about how certain drugs can make us feel and look better. While most of these ads deal with proprietary drugs, the belief created is that drugs are a legitimate and effective way to help us cope with everyday problems. Certainly drugs can have a profound effect on how we feel and act, but research has also demonstrated that our mind plays a major role in the healing process. For many people, it's easier to take a drug than to adopt a healthier lifestyle.

Growing up, most of us probably had a medicine cabinet full of prescription and over-the-counter (OTC) drugs, freely dispensed to family members to treat a variety of ailments. This familiarity with drugs, coupled with rising health-care costs, has prompted many people to diagnose and medicate themselves with OTC medications without sufficient knowledge of the possible side effects. Although most of these preparations have little potential for abuse, it does not mean that they are innocuous. Generally speaking, OTC drugs are relatively safe if taken at the recommended dosage by healthy people, but the risk of dangerous side effects rises sharply when people exceed the recommended dosage. Another potential danger associated with the use of OTC drugs is the drug interactions that can occur when they are taken in conjunction with prescription medications. The gravest danger associated with the use of OTC drugs is that an individual may use them to control symptoms of an underlying disease and thus prevent its early diagnosis and treatment.

While OTC drugs can be abused, an increasing number of drug-related deaths over the past five years have been linked to prescription drugs. These drugs, opiate-based painkillers such as OxyContin, Darvon, and Vicodin are often used as an alternative to an illicit high. Ironically, however, there has been a recent surge in heroin use as these prescription drugs become harder to get.

As a culture, we have grown up believing that there is, or should be, a drug to treat any malady or discomfort that befalls us. Would we have a drug problem if there was no demand for drugs? One drug which is used widely in the United States is alcohol, especially on college campuses. Every year over 1,000 students die from alcohol-related causes, mostly drinking and driving. Other risks associated with students' drinking include missed classes, falling behind in schoolwork, damage to property, and injuries, which occur while under the influence of alcohol.

While alcohol abuse among college students is a serious issue, drinking among pregnant women is also a concern. Women who drink during their pregnancies risk delivering a baby who could suffer from a range of effects including physical, emotional, mental, behavioral, and cognitive abnormalities.

In addition to alcohol, another widely used legal drug is tobacco. Millions still smoke despite all the well-publicized health effects linked to smoking. Many Americans have quit and many others would like to quit. To facilitate this process, some companies have developed programs to help employees stop smoking. Because smoking and its related diseases cost approximately $150 billion each year, the stakes are enormous. A recent introduction, electronic cigarettes are considered controversial relative to their safety. While the research is limited, some smokers use electronic cigarettes to help quit the habit while others use the product to reduce the effects of secondhand smoke. One concern over electronic cigarettes is their appeal to minors. E-cigarettes often come in flavors that appear to be targeted toward children.

Article

Prepared by: Eileen Daniel, *SUNY College at Brockport*

Pot Goes Legit

What the End of Prohibition Looks Like in Colorado

Jacob Sullum

Learning Outcomes

After reading this article, you will be able to:

- Explain the restrictions imposed on marijuana sellers in Colorado.

- Understand the provisions of Colorado's Amendment 64.

- Describe the 70/30 rule regarding marijuana growing and selling.

"What we need," said Norton Arbelaez, a thirty-something attorney and businessman in a suit and tie, "is a vertically integrated, closed-loop regulatory framework." The bureaucrats, politicians, and entrepreneurs crowding the conference room took notes, watched his PowerPoint slides, and furrowed their brows. This was the fourth meeting of a working group set up by a task force appointed by the governor of Colorado, and if you happened to wander by you would think, it sounded as dull as the average subcommittee session anywhere.

Until you discerned the subject of the meeting. "We will be, and are, the cannabis industry in Colorado," Arbelaez proclaimed. "It is our necks that are on the line."

Last November, 75 years after Congress enacted national marijuana prohibition, voters in Colorado and Washington decided to opt out. After Coloradans approved Amendment 64, which legalized the production, possession, and distribution of marijuana for recreational use, Gov. John Hickenlooper appointed the Amendment 64 Implementation Task Force to advise state legislators on how to regulate the nascent cannabis industry, which for years had served patients under Colorado's medical marijuana law but now was authorized to supply any adult 21 or older. And as in all sorts of industries, the incumbents were trying to write the rules in their favor.

"We need to maintain the edifice of what continues to work in Colorado," said Arbelaez, who co-owns two medical marijuana dispensaries in Denver and serves on the board of the Medical Marijuana Industry Group. Among other things, he said that means retaining a rule that requires pot retailers to grow at least 70 percent of what they sell while selling no more than 30 percent of what they grow to other outlets. Arbelaez argued that the 70/30 rule, designed to prevent recreational consumers from obtaining medical marijuana, would help stop diversion of recreational marijuana to minors or other states and thereby discourage federal interference.

The other members of the working group seemed unpersuaded. Liquor stores do not make the distilled spirits they stock, and pharmacies do not produce the drugs they sell. Why should pot stores have to grow their own marijuana?

"I am still left scratching my head about vertical integration and why it's so important," said Denver City Councilman Chris Nevitt. "The 70 percent rule is endlessly complicated and confusing." Nevitt alluded to the financial interests at stake: when the rule took effect in 2011, more than a decade after Colorado voters approved the medical use of marijuana, dispensaries had to invest in growing space and equipment, and they were forced into sometimes awkward business partnerships with growers. "I totally understand the anxiety of an industry that has made all of these investments," Nevitt said. "But I am still scratching my head."

Jessica LeRoux, owner of Twirling Hippy Confections, a Denver business that supplies cannabis-infused chocolates and cheesecakes to medical marijuana centers (MMCs) across the state, concurred. "The 70/30 rule does not work," LeRoux stated flatly. "This is not vertical integration. This is vertical protectionism."

But most MMC owners in the room seemed to support the 70/30 rule. "The current medical marijuana system works for us," said Erica Freeman of Choice Organics in Fort Collins.

"Changing the rules again will force new mergers," warned Tad Bowler of Rocky Road Remedies in Steamboat Springs. "The small centers won't be able to compete." Michael Elliott, executive director of the Medical Marijuana Industry Group, declared "we are united" in supporting the 70/30 rule.

A straw poll of the working group revealed that its members were overwhelmingly opposed to requiring vertical integration, instead favoring a more flexible approach that would allow retailers to grow whatever percentage of their inventory they wanted, including zero. But in the end, after several more weeks of meetings, the dispensaries represented by Elliott's group prevailed. In its March 13 report, the task force recommended that the 70/30 rule remain in effect for at least three years and that new entrants be excluded from the market for 12 months. Two months later, Gov. Hickenlooper signed a marijuana regulation bill that included watered-down versions of both ideas, extending 70/30 until October 2014 and giving MMCs a three-month head start in the licensing process.

"The industry did a really good job of building a coalition" explains University of Denver law professor Sam Kamin, a member of the task force. "They convinced law enforcement and public health that part of keeping the industry in check and part of keeping it diverse and keeping the feds at bay was the current model."

Rob Corry, a Denver attorney and longtime marijuana activist, is less polite, calling the 70/30 rule "completely unworkable and economically illiterate." But Corry sees a bright side to the dispute over vertical integration. "On the one hand," he says, "I'm disappointed at rent seeking behavior and businesses that seek the heavy hand of government to prevent new competition. On the other hand, it means that our industry has grown up and is behaving like every other industry out there."

Conservatives for Cannabis

Normalizing a formerly criminal business is the avowed goal of Amendment 64, which declares that "marijuana should be regulated in a manner similar to alcohol." The initiative will succeed to the extent that it transforms a countercultural symbol into a capitalist commodity. Dutch officials like to say, regarding their policy of tolerating the retail sale of cannabis, that they made marijuana boring by making it legal. Something similar is happening in Colorado, where the head rush of passing Amendment 64 has given way to the headache of implementing it.

That process, which is supposed to culminate in state-licensed pot stores by next January, aims to address the concerns of marijuana's detractors as well as its fans. Among other things, that means trying to avoid a crackdown by the federal government, which cannot force Colorado to ban marijuana but can make trouble for businesses openly selling a product that

remains illegal under the Controlled Substances Act. Wariness of the feds has shaped every aspect of the new legal regime, from the size of store signs to the size of marijuana brownies, from the amount of tax charged on a quarter-ounce of Hidden Valley Kush to the amount of THC allowed in a driver's bloodstream. These are the mundane details that will define Colorado's momentous experiment in pharmacological tolerance. Boring debates about vertical integration could signal the beginning of the end for the war on drugs.

Colorado and Washington are 2 of the 11 states that opted out of alcohol prohibition through ballot initiatives that voters approved in November 1932, more than a year before the 21st Amendment (which repealed alcohol prohibition nationally) was ratified. Eighty years later, Colorado and Washington used the same method to opt out of marijuana prohibition, by surprisingly strong margins of about 10 points in both states. The victory was especially striking in Colorado, which is more Republican than both Washington and California, where a marijuana legalization initiative lost by seven points just two years earlier. Four years before that Colorado voters had resoundingly rejected Amendment 44, which would have merely made it legal to possess up to an ounce of marijuana. Amendment 64 accomplished that while also legalizing home cultivation and authorizing commercial production and distribution. Yet it was supported by 55 percent of voters, compared to the 41 percent who went for Amendment 44 in 2006.

Former Colorado congressman Tom Tancredo, a conservative Republican, supported Amendment 64 but did not expect it to pass. "The only thing I can attribute it to [is that] we presented a case for conservatives to vote for it," Tancredo says. "The exit polling showed that we had a much stronger support from Republicans and conservatives than they ever had in the past." Mason Tvert, who spearheaded both the 2006 and 2012 campaigns, notes that "we won El Paso County, which is insane." El Paso County—which includes Colorado Springs, home of the U.S. Air Force Academy and Focus on the Family—is "considered one of the most conservative parts of the country," he says. "We won it by 10 votes, but if we lost by 5,000 I would still tout it as unbelievable."

In an op-ed piece published by the Colorado Springs Gazette about six weeks before the election, Tancredo announced that "I am endorsing Amendment 64 not despite my conservative beliefs, but because of them." He compared the ban on marijuana to alcohol prohibition, "a misguided big-government policy experiment," and argued that legalizing marijuana would strike a blow against murderous Mexican drug cartels. Tancredo, who had criticized aspects of the war on drugs during his decade in Congress, combined practical arguments with an explicitly libertarian appeal. "Our nation is spending tens of billions of dollars annually in an attempt to prohibit adults from using a substance objectively less harmful than alcohol," he wrote. "Marijuana prohibition is perhaps the oldest and most persistent nanny-state law we have in the U.S. We simply cannot afford a government that tries to save people from themselves. It is not the role of government to try to correct bad behavior, as long as those behaviors are not directly causing physical harm to others."

The wastefulness and unfairness of enforcing marijuana prohibition was underlined by a report released a month later. Queens College sociologist Harry Levine and two co-authors showed that police in Colorado were arresting more than 10,000 pot smokers every year, even though the state legislature supposedly had decriminalized marijuana possession in 1975. Possession of small amounts (initially less than an ounce, raised to two ounces in 2010) remained a crime, albeit a "petty offense." Pot smokers were not doing hard time, but they were still burdened by the cost, inconvenience, and humiliation associated with an arrest, not to mention the lasting disadvantage of a criminal record.

Tvert says several factors help explain why Coloradans decided it was time to treat pot smokers like consumers instead of criminals. Nationwide support for legalization has been rising more or less steadily since the 1980s, hitting 50 percent in the Gallup Poll for the first time in 2011. And unlike in 2006, voters were picking a president in 2012. "We see much greater turnout in presidential election years ('Tvert says') and when there is more turnout, there is virtually always more support for making marijuana legal." He also credits six years of public persuasion emphasizing the theme reflected in the name of the group he co-founded in 2005, SAFER (Safer Alternative for Enjoyable Recreation), and the tide of the 2009 book he co-wrote, *Marijuana Is Safer.* Tvert cites polling data indicating that people who accept that premise are much more likely to support legalization than people who don't. "Our strategy all along," he says, "was to bring that message and break people's fears of marijuana down to the point where they would go ahead and go with their gut feeling on making it legal."

Supporters of Amendment 64 had a big financial advantage in getting their message across (although not as big as the one enjoyed by legalizers in Washington, who outspent their opponents by 400 to 1). According to campaign finance reports, seven groups backing the initiative raised about $2.7 million, the vast majority of it from out-of-state donors, including the Marijuana Policy Project and the Drug Policy Alliance. The opposition, which consisted largely of law enforcement groups, raised about $560,000, half of it from out-of-state donors. The biggest backer of the No on 64 campaign was Save Our Society From Drugs, a Florida-based group cofounded by Mel Sembler, a Republican fundraiser and drug treatment entrepreneur who co-founded Straight Inc., the notorious (and now-defunct) chain of behavior modification centers for troubled teenagers.

Tvert argues that, contrary to what you might expect, the switch from merely decriminalizing use to legalizing the marijuana business improved Amendment 64's prospects because it promised to eliminate the black market and addressed the question of where people would get the pot they were now allowed to smoke. Voters' familiarity with state-regulated medical marijuana centers also helped. "When you talk about legalizing marijuana in the abstract," says Rob Kampia, executive director of the Marijuana Policy Project, "people say, 'I don't understand. What does it look like?' The visual matters. The medical marijuana dispensaries have been regulated since 2010, and there were already hundreds of stores voters would walk past every day."

"Like Any Other Business"

On the first floor of a professional building at the foot of Broadway in Colorado's capital is a black awning displaying the words "Denver Relief" in sans-serif type next to a green cross. Inside you find a waiting room with tan walls and brown leather couches flanking an Oriental rug on which sits a coffee table displaying issues of National Geographic. The shop— which began in May 2009 as a delivery service, making it "the second-oldest continuously operating medical marijuana center in the state of Colorado," according to co-owner Kayvan Khalatbari—is located in the same complex as an urgent care clinic. It looks like a cross between a dentist's office and a law firm. "There are no Bob Marley posters," notes Khalatbari, a 30-year-old Nebraska native who moved to Denver in 2004 for a job in electrical engineering, became an active member of SAFER, and now has a stake in two pizza places as well as the dispensary. "We want to be treated like any other business."

At the intake window, customers have to show their state-issued medical marijuana cards, which indicate that they have "a debilitating medical condition" for which a doctor has recommended cannabis as a treatment. Then they can gain entry to a back room, through two locked steel doors, where they will find a partitioned black granite counter of the sort where people might sit to try on sunglasses or lipstick. Displayed on racks attached to a brick wall behind the counter is an array of marijuana products, including drinks, pastries, lollipops, chocolate bars, sunflower seeds, e-cigarette cartridges, and two dozen varieties of buds in glass jars.

For visitors accustomed to the black market's meager selection, iffy quality, and high prices, the back room at Denver Relief is a revelation. The prices range from $30 to $40 for an eighth of an ounce. Other Denver dispensaries, such as Medicine Man on Nome Street, charge as little as $20, with $25 being fairly typical. According to data collected by the website Price of Weed, Americans commonly spend twice as much, around $50, for the same quantity of high-quality marijuana in the black market.

Denver Relief's grow operation, which produces several hundred pounds of marijuana a year, occupies a nondescript warehouse in an area of the city zoned for light industry. There is a separate room for each stage of growth, each with its own "lighting" scheme, calculated to maximize the production of psychoactive resin. The process, which starts with cuttings from mother plants and ends in a drying room where buds are packed in plastic crates, takes about five months.

The operation produces more than 30 strains of pot, with names like Hashberry, Daywrecker, Durban Poison, Q3 (Purple Urkle crossed with Space Queen), and Blue Dream (DJ Short's Blueberry crossed with Santa Cruze Haze). "There is way more of a difference than most laymen or novices imagine," says Nick Hice, Khalatbari's partner and Denver Relief's cultivation manager. "People think 'it's all green.' That's like someone who doesn't drink beer or wine saying 'it's all beer' or 'it's all wine.' Every one of these strains is different, and there are connoisseurs out there who can pull out the different aromas." Even to my uneducated nose, the strains have distinctive smells, including not just the hops and pine you might expect but surprising fruit notes such as lemon, orange, mango, banana, and pineapple.

The different varieties also have noticeably different psychoactive effects, says Hice, especially when you compare the two major types of marijuana, Cannabis sativa and Cannabis indica. "For medical purposes," he says, "we would usually recommend a sativa for the beginning of the day or early in the day when you still have things to do and you still need to function, whereas the indicas can be more lethargic and give you more of a whole-body high, where your whole body becomes slower and sluggish." According to Denver Relief's website, for example, Ghost Train Haze, a sativa-dominant hybrid, "will keep you active while letting you maintain lucidity." By contrast, Bio-Jesus, an indica-dominant strain, "is recommended for evening pain relief when functionality is not a requirement."

The quality and variety on which connoisseurship depends are an important but rarely mentioned benefit of legalization. While alcohol prohibition may have inspired creative cocktail recipes aimed at disguising the taste of black-market booze, it was hardly conducive to the enjoyment of fine liquor. The difference between black-market pot and the cannabis products available at a shop like Denver Relief is the difference between bathtub gin and the dozens of premium gin brands available today, each with its own aroma and flavor.

The Myth of "Seed-to-Sale" Oversight

While today's medical marijuana centers give you a sense of what fully legal cannabis will look like in Colorado, they operate under restrictions that make little or no sense for businesses serving the recreational market. To begin with, there's that requirement that customers have "a debilitating medical condition." To qualify, a condition must be either listed in Amendment 20, the 2000 initiative that legalized medical use of marijuana, or approved by the Colorado Department of Public Health and Environment, which is charged with maintaining the state's registry of approved patients. Those rules are stricter than California's Compassionate Use Act, which allows people to use marijuana for treatment of six specified conditions (including chronic pain), plus "any other illness for which marijuana provides relief."

Under Colorado law, a medical marijuana center is allowed to grow up to six plants for each patient who designates it as his "provider" in the registry. Denver Relief, for example, has about 400 members, meaning it is allowed to grow around 2,400 plants. Every plant is notionally assigned to a patient, but patients are not limited to pot from "their" plants, and they need not buy exclusively from their designated provider. Furthermore, MMCs can sell marijuana to each other, as long as it's no more than 30 percent of what they grow. MMCs are supposed to account for every last gram they produce and file reports whenever they transport marijuana. The rules are aimed at preventing diversion to people who are not registered patients, whereas in the recreational market the government's main concern will be preventing diversion to minors (defined as people younger than 21) and other states.

Although Colorado's regulations are often credited with allowing dispensaries there to operate relatively unmolested by the federal government, a state audit released in March revealed that all the talk of strict oversight was more aspirational than descriptive. Colorado's vaunted "seed-to-sale" monitoring system, which was supposed to include electronic plant tags, 24-hour video surveillance, and records of every marijuana transfer, was never actually implemented. "The envisioned seed-to-sale model does not currently exist in Colorado," said State Auditor Dianne Ray, and in any case "may not make sense," especially with the legal marijuana market expanding to include recreational users.

As a result of inadequate manpower, funding shortages, and poor financial management, Ray said, the Medical Marijuana Enforcement Division (MMED) not only had failed to create the planned high-tech tracking system; it did not even "review forms designed to track medical marijuana activities and inventories and ensure that medical marijuana is not being diverted from the system." That's right: although medical marijuana businesses were required to file forms whenever they moved any of their product, no one ever looked at them.

Furthermore, state inspectors would visit medical marijuana businesses during the application process but generally did not check in again after they were up and running, so it was hard to say how many of 1,440 or so operations officially overseen by the MMED (including dispensaries, their growing operations, and producers of cannabis edibles) were actually complying with regulations such as the 70/30 rule or the limit of six plants per patient. "The current code is extremely difficult to regulate," MMED Director Laura Harris, now head of the repurposed Marijuana Enforcement Division, told me in January. "What you will hear from many in industry is that this works. Well, I'm not as optimistic about it working."

Harris said enforcement was "complaint-driven," although "we have to prioritize our complaints because we have a limited number of investigators whose primary mission at this point has to be conducting pre-licensing inspections." The auditor's report recommended discontinuing those inspections in favor of "risk-based on-site inspections of the licensed businesses as part of a comprehensive monitoring program." The report estimated that pre-approval inspections of all 2,400 applicants who sought state licenses prior to a two-year moratorium that began in August 2010 "would take about 12,300 hours, which equals the work of six full-time equivalent staff in a year." It added that "the number of Division staff available to perform these on-site inspections has been as high as 19 but has been reduced to 10 as of February 2013." You can start to see why it took so long to obtain a license. According to the audit, "The shortest approval time was 436 days, while the longest approval time was 807 days." The average was about two years. "Out of about 2,400 pre-moratorium applications," the report said, "the Division has approved or denied only 622, or about 26 percent [as of October 2012]. The rest of the applications were still pending (41 percent) or were voluntarily withdrawn by the applicant (33 percent)." Pre-moratorium cannabis businesses were allowed to continue operating in the meantime.

Marijuana taxes are supposed to change all this, giving Harris' agency the resources to regulate in reality as well as theory. In addition to existing state and local sales taxes (which total 7.6 percent in Denver), a bill signed by Gov. Hickenlooper in May would impose an excise tax of 15 percent, as envisioned by Amendment 64, and a special sales tax of 10 percent. Both levies are subject to approval by voters this fall, as required by Colorado's constitution. An April report by researchers at Colorado State University estimated that, together with the standard state sales tax of 2.9 percent, a 15 percent excise tax and a 15 percent special sales tax (which legislators were considering at the time) would add $34 or so to the retail price of an ounce, making it about 23 percent higher than it would otherwise be. The estimated final price, based on a production cost of $600 a pound, was $185 an ounce, about the same as the price many dispensaries currently charge. The report's estimate of total state revenue, which hinged on various questionable assumptions about total consumption and other factors, was

$131 million a year, which would go mainly to the Department of Revenue and a school construction fund.

Legalize It, but Don't Advertise It

In addition to the taxes, the legislature enacted various restrictions on the production and sale of marijuana, many of them suggested by the Amendment 64 Implementation Task Force. While visitors to Colorado will be allowed to buy marijuana, for instance, they will be limited to a quarter of an ounce per transaction. Residents, by contrast, can buy up to an ounce at a time. The idea is to discourage interstate smuggling by making it more difficult to accumulate large quantities. But the residence-based restriction may be vulnerable to challenge under both the state and federal constitutions.

One regulation approved by the legislature was so clearly unconstitutional that the state decided not to enforce it. A provision introduced by state Rep. Bob Gardner (R-Colorado Springs) would have required that "magazines whose primary focus is marijuana or marijuana businesses" be kept out of sight in stores open to people younger than 21. Gardner, who likened marijuana magazines to pornography, imagined that his rule would be upheld as reasonable restriction on commercial speech. But as the American Civil Liberties Union of Colorado pointed out in a federal lawsuit it filed on behalf of bookstores and newsstands, "the government's content-based restriction on non-commercial truthful information cannot pass constitutional muster" because marijuana magazines "are not within a recognized category of unprotected speech." Colorado Attorney General John Suthers agreed in a June 5 memo advising the Department of Revenue to refrain from enforcing Gardner's amendment in light of its conflict with the free speech guarantees of the state and federal constitutions. Denver attorney David Lane, who represented High Times in another lawsuit challenging the magazine rule, told Westword, "You would think a responsible adult in the legislature would have spoken up."

Other restrictions on marijuana-related speech may also be constitutionally vulnerable. The new marijuana law requires state regulators to ban "mass-market campaigns that have a high likelihood of reaching minors," for instance. The U.S. Supreme Court has rejected more modest restrictions on tobacco advertising that were likewise aimed at shielding minors from messages about products they are not allowed to buy. In the 2001 case *Lorillard Tobacco v. Reilly,* the Court overturned a Massachusetts ban on tobacco billboards within 1,000 feet of a school or playground, saying the rule banned outdoor tobacco advertising from "a substantial portion of Massachusetts' largest cities" and in some places amounted to "nearly a complete ban on the communication of truthful information about smokeless tobacco and cigars to adult consumers." Although it's not clear how federal courts would view restrictions on ads for products banned by federal law, Colorado courts traditionally have read the state constitution's free speech guarantee even more broadly than the Supreme Court has read the First Amendment.

Child protection is also the rationale for a provision calling upon the Marijuana Enforcement Division to create "requirements similar to the federal Poison Prevention Packaging Act of 1970," which describes "special packaging" that is "designed or constructed to be significantly difficult for children under five years of age to open or obtain a toxic or harmful amount of the substance contained therein within a reasonable time and not difficult for normal adults to use properly." But while it may be relatively straightforward to put marijuana buds in bottles with childproof caps, it's not clear how "special packaging" for cannabis-infused brownies or candy bars will work. Laura Harris, head of the Marijuana Enforcement Division, notes that legislators contemplated a similar requirement for medical marijuana. "They said you create a rule that describes a kind of packaging we want that will be child resistant" ["Harris says"]. It was never done, she adds, because "that's a thorny issue. What does that look like?"

Although the childproof packaging mandate will raise prices and may cause some inconvenience, the rules about what you can do inside a pot shop are more significant from a consumer's point of view. Customers will not be able to buy alcohol, tobacco, or cannabis-free snacks or drinks, and they will not be allowed to consume marijuana on the premises. The latter rule apparently puts the kibosh on dreams of Amsterdam-style cannabis cafes sprouting on the streets of Denver and Fort Collins. But what if you buy marijuana in a pot shop and take it with you to a bar or restaurant? In an effort to forestall such BYOW arrangements, legislators added marijuana to Colorado's Clean Indoor Air Act, which bans smoking in bars and restaurants. But as amended, the law applies only to "combustible marijuana" and "marijuana smoke," leaving open the possibility that bars and restaurants could allow patrons to use vaporizers or consume cannabis-infused foods purchased elsewhere.

There may be other legal options for people who want to consume marijuana in a social environment similar to a cafe or tavern. Last New Year's Eve, after the Amendment 64 provisions protecting possession and home cultivation took effect, Rob Corry, the attorney and marijuana activist, held the first meeting of a floating pot party he dubbed Club 64 at a hemp clothing store in Denver. "We had a DJ, lights, dancing, good music," Corry says. "We did serve alcohol, [but] we gave it away because we didn't have a liquor license for that event. We also had marijuana that we were giving away. We weren't selling it. The main way we raised revenue was with an event fee of $30." A variation on this theme would be charging for food and coffee but giving pot away, which could result in something like Amsterdam's so-called coffee shops.

Either operation seems to satisfy Amendment 64's requirements, although much depends on how the initiative's ban on consuming marijuana "openly and publicly" is interpreted. Corry argues that the phrase imposes two distinct conditions: to be prohibited, marijuana use must be "open" (visible to passers-by) and "public" (occurring on public property). Smoking pot while walking down a crowded sidewalk would be the paradigmatic example. But according to Corry's reading of the law, smoking pot in a secluded area of a park would be public without being open, while smoking pot on your front porch or on the patio of a restaurant (where the Clean Indoor Air Act does not apply) would be open without being public.

Denver Relief's Kayvan Khalatbari takes a different view. "On-site consumption is not going to happen," he asserts. "This is not going to be an Amsterdam. It's supposed to be done in the privacy of your own home behind drawn shades. You're not supposed to use it in front of anybody in public. Period."

Free Pot! (Donation Encouraged)

Another gray area is the nonprofit production and distribution of marijuana. Under Amendment 64, Coloradans may privately grow up to six plants and possess the marijuana from them (which could be a lot more than an ounce) on the premises where it was produced. They are also allowed to "assist" others in growing and possessing marijuana, and they can legally transfer up to an ounce at a time "without remuneration." These provisions seem to leave considerable leeway for various cooperative arrangements. Corry advises clients that seeking compensation for the costs they incur in growing marijuana, including rent, supplies, and utilities, is perfectly legal. Even seeking compensation for one's time should be acceptable, he says, although it is risky because that could be interpreted as "remuneration."

Last January police in Colorado Springs busted three guys for running Billygoatgreen MMJ, which was giving away marijuana while accepting "suggested donation[s] toward researching [marijuana] and improving our cultivation operation." The suggested donation for a quarterounce of Sour Kush, for instance, was $55. A spokeswoman for Attorney General Suthers told the The Denver Post such operations were clearly illegal, since "distributing marijuana in exchange for suggested donations is a scam to get around the laws against the sale of marijuana." Colorado Springs Police Lt. Mark Comte, who works in the Metro Vice, Narcotics, and Intelligence Division, seemed to disagree in an interview with The Colorado Springs Independent: "If I show up at your house with less than an ounce of marijuana, I'm 21, you're 21, and I say, 'Hey dude, it cost me 50 bucks in gas to get over here,' and you give me 50 bucks for my gas, there's nothing illegal. I mean, you and I both know what's going on with it, but they know what the loopholes are right now." Comte nevertheless defended the Billygoatgreen arrests, saying those guys were transferring more than an ounce at a time.

In May, The Denver Post reported that "an untold number" of cannabis collectives "have formed in Colorado since Amendment 64's passage." They included MJ Proper, a 501(c)(3) organization that sought to "foster the charitable [activity], scientific investigation, and education necessary to safely grow and consume recreational cannabis responsibly." According to MJ Proper's website, the benefits of joining the organization included eighth-ounce bags of Dark Star buds and six packs of cannabis-infused beer, both delivered for $37.50 each. Offended by such creative interpretations of the law, state legislators banned distribution of marijuana by any unlicensed "business or non-profit, including but not limited to a sole proprietorship, corporation, or other business enterprise." Although that provision led MJ Proper to suspend operations, it apparently does not apply to less formally organized efforts. In any case, it is hard to see how the legislature can ban cooperative cultivation without violating Amendment 64, which is now part of the state constitution.

The provisions allowing home cultivation and nonprofit transfers, which cops tend to view as dangerous loopholes, are actually a pretty clever insurance policy. If state-licensed pot shops open as planned, the do-it-yourself sector will account for a tiny share of marijuana consumption, just as home brewing accounts for a tiny share of beer consumption. Why grow your own if retailers are offering a nice selection of high-quality marijuana at reasonable prices? But unless and until that scenario materializes, the allowance for noncommercial production provides an alternative.

In a Brookings Institution paper published last April, legal analyst Stuart Taylor cites that alternative as a reason for federal drug warriors to think twice before trying to stop legalization in Colorado. Taylor warns that "a federal crackdown would backfire by producing an atomized, anarchic, state-legalized but unregulated marijuana market that federal drug enforcers could neither contain nor force the states to contain." The feds could use threats of prosecution and forfeiture to shut down state-licensed stores or prevent them from opening. That approach worked well for John Walsh, the U.S. attorney in Colorado, who last year sent threatening letters to the landlords and operators of more than 50 medical marijuana centers he deemed too close to schools. According to Laura Harris, all of them closed, with nary a raid or arrest. But if the Justice Department succeeded in blocking recreational pot shops, it would be confronted by thousands of small, inconspicuous growers instead of a few hundred openly operating retailers. Taylor argues that if the feds cooperate with Colorado officials to prevent diversion of marijuana, they will have a better chance of limiting the impact on states that continue to treat cannabis as contraband.

For those who favor confrontation, aggressive enforcement is not the only option. Opponents of legalization, including anti-drug activists, former heads of the Drug Enforcement Administration, and several members of Congress, want the Justice Department to fight it in court. They argue that Colorado's marijuana laws are invalid under the Constitution's Supremacy Clause (which says federal statutes are "the supreme law of the land") because they are pre-empted by the Controlled Substances Act (CSA). They note that the Supreme Court, based on a very broad interpretation of the power to regulate interstate commerce, has upheld enforcement of the CSA's ban on marijuana even in states that allow medical use.

But the fact that the feds can continue to enforce marijuana prohibition in Colorado does not mean they can compel Colorado to help. Under our federal system, states have no obligation to punish every action that Congress decides to treat as a crime, and Congress cannot command state officials to enforce its laws. Furthermore, the CSA itself expressly limits pre-emption to situations where there is "a positive conflict" between state and federal law "so that the two cannot consistently stand together."

As Vanderbilt University law professor Robert Mikos explains in a Cato Institute paper published last December, "a positive conflict would seem to arise anytime a state engages in, or requires others to engage in, conduct or inaction that violates the CSA." If state officials grew medical marijuana or distributed it to patients, for example, they would be violating the CSA, and the law establishing that program would be pre-empted. But specifying the criteria for exemption from state penalties does not require anyone to violate the CSA. Mikos concludes that Congress "has left [states] free to regulate marijuana, so long as their regulations do not positively conflict with the CSA."

It is notable that in the 17 years since states began legalizing marijuana for medical use, the Justice Department has never tried to overturn those laws in court with a pre-emption argument, even though it has interfered with the distribution of cannabis to patients in various other ways. "They know they can't force a state to criminalize a given behavior, which is why the federal government has never tried to push a pre-emption argument [against] these medical marijuana laws," Alex Kreit, a professor at the Thomas Jefferson School of Law who has studied the pre-emption issue, told the Drug War Chronicle last year. "Opponents of these laws would love nothing more than to be able to preempt them, but there is not a viable legal theory to do that. The federal government recognizes that's a losing battle. I would be surprised if they filed suit against Colorado or Washington saying their state laws are pre-empted. It would be purely a political maneuver because they would know they would lose in court."

A Yellow Light for Legalization

At the end of August, nearly 10 months after Colorado and Washington voters decided to legalize marijuana, the Justice Department finally responded. In a memo to U.S. attorneys, Deputy Attorney General James Cole indicated that if the two states adequately address federal concerns about issues such as drugged driving, sales to minors, and diversion to other states, the feds will allow their experiments to proceed. But if regulation and enforcement are not strict enough, he said, the Justice Department may yet decide to prosecute growers and sellers who comply with the new marijuana laws or challenge the laws themselves in federal court.

A bill introduced by Rep. Dana Rohrabacher (R-Calif.) in April would take the decision away from the Obama administration by barring federal prosecution of people who grow, possess, transport, or sell marijuana in compliance with state laws. The Respect State Marijuana Laws Act of 2013 has 18 cosponsors, including three Republicans in addition to Rohrabacher: Justin Amash and Dan Benishek of Michigan, which has a medical marijuana law, and Don Young of Alaska, where it is legal to possess less than four ounces of cannabis in your home.

A more modest bill introduced last November by Rep. Diana DeGette (D-Colo.), clarifying that state regulation of marijuana does not violate the Controlled Substances Act, attracted the support of another Republican, Mike Coffman, a conservative who succeeded Tom Tancredo as representative of Colorado's 6th Congressional District in 2009. Coffman had never before shown any inclination to favor drug policy reform. But Amendment 64 won about 52 percent of the vote in Adams, Arapahoe, and Douglas counties, which make up Coffman's district. That's 4 percent points more than Coffman, who was re-elected with a 48 percent plurality. "I think he's a smart guy," says Christian Sederberg, a Denver lawyer who was involved in passing and implementing Amendment 64. Coffman, Sederberg suggests, realized that "if this issue got more votes than I did, that's a very clear signal that it's time to evolve." Amendment 64, incidentally, also received more votes in Colorado than Barack Obama did.

Wanda James, co-owner of a marijuana edibles business in Denver called Simply Pure, argues that politicians ignore growing public support for legalization at their peril. "Three million people in America on election night voted to legalize marijuana," says James, who plans on jumping into the recreational market with both feet. "I can't imagine the United States government starting some arrest campaign on people who are compliant with their state laws. I just can't see the American government doing this when the will of the people is saying 'enough.'" Anyway, she says, "What court in Colorado is going to convict me?"

Critical Thinking

1. Will the restrictions imposed by Amendment 64 adequately prevent the sale of marijuana to minors?

2. Should marijuana be regulated in a manner similar to alcohol?

3. Why do many conservatives support the legal sale of marijuana?

Create Central

www.mhhe.com/createcentral

Internet References

Norml
  http://www.norml.org
State Marijuana Laws Map
  http://www.governing.com

JACOB SULLUM is a nationally syndicated columnist and the author of *Saying Yes: In Defense of Drug Use* (Tarcber Penguin).

Article   Prepared by: Eileen L. Daniel, *SUNY Brockport*

Rethinking Drug Policy Assumptions

JEFFERSON M. FISH

Learning Outcomes

After reading this article, you will be able to:

- Explain why the war on drugs has not been successful.
- Describe drug legalization options.
- Describe why therapy for substance abuse is less successful than treatment for anxiety and depression.

The so-called war on drugs has lasted more than four decades and increasing numbers of people are convinced that it is not only unwinnable but also misguided. From foreign policy to domestic policy to drug treatment, U.S. drug policy has been based on inaccurate assumptions and incorrect causal models that have led to an ever-escalating failure. The attempt here is to identify some of the principal errors, point out their shortcomings, and offer more plausible assumptions and models in their stead. These alternatives point not simply to downsizing the war and decriminalizing marijuana, as voters in Colorado and Washington State recently did, but to ending the war on drugs altogether by considering a range of legalization options.

Attacking Drugs vs. the Black Market

Current U.S. policy is based on the assumption that drugs cause crime, corruption, and disease. Hence, we label and ban some substances as "dangerous drugs." It follows that bad people supply these drugs, so we lock them up, but the supply keeps getting through. Engagement between police and criminal suppliers ramps up, leading only to more crime, corruption, and disease at home, while the battle spreads around the world.

It looks as if the more we clamp down, the worse the problem gets. Up until now the response has been not to question the underlying assumption, but to further escalate the war, hoping the right side will eventually achieve victory. There seems to be no consideration of the possibility that it's the policy itself that's making matters worse.

Here's an alternative causal model, one that actually explains the failure of our longstanding policy: drug prohibition—that is, the war on drugs—causes an illegal, or black market, which in turn causes crime, corruption, and disease. With this model, the goal of drug policy should be to attack the black market instead of attacking drugs because the market undermines the stability of friendly countries (witness Colombia and Mexico) and finances our enemies (al-Qaeda and the Taliban, for example). Attempts to suppress the black market by force merely spread it, from one country to another or, in response to local police crackdowns, from one neighborhood to another.

The way to attack an illegal market is to create a legal one. As we learned when Prohibition ended and it became possible to buy alcohol legally, crime, corruption, and disease (such as blindness or even death from contaminated or substitute products sold as alcohol) fell dramatically.

Decriminalization won't work—even though not locking people up for using a substance is a more humane policy—because it does nothing about the black market. Most people are unaware that Prohibition, with its rampant crime and gang violence, was actually a decriminalization regime for alcohol. The Eighteenth Amendment criminalized "the manufacture, sale, or transportation of intoxicating liquors" but not possession for personal use.

Degrees and Types of Legalization

The question of *how* to legalize drugs (as opposed to whether to legalize) is a complex one that I have dealt with in three separate works offering a wide range of policy alternatives. While the question is too broad to be settled here, let me at least call attention to two of the most important issues that need to be addressed. First, for each substance, one has to consider whether it should be as legal as tomatoes, or if it should be regulated akin to aspirin, or as alcohol and tobacco, or as antibiotics. That is, there are many forms of "legalization," and the term has different meanings for agricultural products, over-the-counter medications, legal psychoactive substances, and prescription medications.

Second, there are two basic approaches to legalization. The first, a rights-based, civil liberties, or libertarian approach, argues that individuals should be free, in private, to have control over their own bodies as long as they don't directly harm other people. This approach tends to be favored by lawyers, judges, police, and others in the criminal justice system because it makes the rules of the game clear to all. The second approach, considered a public health or harm reduction, cost-benefit approach, emphasizes preventing the spread of disease and protecting the health of users. It attempts to devise a different strategy for each substance based on the best scientific knowledge available, and tends to be favored by physicians, psychologists, and those in the biomedical and social sciences. There are many varieties of each kind of approach, and many instances where they agree—but there are also points at which they propose quite different policies; and these differences would need to be addressed in any debate over legalization legislation.

Another key assumption underlying drug prohibition is that drugs "hook" victims, so that making drugs illegal will prevent addiction and the spread of associated diseases. There are many problems with this assumption, but I will only discuss a few. First of all, to simply focus on "drugs" while ignoring dosage level and mode of administration is a mistake. (Other relevant variables include the situation in which the substance is used and the effects users expect it to have.) Higher dosage levels are associated with an increased risk of more serious problems, from dependency to death. Similarly, administering a substance by injecting it is a very efficient means of getting it into your system, but also a dangerous one because of the increased risk of transmitting diseases like HIV and hepatitis through shared needles.

Contrary to the above assumption, the "Iron Law of Prohibition" states that prohibition leads to higher dosage levels and more dangerous modes of administration. These consequences follow naturally from the illegal market. Black marketeers want to pack as much of an outlawed substance as possible into the minimum volume, which is the definition of a high-dosage level; and purchasers, because of the inflated black market price, want the biggest bang for their buck. Similarly, because injecting is so efficient a way of using an expensive substance, there is an economic motivation to use this more dangerous means of administration.

Under Prohibition, the United States went from a nation of drinkers of safe beer (low-dosage alcohol) to drinkers of higher-dosage and often contaminated whiskey. After Prohibition the country gradually returned to its preference for beer. Similarly, over time users have gone from smoked opium to injected heroin; from low-dosage cocaine in the original Coca-Cola to inhaled powdered cocaine to crack; and from lower THC levels in marijuana to higher levels. In addition, because marijuana is bulky and has a strong odor it has the black market disadvantages of taking up a lot of space and being relatively easy to detect. This drives up the price of marijuana relative to cocaine and heroin, and creates an economic incentive for users to switch from soft to hard drugs.

A major study published in *American Psychologist* back in 1990 contradicted the assumption that drugs "hook" victims. Its findings, summarized in the study's Abstract, have long been known, but are startling to many non-experts, and are worth quoting here:

The relation between psychological characteristics and drug use was investigated in subjects studied longitudinally, from preschool through age 18. Adolescents who had engaged in some drug experimentation (primarily with marijuana) were the best-adjusted in the sample. Adolescents who used drugs frequently were maladjusted, showing a distinct personality syndrome marked by interpersonal alienation, poor impulse control, and manifest emotional distress. Adolescents who, by age 18, had never experimented with any drug were relatively anxious, emotionally constricted, and lacking in social skills. Psychological differences between frequent drug users, experimenters, and abstainers could be traced to the earliest years of childhood and related to the quality of parenting received. The findings indicate that (a) problem drug use is a symptom, not a cause, of personal and social maladjustment, and (b) the meaning of drug use can be understood only in the context of an individual's personality structure and developmental history. It is suggested that current efforts at drug prevention are misguided to the extent that they focus on symptoms, rather than on the psychological syndrome underlying drug abuse.

In other words, instead of saying that drugs hook victims, a better causal model for drug abuse is to say that people with significant problems self-medicate. In addition, this description of drug use fits with what we know about adolescence. That is, in our individualistic culture, adolescence is a time of experimentation with different options during the transition from childhood to adulthood. Teenagers work summer or part-time jobs, and they are exposed to courses in a variety of disciplines so that they can make informed career decisions. Dating is an institution that provides young people with experience in forming, maintaining, and dissolving intimate relationships, so that they have a basis for selecting a life partner. In a similar way, teen experimentation with forbidden psychoactive substances can be seen as a way of learning their effects so that people can decide whether to use them in the future.

Punishment vs. Reintegration and Mandatory vs. Voluntary Treatment

Another set of mistaken assumptions underlies current policy regarding prevention and treatment. When it comes to illegal substances, current policy argues that (1) all use is abuse; (2) zero tolerance will discourage use and therefore abuse; (3) punishing users will send a powerful message to others and prevent them from going down the wrong path; and (4) mandatory drug treatment, offered by the courts as an alternative to imprisonment, is an effective and enlightened policy.

An alternative set of assumptions is that (1) only some use, when it is out of control and self-destructive, is abuse; (2) for many individuals and many psychoactive substances, both legal and illegal, controlled, non-problematic use is possible; (3) marginalizing problem users is counterproductive—a more effective strategy is to reduce the harm they do to themselves and others and attempt to reintegrate them into society; and (4) mandatory treatment (for example, in drug courts) undermines the institution of psychotherapy, and is less effective than voluntary treatment.

Tolerance is a virtue, so it's unfortunate that a slogan like "zero tolerance" has become part of the world of prevention and treatment. A better slogan might be "get a life."

When the Vietnam War ended and the troops came home, there was great anxiety in the law enforcement community. Tens of thousands of drug-addicted, trained killers were about to descend on American society. The fear was that their cravings for illegal substances, such as marijuana and heroin, would lead to an unprecedented crime wave as their addictions forced them to come up with the money to support their habits.

It never happened. Yes, some continued to have drug problems and others sought treatment, but for the great majority of problem users, they simply stopped. On their own. With no professional help.

This non-crime wave makes no sense according to the "drugs hook victims" ideology, but it is easily understandable if you employ the point of view that people with significant problems self-medicate. In Vietnam, soldiers faced constant danger and staying high made them feel better. Back home, staying high interfered with their reintegration into society. Work, family, love, a better future—all of these depended on attending to and living in reality, not blotting it out.

Years ago, I had a conversation with a marijuana activist. He was an intelligent, college-educated young man who could have earned much more in another line of work, but whose revulsion at our drug policy led him to sacrifice income for what he viewed as a worthy cause. "You know," he said, "I've actually been smoking very little these days." He described his situation—he worked long hours and needed to keep a clear head; he was in a serious relationship with a woman and wanted to focus his attention on her when they were together; and as a single adult he had responsibilities for feeding himself and maintaining his apartment. In essence, he had a life and was involved with highly valued activities, so that marijuana functioned for him the way alcohol functions for occasional users of that substance—now and then providing a few hours of an altered state of consciousness, integrated responsibly as part of a fulfilling life.

By criminalizing all use we marginalize problem users, which diminishes their likelihood of recovery; and we also marginalize non-problem users who've had the bad luck to get caught up in the criminal justice system—thereby creating serious problems for them where none existed before.

Supposedly, mandatory drug treatment offers an enlightened option for users who've been arrested. To understand why this is not the case, it's necessary to have a basic understanding of the way therapy works. To begin with, therapy is based on trust. In voluntary therapy, the therapist is working for the client, and what happens in therapy is protected by confidentiality, which allows the client to candidly discuss anything, including illegal drug use. If the client feels that therapy isn't working, that client is free to leave altogether, or to seek another therapist. In mandatory drug treatment, the therapist is working for the court, and a client seeking to leave therapy can be labeled as uncooperative, which can result in imprisonment.

For non-problem users, therapy turns into a charade. The individual has to pretend he or she has a drug problem to avoid going to jail. The user then has to pretend to cooperate with the therapist, since lack of cooperation could result in jail time. In this situation, therapists get paid for their time, which provides an incentive to maintain the charade. Eventually, the client is deemed cured and has succeeded in avoiding jail by undergoing the lesser punishment of pretend therapy. (Some people may actually benefit from the process by dealing better with various aspects of their lives, but this is hardly a justification for undermining the institution of therapy by making therapist and client co-conspirators in a lie.)

In order to understand the situation for problem users it's necessary to consider the role of motivation in therapy. ("How many therapists does it take to change a light bulb?" the relevant joke goes. "Only one, but the light bulb has to *want* to change.") Why is it that the success rates in therapy are so much better for anxiety and depression than they are for substance abuse? The reason is that anxiety and depression are unpleasant, so clients are motivated to change. They are likely to cooperate with therapists because they want to experience less of those unpleasant feelings, and more positive feelings instead. The situation is the opposite for overeating, risky sexual behavior, gambling, and substance abuse. These are pleasurable activities, so change—even if it is clearly better for the client—entails a loss of an important source of pleasure. Thus, when clients are self-motivated to change, because they see that they are headed in a bad direction, they are more likely to cooperate with a therapist who suggests difficult or unpleasant tasks than they are with a court-ordered therapist who says "Change, or else!" This is one reason for the slogan "drug treatment on demand." You'll get better results with people who want to change than with those who are forced to change against their will.

One form of brief therapy, known as solution-focused therapy, describes three kinds of therapeutic relationships. In a customer relationship, the individual wants to change (technically, the individual is "willing to construct a solution"), and the therapist helps that person to change. In a complainant relationship, the client wants to complain but is unwilling to change (one who might say, "I'd be fine if only my spouse would change"). In a visitor relationship, the individual has neither a complaint nor an interest in changing (such as a child who has problems at school, whose mother brings him or her for therapy, and whose father [the visitor] comes because the therapist asked him to, although he isn't sure what he's doing there). In general, solution-focused therapists work directly toward change with customers, and try to convert complainants and visitors into customers.

A colleague of mine suggested that mandatory treatment deserved a separate label as a fourth kind of relationship—a hostage relationship.

In short, replacing the inaccurate assumptions and causal models underlying the war on drugs with better alternatives points to a different way of understanding drug use and abuse and to different drug policy options. These alternatives include shifting our primary aim from attacking drugs to shrinking the black market through a targeted policy of legalization for adults, and differentiating between problem users (who should be offered help) and non-problem users (who should be left alone). We must also shift from a policy of punishing and marginalizing problem users to one of harm reduction and reintegration into society, while shifting from a mandatory treatment policy to one of voluntary treatment. Moreover, abstention need not be the only acceptable treatment outcome—we must recognize that many (but not all) problem users can become occasional, non-problematic users. Finally, moving away from a near-exclusive treatment focus on the substance itself to building on positive aspects of people's lives, such as work, family, friends, and interests, will enable us to forge a more successful, more humanistic approach to drug use.

Critical Thinking

1. Why is the war on drugs considered unwinnable?
2. What are some of the ranges of legalized options relative to drug legalization?
3. Why are the success rates in therapy so much better for anxiety and depression than they are for substance abuse?

Create Central

www.mhhe.com/createcentral

Internet References

Food and Drug Administration (FDA)
   www.fda.gov
National Institute on Drug Abuse (NIDA)
   www.nida.nih.gov

JEFFERSON M. FISH *is professor emeritus, former Psychology Department chair, and former director of clinical psychology at St. John's University, New York City. He is the author or editor of twelve books, most recently* **The Myth of Race.** *His* Psychology Today *blog is called "**Looking in the Cultural Mirror**" and his website is **www. jeffersonfish.com.** You can also find him on **Facebook** and **Twitter**.*

Article

Prepared by: Eileen L. Daniel, *SUNY College at Brockport*

When It Comes to E-cigs, Big Tobacco Is Concerned for Your Health

MARTINNE GELLER

Learning Outcomes

After reading this article, you will be able to:

- Understand why tobacco companies support more stringent labeling on e-cigarettes.

- Describe what types of controls tobacco companies support relative to e-cigarettes.

The health warning on a MarkTen electronic cigarette package is 116 words long.

That's much longer than the warnings on traditional cigarette packs in the United States. Nicotine, the e-cigarette warning says, is "addictive and habit-forming, and it is very toxic by inhalation, in contact with the skin, or if swallowed." It is not intended for women who are pregnant or breast-feeding, or people . . . who take medicine for depression or asthma. "Nicotine can increase your heart rate and blood pressure and cause dizziness, nausea and stomach pain," says MarkTen, a leading brand in the United States. The ingredients can be "poisonous."

MarkTen's parent company Altria, maker of Marlboro cigarettes, said the language seemed appropriate. There is no required health warning on electronic cigarettes in the United States, so "we had to do what we thought was right," said a spokesman for Altria Client Services.

The company's frankness about the perils of nicotine dates back to the late 1990s, when it led a campaign for cigarettes to be regulated by the U.S. Food and Drug Administration (FDA). Small tobacco companies at the time said the big guys would use regulation to seal their dominance. Today, small e-cigarette makers are saying the same thing. Many argue that firms like Altria and Reynolds American want hefty rules to help neutralize the threat that e-cigarettes pose to their businesses. By accentuating the risks of "vaping," they say, big firms may deter smokers from trying the new devices, even though most scientists agree they are safer.

"If you read that (warning) as a smoker, you might think 'Oh, I'll just stick with a cigarette,'" said Oliver Kershaw, a former 15-a-day-smoker who quit through e-cigarettes and founded websites that advocate them.

Big tobacco companies have pushed for a range of controls on e-cigarettes. These include lengthy health warnings, reduced product ranges, restricted sales, and scientific testing requirements. Kershaw and others say such efforts risk squeezing small players. Too many rules would stifle innovation and reduce the range of products to "a very simple, utilitarian e-cigarette," said Fraser Cropper, CEO of Totally Wicked, an independent e-cigarette company based in the UK.

Big tobacco companies say their goal in pushing for firm control is not to hurt smaller competitors. Regulation will benefit consumers and e-cigarette companies alike by ensuring safety and quality standards and boosting confidence, they say. Small companies should not be exempt from responsible behavior.

"Our stated goal is to get to e-vapor leadership, to have the strongest brands in the marketplace," said the Altria spokesman. He could not predict the impact of increased regulation on smaller firms. "I don't know how they run their businesses and what it would cost them to meet those requirements."

Most anti-tobacco campaigners agree that e-cigarettes should be regulated. But some believe that they deserve a lighter touch than tobacco because they can help smokers quit and may be less harmful than smoking.

Measures that make e-cigarettes less appealing or hard to come by may keep people smoking, these people say. Clive Bates, a former head of UK charity Action on Smoking and Health (ASH), thinks public health officials who advocate tough controls end up helping Big Tobacco's conventional brands.

"They really are all doing their utmost to protect the cigarette trade," Bates said. "They just don't realize it." He thinks that regulations should encourage smokers to quit, or switch.

The image of e-cigarettes is already changing. The proportion of people in Britain who think vaping is just as harmful as smoking doubled last year to 15 percent, according to a survey by ASH. In the United States, a similar picture is emerging. The growth in U.S. sales of e-cigarettes slowed to 5 percent in the fourth quarter last year from 19 percent a year earlier, according to Wells Fargo analyst Bonnie Herzog. She attributes that partly to increased uncertainty about the products.

Derek Yach, a director at Vitality Institute, a health research company, doubts that there is any "conspiratorial effort" to crush the new business. But he says that "if the dominant message is one of doubt, then the status quo gets maintained." Yach once headed tobacco control at the World Health Organization and worked at PepsiCo.

Japan Tobacco International, the world's third-largest tobacco company, thinks that strict regulations could hurt young firms. "If you make it extremely hard (to comply), you would drive small companies out of business," said Ian Jones, JTI's head of scientific and regulatory affairs for emerging products. "You would lose the value of the category, you would lose the spark."

"Open Systems"

E-cigarettes came onto the market a decade ago promising a safer nicotine fix. The devices heat nicotine-laced liquid to create an inhalable vapor, rather than burn tobacco. That gives smokers the traditional hand-to-mouth ritual without the deadly smoke.

The global vaping market, which could top $7 billion this year, is evenly split between cigarette look-alikes, often sold by tobacco companies, and refillable "vapors, tanks, and mods"—devices which users modify to suit their needs. These are often made by smaller firms. Demand for them is growing three times as fast as the overall market, as users say they find them more satisfying than early all-in-one models.

Serious devotees favor such refillable "open systems" that let them mix and match liquids and batteries to vary their nicotine intake. Open systems are often sold in vape shops and lend an edgy, do-it-yourself creativity to the vaping community. According to Wells Fargo, there are now around 8,500 vape shops in the United States and 19,400 globally. Vape shops account for about one-third of all U.S. sales, while the Internet accounts for another third.

In August, Reynolds—which does not produce mods—urged the FDA to "ban open system e-cigarettes, including all component parts." Such systems, Reynolds wrote, present a "unique risk for adulteration, tampering and quality control."

If the FDA does not want a ban, Reynolds suggested, it should regulate vape shops as manufacturers. That would subject them to FDA inspection, registration, manufacturing standards, and product clearance requirements.

Vape shops often mix nicotine and flavoring, just as pharmacies compound drugs, said Richard Smith, communications manager at Reynolds. This means that "the vape shop seller is a manufacturer under the applicable laws and regulations."

E-cigarette independents say such a move targets them; analysts note that the business model of big tobacco firms depends on mass production, not mix-and-match.

"I think they (Reynolds) probably want that snuffed out before it gains traction," said Philip Gorham, an Amsterdam-based tobacco analyst at Morningstar.

Reynolds says that's not true. "We fully support innovation in tobacco products, including vapor products," said Smith. The company wants "a level playing-field where all manufacturers are subject to equal treatment."

Doing Their Duty

Shane MacGuill, a tobacco analyst at market research firm Euromonitor International, said Reynolds' move may seem zealous, but companies have a duty to shareholders: "It would be remiss . . . of them not to try and push for the competitive environment that is as favorable to them as possible."

Steven Parrish, a former Altria executive who retired in 2008, said that as long as people are honest, there's nothing wrong with advocating to protect their interests. And embracing regulation can help the tobacco industry win trust.

"I think one of the things the industry would like to see . . . is a world in which the tobacco industry is much more like the pharmaceutical industry in terms of how it operates," he said: "Very heavily regulated and maybe not loved and admired, but at least acknowledged as a legitimate business."

That makes young people a particularly sensitive point of tension.

Most e-cigarette companies want tighter controls on who can buy, such as a minimum age. Altria's NuMark goes further. It says U.S. purchases should also be "clerk-assisted or conducted in an otherwise non-self-service environment."

Smaller e-cigarette makers say that would hand a big advantage to tobacco companies.

U.S. convenience stores are the main outlets for tobacco products. Tobacco firms offer the stores rich incentives to promote their brands, and according to Morningstar, tobacco can provide more than a third of stores' profit. Cigarettes can only be sold behind the counter. They are displayed on heavily branded shelving which the tobacco firms often provide.

Putting e-cigarettes behind the counter would force the products to compete for consumer attention in space that tobacco firms influence, small companies say.

"As long as you say it has to be 12 feet from a child's hand at the counter, it guarantees (the e-cigarette) gets onto their wall," said Jan Verleur, CEO and co-founder of VMR, a Miami-based e-cigarette company.

Altria says retailers choose how and where to display products.

Early Warnings

Some small e-cig firms are pushing back. Totally Wicked is challenging Europe's Tobacco Products Directive (TPD), which was adopted in 2014 and comes into force in 2016.

It's up to member states to apply the EU rules in their own way, but the directive says manufacturers must tell regulators what's in a new product six months before launch. Producers will have to list ingredients, emissions, toxicological data, and nicotine doses and uptake, as well as health effects. A new notification is required for every big change.

Totally Wicked is fighting the TPD in the EU Court of Justice in Luxembourg. Such detailed reporting is more onerous even than for traditional cigarettes, the company argues. It says it is disproportionate, considering that e-cigarettes are probably less harmful. Its CEO says the six-month notification would slow innovation in an industry where manufacturers can move from concept to shelf in 10 weeks.

British American Tobacco's Nicoventures unit agrees with Totally Wicked that the six-month notice period "runs the risk of stifling innovation," according to a spokeswoman.

But global tobacco leader Philip Morris International—which used to be part of Altria—said it thinks this kind of advance notification is appropriate to ensure standards. Its own tests already go beyond the TPD rules, a spokeswoman said. Robust scientific research is "something we believe in as the core of our work in this new product category."

In the United States, the FDA aims to deliver its final ruling on e-cigarettes in June. E-cigarette firms that there say anything that requires lengthy and costly trials could be manageable for big business but may hurt smaller companies. "The more science that's required, the more expensive it becomes," said Sanjiv Desai, general counsel of U.S. e-cigarette firm VMR.

A spokesman for the FDA said it was weighing the burden on everyone, including small manufacturers. It plans to help small companies by phasing in new rules. The European Union also plans to give firms time to adapt. It has said clear rules will help smaller firms; it plans to assess the costs of notification.

For Yach, the former WHO tobacco official, regulators should remember that e-cigarettes are more than a new business. "A heavy smoker has a 20 times greater risk of lung cancer," Yach said. "Switch to e-cigarettes and that risk is virtually going to zero."

Critical Thinking

1. Why do tobacco companies try to impose more stringent labeling on e-cigarettes?
2. Why is the image of e-cigarettes changing?

Internet References

Food and Drug Administration
www.fda.gov
National Institutes of Health
www.nih.gov

Article   Prepared by: Eileen L. Daniel, *SUNY Brockport*

Drowned in a Stream of Prescriptions

Before his addiction, Richard Fee was a popular college class president and aspiring medical student. "You keep giving Adderall to my son, you're going to kill him," said Rick Fee, Richard's father, to one of his son's doctors.

ALAN SCHWARZ

Learning Outcomes

After reading this article, you will be able to:

- Explain the risks associated with the use of non-prescribed prescription drugs.

- Describe the mechanisms in which drugs such as Ritalin and Adderall work.

- Understand the reasons for the widespread use of these drugs among college students.

Virginia beach—Every morning on her way to work, Kathy Fee holds her breath as she drives past the squat brick building that houses Dominion Psychiatric Associates.

It was there that her son, Richard, visited a doctor and received prescriptions for Adderall, an amphetamine-based medication for attention deficit hyperactivity disorder. It was in the parking lot that she insisted to Richard that he did not have A.D.H.D., not as a child and not now as a 24-year-old college graduate, and that he was getting dangerously addicted to the medication. It was inside the building that her husband, Rick, implored Richard's doctor to stop prescribing him Adderall, warning, "You're going to kill him."

It was where, after becoming violently delusional and spending a week in a psychiatric hospital in 2011, Richard met with his doctor and received prescriptions for 90 more days of Adderall. He hanged himself in his bedroom closet two weeks after they expired.

The story of Richard Fee, an athletic, personable college class president and aspiring medical student, highlights widespread failings in the system through which five million Americans take medication for A.D.H.D., doctors and other experts said.

Medications like Adderall can markedly improve the lives of children and others with the disorder. But the tunnel-like focus the medicines provide has led growing numbers of teenagers and young adults to fake symptoms to obtain steady prescriptions for highly addictive medications that carry serious psychological dangers. These efforts are facilitated by a segment of doctors who skip established diagnostic procedures, renew prescriptions reflexively and spend too little time with patients to accurately monitor side effects.

Richard Fee's experience included it all. Conversations with friends and family members and a review of detailed medical records depict an intelligent and articulate young man lying to doctor after doctor, physicians issuing hasty diagnoses, and psychiatrists continuing to prescribe medication—even increasing dosages—despite evidence of his growing addiction and psychiatric breakdown.

Very few people who misuse stimulants devolve into psychotic or suicidal addicts. But even one of Richard's own physicians, Dr. Charles Parker, characterized his case as a virtual textbook for ways that A.D.H.D. practices can fail patients, particularly young adults. "We have a significant travesty being done in this country with how the diagnosis is being made and the meds are being administered," said Dr. Parker, a psychiatrist in Virginia Beach. "I think it's an abnegation of trust. The public needs to say this is totally unacceptable and walk out."

Young adults are by far the fastest-growing segment of people taking A.D.H.D medications. Nearly 14 million monthly prescriptions for the condition were written for Americans ages 20 to 39 in 2011, two and a half times the 5.6 million just four years before, according to the data company I.M.S. Health. While this rise is generally attributed to the maturing of adolescents who have A.D.H.D. into young adults—combined with a greater recognition of adult A.D.H.D. in general—many experts caution that savvy college graduates, freed of parental oversight, can legally and easily obtain stimulant prescriptions from obliging doctors.

"Any step along the way, someone could have helped him—they were just handing out drugs," said Richard's father. Emphasizing that he had no intention of bringing legal action against any of the doctors involved, Mr. Fee said: "People have to know that kids are out there getting these drugs and getting addicted to them. And doctors are helping them do it."

" . . .when he was in elementary school he fidgeted, daydreamed and got A's. he has been an A-B student until mid college when he became scattered and he wandered while reading He never had to study. Presently without medication, his mind thinks most of the time, he procrastinated, he multitasks not finishing in a timely manner."

Dr. Waldo M. Ellison
Richard Fee initial evaluation
Feb. 5, 2010

Richard began acting strangely soon after moving back home in late 2009, his parents said. He stayed up for days at a time, went from gregarious to grumpy and back, and scrawled compulsively in notebooks. His father, while trying to add Richard to his health insurance policy, learned that he was taking Vyvanse for A.D.H.D.

Richard explained to him that he had been having trouble concentrating while studying for medical school entrance exams the previous year and that he had seen a doctor and received a diagnosis. His father reacted with surprise. Richard had never shown any A.D.H.D. symptoms his entire life, from nursery school through high school, when he was awarded a full academic scholarship to Greensboro College in North Carolina. Mr. Fee also expressed concerns about the safety of his son's taking daily amphetamines for a condition he might not have.

"The doctor wouldn't give me anything that's bad for me," Mr. Fee recalled his son saying that day. "I'm not buying it on the street corner."

Richard's first experience with A.D.H.D. pills, like so many others', had come in college. Friends said he was a typical undergraduate user—when he needed to finish a paper or cram for exams, one Adderall capsule would jolt him with focus and purpose for six to eight hours, repeat as necessary.

So many fellow students had prescriptions or stashes to share, friends of Richard recalled in interviews, that guessing where he got his was futile. He was popular enough on campus—he was sophomore class president and played first base on the baseball team—that they doubted he even had to pay the typical $5 or $10 per pill.

"He would just procrastinate, wait till the last minute and then take a pill to study for tests," said Ryan Sykes, a friend. "It got to the point where he'd say he couldn't get anything done if he didn't have the Adderall."

Various studies have estimated that 8 percent to 35 percent of college students take stimulant pills to enhance school performance. Few students realize that giving or accepting even one Adderall pill from a friend with a prescription is a federal crime. Adderall and its stimulant siblings are classified by the Drug Enforcement Administration as Schedule II drugs, in the same category as cocaine, because of their highly addictive properties.

"It's incredibly nonchalant," Chris Hewitt, a friend of Richard, said of students' attitudes to the drug. "It's: 'Anyone have any Adderall? I want to study tonight,'" said Mr. Hewitt, now an elementary school teacher in Greensboro.

After graduating with honors in 2008 with a degree in biology, Richard planned to apply to medical schools and stayed in Greensboro to study for the entrance exams. He remembered how Adderall had helped him concentrate so well as an undergraduate, friends said, and he made an appointment at the nearby Triad Psychiatric and Counseling Center.

According to records obtained by Richard's parents after his death, a nurse practitioner at Triad detailed his unremarkable medical and psychiatric history before recording his complaints about "organization, memory, attention to detail." She characterized his speech as "clear," his thought process "goal directed" and his concentration "attentive."

Richard filled out an 18-question survey on which he rated various symptoms on a 0-to-3 scale. His total score of 29 led the nurse practitioner to make a diagnosis of "A.D.H.D., inattentive-type"—a type of A.D.H.D. without hyperactivity. She recommended Vyvanse, 30 milligrams a day, for three weeks.

Phone and fax requests to Triad officials for comment were not returned.

Some doctors worry that A.D.H.D. questionnaires, designed to assist and standardize the gathering of a patient's symptoms, are being used as a shortcut to diagnosis. C. Keith Conners, a longtime child psychologist who developed a popular scale similar to the one used with Richard, said in an interview that scales like his "have reinforced this tendency for quick and dirty practice."

Dr. Conners, an emeritus professor of psychiatry and behavioral sciences at Duke University Medical Center, emphasized that a detailed life history must be taken and other sources of information—such as a parent, teacher or friend—must be pursued to learn the nuances of a patient's difficulties and to rule out other maladies before making a proper diagnosis of A.D.H.D. Other doctors interviewed said they would not prescribe medications on a patient's first visit, specifically to deter the faking of symptoms.

According to his parents, Richard had no psychiatric history, or even suspicion of problems, through college. None of his dozen high school and college acquaintances interviewed for this article said he had ever shown or mentioned behaviors related to A.D.H.D.—certainly not the "losing things" and "difficulty awaiting turn" he reported on the Triad questionnaire—suggesting that he probably faked or at least exaggerated his symptoms to get his diagnosis.

That is neither uncommon nor difficult, said David Berry, a professor and researcher at the University of Kentucky. He is a co-author of a 2010 study that compared two groups of college students—those with diagnoses of A.D.H.D. and others who were asked to fake symptoms—to see whether standard symptom questionnaires could tell them apart. They were indistinguishable.

"With college students," Dr. Berry said in an interview, "it's clear that it doesn't take much information for someone who wants to feign A.D.H.D. to do so."

Richard Fee filled his prescription for Vyvanse within hours at a local Rite Aid. He returned to see the nurse three weeks later and reported excellent concentration: "reading books—read 10!" her notes indicate. She increased his dose to 50 milligrams a day. Three weeks later, after Richard left a message for her asking for the dose to go up to 60, which is on the high end of normal adult doses, she wrote on his chart, "Okay rewrite."

Richard filled that prescription later that afternoon. It was his third month's worth of medication in 43 days.

"The patient is a 23-year-old Caucasian male who presents for refill of vyvanse—recently started on this while in NC b/c of lack of motivation/loss of drive. Has moved here and wants refill"

Dr. Robert M. Woodard
Notes on Richard Fee
Nov. 11, 2009

Richard scored too low on the MCAT in 2009 to qualify for a top medical school. Although he had started taking Vyvanse for its jolts of focus and purpose, their side effects began to take hold. His sleep patterns increasingly scrambled and his mood darkening, he moved back in with his parents in Virginia Beach and sought a local physician to renew his prescriptions.

A friend recommended a family physician, Dr. Robert M. Woodard. Dr. Woodard heard Richard describe how well Vyvanse was working for his A.D.H.D., made a diagnosis of "other malaise and fatigue" and renewed his prescription for one month. He suggested that Richard thereafter see a trained psychiatrist at Dominion Psychiatric Associates—only a five-minute walk from the Fees' house.

With eight psychiatrists and almost 20 therapists on staff, Dominion Psychiatric is one of the better-known practices in Virginia Beach, residents said. One of its better-known doctors is Dr. Waldo M. Ellison, a practicing psychiatrist since 1974.

In interviews, some patients and parents of patients of Dr. Ellison's described him as very quick to identify A.D.H.D. and prescribe medication for it. Sandy Paxson of nearby Norfolk said she took her 15-year-old son to see Dr. Ellison for anxiety in 2008; within a few minutes, Mrs. Paxson recalled, Dr. Ellison said her son had A.D.H.D. and prescribed him Adderall.

"My son said: 'I love the way this makes me feel. It helps me focus for school, but it's not getting rid of my anxiety, and that's what I need,'" Mrs. Paxson recalled. "So we went back to Dr. Ellison and told him that it wasn't working properly, what else could he give us, and he basically told me that I was wrong. He basically told me that I was incorrect."

Dr. Ellison met with Richard in his office for the first time on Feb. 5, 2010. He took a medical history, heard Richard's complaints regarding concentration, noted how he was drumming his fingers and made a diagnosis of A.D.H.D. with "moderate symptoms or difficulty functioning." Dominion Psychiatric records of that visit do not mention the use of any A.D.H.D.

symptom questionnaire to identify particular areas of difficulty or strategies for treatment.

As the 47-minute session ended, Dr. Ellison prescribed a common starting dose of Adderall: 30 milligrams daily for 21 days. Eight days later, while Richard still had 13 pills remaining, his prescription was renewed for 30 more days at 50 milligrams.

Through the remainder of 2010, in appointments with Dr. Ellison that usually lasted under five minutes, Richard returned for refills of Adderall. Records indicate that he received only what was consistently coded as "pharmacologic management"—the official term for quick appraisals of medication effects—and none of the more conventional talk-based therapy that experts generally consider an important component of A.D.H.D. treatment.

His Adderall prescriptions were always for the fast-acting variety, rather than the extended-release formula that is less prone to abuse.

"Patient doing well with the medication, is calm, focused and on task, and will return to office in 3 months"

Dr. Waldo M. Ellison
Notes on Richard Fee
Dec. 11, 2010

Regardless of what he might have told his doctor, Richard Fee was anything but well or calm during his first year back home, his father said.

Blowing through a month's worth of Adderall in a few weeks, Richard stayed up all night reading and scribbling in notebooks, occasionally climbing out of his bedroom window and on to the roof to converse with the moon and stars. When the pills ran out, he would sleep for 48 hours straight and not leave his room for 72. He got so hot during the day that he walked around the house with ice packs around his neck—and in frigid weather, he would cool off by jumping into the 52-degree backyard pool.

As Richard lost a series of jobs and tensions in the house ran higher—particularly when talk turned to his Adderall—Rick and Kathy Fee continued to research the side effects of A.D.H.D. medication. They learned that stimulants are exceptionally successful at mollifying the impulsivity and distractibility that characterize classic A.D.H.D., but that they can cause insomnia, increased blood pressure and elevated body temperature. Food and Drug Administration warnings on packaging also note "high potential for abuse," as well as psychiatric side effects such as aggression, hallucinations and paranoia.

A 2006 study in the journal Drug and Alcohol Dependence claimed that about 10 percent of adolescents and young adults who misused A.D.H.D. stimulants became addicted to them. Even proper, doctor-supervised use of the medications can trigger psychotic behavior or suicidal thoughts in about 1 in 400 patients, according to a 2006 study in The American Journal of Psychiatry. So while a vast majority of stimulant users will not experience psychosis—and a doctor may never encounter it in decades of careful practice—the sheer volume of prescriptions leads to thousands of cases every year, experts acknowledged.

When Mrs. Fee noticed Richard putting tape over his computer's camera, he told her that people were spying on him. (He put tape on his fingers, too, to avoid leaving fingerprints.) He cut himself out of family pictures, talked to the television and became increasingly violent when agitated.

In late December, Mr. Fee drove to Dominion Psychiatric and asked to see Dr. Ellison, who explained that federal privacy laws forbade any discussion of an adult patient, even with the patient's father. Mr. Fee said he had tried unsuccessfully to detail Richard's bizarre behavior, assuming that Richard had not shared such details with his doctor.

"I can't talk to you," Mr. Fee recalled Dr. Ellison telling him. "I did this one time with another family, sat down and talked with them, and I ended up getting sued. I can't talk with you unless your son comes with you."

Mr. Fee said he had turned to leave but distinctly recalls warning Dr. Ellison, "You keep giving Adderall to my son, you're going to kill him."

Dr. Ellison declined repeated requests for comment on Richard Fee's case. His office records, like those of other doctors involved, were obtained by Mr. Fee under Virginia and federal law, which allow the legal representative of a deceased patient to obtain medical records as if he were the patient himself.

As 2011 began, the Fees persuaded Richard to see a psychologist, Scott W. Sautter, whose records note Richard's delusions, paranoia and "severe and pervasive mental disorder." Dr. Sautter recommended that Adderall either be stopped or be paired with a sleep aid "if not medically contraindicated."

Mr. Fee did not trust his son to share this report with Dr. Ellison, so he drove back to Dominion Psychiatric and, he recalled, was told by a receptionist that he could leave the information with her. Mr. Fee said he had demanded to put it in Dr. Ellison's hands himself and threatened to break down his door in order to do so.

Mr. Fee said that Dr. Ellison had then come out, read the report and, appreciating the gravity of the situation, spoke with him about Richard for 45 minutes. They scheduled an appointment for the entire family.

"meeting with parents—concern with 'metaphoric' speaking that appears to be outside the realm of appropriated one to one conversation. Richard says he does it on purpose—to me some of it sounds like pre-psychotic thinking."

Dr. Waldo M. Ellison
Notes on Richard Fee
Feb. 23, 2011

Dr. Ellison stopped Richard Fee's prescription—he wrote "no Adderall for now" on his chart and the next day refused Richard's phone request for more. Instead he prescribed Abilify

and Seroquel, antipsychotics for schizophrenia that do not provide the bursts of focus and purpose that stimulants do. Richard became enraged, his parents recalled. He tried to back up over his father in the Dominion Psychiatric parking lot and threatened to burn the house down. At home, he took a baseball bat from the garage, smashed flower pots and screamed, "You're taking my medicine!"

Richard disappeared for a few weeks. He returned to the house when he learned of his grandmother's death, the Fees said.

The morning after the funeral, Richard walked down Potters Road to what became a nine-minute visit with Dr. Ellison. He left with two prescriptions: one for Abilify, and another for 50 milligrams a day of Adderall.

According to Mr. Fee, Richard later told him that he had lied to Dr. Ellison—he told the doctor he was feeling great, life was back on track and he had found a job in Greensboro that he would lose without Adderall. Dr. Ellison's notes do not say why he agreed to start Adderall again.

Richard's delusions and mood swings only got worse, his parents said. They would lock their bedroom door when they went to sleep because of his unpredictable rages. "We were scared of our own son," Mr. Fee said. Richard would blow through his monthly prescriptions in 10 to 15 days and then go through hideous withdrawals. A friend said that he would occasionally get Richard some extra pills during the worst of it, but that "it wasn't enough because he would take four or five at a time."

One night during an argument, after Richard became particularly threatening and pushed him over a chair, Mr. Fee called the police. They arrested Richard for domestic violence. The episode persuaded Richard to see another local psychiatrist, Dr. Charles Parker.

Mrs. Fee said she attended Richard's initial consultation on June 3 with Dr. Parker's clinician, Renee Strelitz, and emphasized his abuse of Adderall. Richard "kept giving me dirty looks," Mrs. Fee recalled. She said she had later left a detailed message on Ms. Strelitz's voice mail, urging her and Dr. Parker not to prescribe stimulants under any circumstances when Richard came in the next day.

Dr. Parker met with Richard alone. The doctor noted depression, anxiety and suicidal ideas. He wrote "no meds" with a box around it—an indication, he explained later, that he was aware of the parents' concerns regarding A.D.H.D. stimulants.

Dr. Parker wrote three 30-day prescriptions: Clonidine (a sleep aid), Venlafaxine (an antidepressant) and Adderall, 60 milligrams a day.

In an interview last November, Dr. Parker said he did not recall the details of Richard's case but reviewed his notes and tried to recreate his mind-set during that appointment. He said he must have trusted Richard's assertions that medication was not an issue, and must have figured that his parents were just philosophically anti-medication. Dr. Parker recalled that he had been reassured by Richard's intelligent discussions of the ins and outs of stimulants and his desire to pursue medicine himself.

"He was smart and he was quick and he had A's and B's and wanted to go to medical school—and he had all the deportment of a guy that had the potential to do that," Dr. Parker said. "He didn't seem like he was a drug person at all, but rather a person that was misunderstood, really desirous of becoming a physician. He was very slick and smooth. He convinced me there was a benefit."

Mrs. Fee was outraged. Over the next several days, she recalled, she repeatedly spoke with Ms. Strelitz over the phone to detail Richard's continued abuse of the medication (she found nine pills gone after 48 hours) and hand-delivered Dr. Sautter's appraisal of his recent psychosis. Dr. Parker confirmed that he had received this information.

Richard next saw Dr. Parker on June 27. Mrs. Fee drove him to the clinic and waited in the parking lot. Soon afterward, Richard returned and asked to head to the pharmacy to fill a prescription. Dr. Parker had raised his Adderall to 80 milligrams a day.

Dr. Parker recalled that the appointment had been a 15-minute "med check" that left little time for careful assessment of any Adderall addiction. Once again, Dr. Parker said, he must have believed Richard's assertions that he needed additional medicine more than the family's pleas that it be stopped.

"He was pitching me very well—I was asking him very specific questions, and he was very good at telling me the answers in a very specific way," Dr. Parker recalled. He added later, "I do feel partially responsible for what happened to this kid."

"Paranoid and psychotic . . . thinking that the computer is spying on him. He has also been receiving messages from stars at night and he is unable to be talked to in a reasonable fashion . . . The patient denies any mental health problems . . . fairly high risk for suicide."

Dr. John Riedler
Admission note for Richard Fee
Virginia Beach Psychiatric Center
July 8, 2011

The 911 operator answered the call and heard a young man screaming on the other end. His parents would not give him his pills. With the man's language scattered and increasingly threatening, the police were sent to the home of Rick and Kathy Fee.

The Fees told officers that Richard was addicted to Adderall, and that after he had received his most recent prescription, they allowed him to fill it through his mother's insurance plan on the condition that they hold it and dispense it appropriately. Richard was now demanding his next day's pills early.

Richard denied his addiction and threats. So the police, noting that Richard was an adult, instructed the Fees to give him the bottle. They said they would comply only if he left the house for good. Officers escorted Richard off the property.

A few hours later Richard called his parents, threatening to stab himself in the head with a knife. The police found him and took him to the Virginia Beach Psychiatric Center.

Described as "paranoid and psychotic" by the admitting physician, Dr. John Riedler, Richard spent one week in the hospital denying that he had any psychiatric or addiction issues. He was placed on two medications: Seroquel and the antidepressant Wellbutrin, no stimulants. In his discharge report, Dr. Riedler noted that Richard had stabilized but remained severely depressed and dependent on both amphetamines and marijuana, which he would smoke in part to counter the buzz of Adderall and the depression from withdrawal.

(Marijuana is known to increase the risk for schizophrenia, psychosis and memory problems, but Richard had smoked pot in high school and college with no such effects, several friends recalled. If that was the case, "in all likelihood the stimulants were the primary issue here," said Dr. Wesley Boyd, a psychiatrist at Children's Hospital Boston and Cambridge Health Alliance who specializes in adolescent substance abuse.)

Unwelcome at home after his discharge from the psychiatric hospital, Richard stayed in cheap motels for a few weeks. His Adderall prescription from Dr. Parker expired on July 26, leaving him eligible for a renewal. He phoned the office of Dr. Ellison, who had not seen him in four months.

"moved out of the house—doesn't feel paranoid or delusional. Hasn't been on meds for a while—working with a friend wiring houses rto 3 months—doesn't feel he needs the abilify or seroquel for sleep."

Dr. Waldo M. Ellison
Notes on Richard Fee
July 25, 2011

The 2:15 p.m. appointment went better than Richard could have hoped. He told Dr. Ellison that the pre-psychotic and metaphoric thinking back in March had receded, and that all that remained was his A.D.H.D. He said nothing of his visits to Dr. Parker, his recent prescriptions or his week in the psychiatric hospital.

At 2:21 p.m., according to Dr. Ellison's records, he prescribed Richard 30 days' worth of Adderall at 50 milligrams a day. He also gave him prescriptions postdated for Aug. 23 and Sept. 21, presumably to allow him to get pills into late October without the need for follow-up appointments. (Virginia state law forbids the dispensation of 90 days of a controlled substance at one time, but does allow doctors to write two 30-day prescriptions in advance.)

Virginia is one of 43 states with a formal Prescription Drug Monitoring Program, an online database that lets doctors check a patient's one-year prescription history, partly to see if he or she is getting medication elsewhere. Although pharmacies are required to enter all prescriptions for controlled substances into the system, Virginia law does not require doctors to consult it.

Dr. Ellison's notes suggest that he did not check the program before issuing the three prescriptions to Richard, who filled the first within hours.

The next morning, during a scheduled appointment at Dr. Parker's clinic, Ms. Strelitz wrote in her notes: "Richard is progressing. He reported staying off of the Adderall and on no meds currently. Focusing on staying healthy, eating well and exercising."

About a week later, Richard called his father with more good news: a job he had found overseeing storm cleanup crews was going well. He was feeling much better.

But Mr. Fee noticed that the more calm and measured speech that Richard had regained during his hospital stay was gone. He jumped from one subject to the next, sounding anxious and rushed. When the call ended, Mr. Fee recalled, he went straight to his wife.

"Call your insurance company," he said, "and find out if they've filled any prescriptions for Adderall."

"spoke to father—richard was in VBPC [Virginia Beach Psychiatric Center] and OD on adderall—NO STIMULANTS—HE WAS ALSO SEEING DR. PARKER"

Dr. Waldo M. Ellison
Interoffice e-mail
Aug. 5, 2011

An insurance representative confirmed that Richard had filled a prescription for Adderall on July 25. Mr. Fee confronted Dr. Ellison in the Dominion Psychiatric parking lot.

Mr. Fee told him that Richard had been in the psychiatric hospital, had been suicidal and had been taking Adderall through June and July. Dr. Ellison confirmed that he had written not only another prescription but two others for later in August and September.

"He told me it was normal procedure and not 90 days at one time," Mr. Fee recalled. "I flipped out on him: 'You gave my son 90 days of Adderall? You're going to kill him!'"

Mr. Fee said he and Dr. Ellison had discussed voiding the two outstanding scripts. Mr. Fee said he had been told that it was possible, but that should Richard need emergency medical attention, it could keep him from getting what would otherwise be proper care or medication. Mr. Fee confirmed that with a pharmacist and decided to drive to Richard's apartment and try to persuade him to rip up the prescriptions.

"I know that you've got these other prescriptions to get pills," Mr. Fee recalled telling Richard. "You're doing so good. You've got a job. You're working. Things with us are better. If you get them filled, I'm worried about what will happen."

"You're right," Mr. Fee said Richard had replied. "I tore them up and threw them away."

Mr. Fee spent two more hours with Richard making relative small talk—increasingly gnawed, he recalled later, by the sense that this was no ordinary conversation. As he looked at Richard he saw two images flickering on top of each other—the boy he had raised to love school and baseball, and the desperate addict he feared that boy had become.

Before he left, Mr. Fee made as loving a demand as he could muster.

"Please. Give them to me," Mr. Fee said.

Richard looked his father dead in the eye.

"I destroyed them," he said. "I don't have them. Don't worry."

"Richard said that he has stopped adderall and wants to work on continuing to progress."

Renee Strelitz
Session notes
Sept. 13, 2011

Richard generally filled his prescriptions at a CVS on Laskin Road, less than three miles from his parents' home. But on Aug. 23, he went to a different CVS about 11 miles away, closer to Norfolk and farther from the locations that his father might have called to alert them to the situation. For his Sept. 21 prescription he traveled even farther, into Norfolk, to get his pills.

On Oct. 3, Richard visited Dr. Ellison for an appointment lasting 17 minutes. The doctor prescribed two weeks of Strattera, a medication for A.D.H.D. that contains no amphetamines and, therefore, is neither a controlled substance nor particularly prone to abuse. His records make no mention of the Adderall prescription Richard filled on Sept. 21; they do note, however, "Father says that he is crazy and abusive of the Adderall—has made directives with regard to giving Richard anymore stimulants—bringing up charges—I explained this to Richard."

Prescription records indicate that Richard did not fill the Strattera prescription before returning to Dr. Ellison's office two weeks later to ask for more stimulants.

"Patient took only a few days of Strattera 40 mg—it calmed him but not focusing," the doctor's notes read. "I had told him not to look for much initially—He would like a list of MD who could rx adderall."

Dr. Ellison never saw Richard again. Given his patterns of abuse, friends said, Richard probably took his last Adderall pill in early October. Because he abruptly stopped without the slow and delicate reduction of medication that is recommended to minimize major psychological risks, especially for instant-release stimulants, he crashed harder than ever.

Richard's lifelong friend Ryan Sykes was one of the few people in contact with him during his final weeks. He said that despite Richard's addiction to Adderall and the ease with which it could be obtained on college campuses nearby, he had never pursued it outside the doctors' prescriptions.

"He had it in his mind that because it came from a doctor, it was O.K.," Mr. Sykes recalled.

On Nov. 7, after arriving home from a weekend away, Mrs. Fee heard a message on the family answering machine from Richard, asking his parents to call him. She phoned back at 10 that night and left a message herself.

Not hearing back by the next afternoon, Mrs. Fee checked Richard's cellphone records—he was on her plan—and saw no calls or texts. At 9 p.m. the Fees drove to Richard's apartment in Norfolk to check on him. The lights were on; his car was in the driveway. He did not answer. Beginning to panic, Mr. Fee found the kitchen window ajar and climbed in through it.

He searched the apartment and found nothing amiss.

"He isn't here," Mr. Fee said he had told his wife.

"Oh, thank God," she replied. "Maybe he's walking on the beach or something."

They got ready to leave before Mr. Fee stopped.

"Wait a minute," he said. "I didn't check the closet."

"Spoke with Richard's mother, Kathy Fee, today. She reported that Richard took his life last November. Family is devasted and having a difficult time. Offerred assistance for family."

Renee Strelitz
Last page of Richard Fee file
June 21, 2012

Friends and former baseball teammates flocked to Richard Fee's memorial service in Virginia Beach. Most remembered only the funny and gregarious guy they knew in high school and college; many knew absolutely nothing of his last two years. He left no note explaining his suicide.

At a gathering at the Fees' house afterward, Mr. Fee told them about Richard's addiction to Adderall. Many recalled how they, too, had blithely abused the drug in college—to cram, just as Richard had—and could not help but wonder if they had played the same game of Russian roulette.

"I guarantee you a good number of them had used it for studying—that shock was definitely there in that room," said a Greensboro baseball teammate, Danny Michael, adding that he was among the few who had not. "It's so prevalent and widely used. People had no idea it could be abused to the point of no return."

Almost every one of more than 40 A.D.H.D. experts interviewed for this article said that worst-case scenarios like Richard Fee's can occur with any medication—and that people who do have A.D.H.D., or parents of children with the disorder, should not be dissuaded from considering the proven benefits of stimulant medication when supervised by a responsible physician.

Other experts, however, cautioned that Richard Fee's experience is instructive less in its ending than its evolution—that it underscores aspects of A.D.H.D. treatment that are mishandled every day with countless patients, many of them children.

"You don't have everything that happened with this kid, but his experience is not that unusual," said DeAnsin Parker, a clinical neuropsychologist in New York who specializes in young adults. "Diagnoses are made just this quickly, and medication is filled just this quickly. And the lack of therapy is really sad. Doctors are saying, 'Just take the meds to see if they help,' and if they help, 'You must have A.D.H.D.'"

Dr. Parker added: "Stimulants will help anyone focus better. And a lot of young people like or value that feeling, especially those who are driven and have ambitions. We have to realize that these are potential addicts—drug addicts don't look like they used to."

The Fees decided to go. The event was sponsored by the local chapter of Children and Adults with Attention Deficit Disorder (Chadd), the nation's primary advocacy group for A.D.H.D. patients. They wanted to attend the question-and-answer session afterward with local doctors and community college officials.

The evening opened with the local Chadd coordinator thanking the drug company Shire—the manufacturer of several A.D.H.D. drugs, including Vyvanse and extended-release Adderall—for partly underwriting the event. An hourlong film directed and narrated by two men with A.D.H.D. closed by examining some "myths" about stimulant medications, with several doctors praising their efficacy and safety. One said they were "safer than aspirin," while another added, "It's O.K.—there's nothing that's going to happen."

Sitting in the fourth row, Mr. Fee raised his hand to pose a question to the panel, which was moderated by Jeffrey Katz, a local clinical psychologist and a national board member of Chadd. "What are some of the drawbacks or some of the dangers of a misdiagnosis in somebody," Mr. Fee asked, "and then the subsequent medication that goes along with that?"

Dr. Katz looked straight at the Fees as he answered, "Not much."

Adding that "the medication itself is pretty innocuous," Dr. Katz continued that someone without A.D.H.D. might feel more awake with stimulants but would not consider it "something that they need."

"If you misdiagnose it and you give somebody medication, it's not going to do anything for them," Dr. Katz concluded. "Why would they continue to take it?"

Mr. Fee slowly sat down, trembling. Mrs. Fee placed her hand on his knee as the panel continued.

Critical Thinking

1. Discuss the risk of addiction, dependence, and overdose from prescription drug abuse.

2. What are reasons college students use prescription drugs they don't need and were not prescribed for them?

Create Central

www.mhhe.com/createcentral

Internet References

Food and Drug Administration (FDA)
    www.fda.gov
National Institute on Drug Abuse (NIDA)
    www.nida.nih.gov

ALAN SCHWARZ is a Pulitzer-Prize nominated reporter for the *New York Times*.

Article   Prepared by: Eileen L. Daniel, *SUNY College at Brockport*

Smoking with Mom

RALPH KEYES

Learning Outcomes

After reading this article, you will be able to:

- Describe how smoking became mainstream among women.

- Discuss the health risks of smoking.

When I try to recall the scent of my mother, what comes to mind is burning tobacco. As she held my little body closely, I could smell its residue on her fingers, and lingering around her lips. If she'd just drawn on a cigarette before hugging me, our bond was confirmed with a puff of smoke. Perhaps that's why the smell of cigarette smoke bothers me less than it does many non-smokers. I detect love in its odor.

Since Mom breast-fed her four children, it's easy to imagine my tiny nose inhaling smoke from her cigarette even as my mouth sucked milk from her nipple. She herself once composed a ditty that went:

> *Here I lie,*
> *On mama's breast*
> *When she smokes*
> *She is a pest.*

When not in her mouth, a cigarette was like a sixth finger on my mother's hand. It's hard to picture her without one. In the most vivid image I can conjure, a white tube juts from my mother's tightly clenched jaw—straight as an archer's arrow—while she scrapes a match across a matchbook's sandy strip to ignite its glow.

On Sunday mornings, Mom couldn't wait to break the spiritual fast of silent worship by stepping outside to light up a cigarette. Although nominally Jewish, she attended Friends Meeting for Worship with my Quaker father. Her favorite Quakers were the ones who joined her in the semi-sacred ritual of lighting each other's cigarettes from matches cupped in hands. Smokers were excellent company, Mom told us. She said that the most congenial passengers on long train rides could always be found in the club car, passing around packages of cigarettes and holding fire to each other's lips. That's where my mother liked to be. Cigarettes were her letter of introduction, an icebreaker, a social lubricant, and a first-rate smokescreen.

While growing up, it never occurred to me to wish my mother wasn't a smoker. Weren't all mothers? I may also have sensed that smoking made her *happy*. Later I would say *less unhappy*. But as a child I didn't think that way. Then I only saw her as a warm woman with huge gray-blue eyes, frizzy brown hair, and a wide mouth from which words and laughter continually spilled, like balls of gum pouring from a broken gumball machine. As an adult, I wondered what lay beneath that exuberance. As I child I didn't wonder. My mother was simply a woman who greeted me with hugs and cookies after school, then sat me beside her at the dining room table so we each could *write*.

I wrote with crayon on newsprint. Mom wrote with a mechanical pencil on lined pages of a spiral-bound notebook. A gleaming cigarette usually nestled between the index and middle fingers of her left hand, or sat smoldering in the ashtray beside her. As she wrote and smoked, my mother talked about her childhood. She told me how she and her friend Pat Glasgow used to rub cigarette ashes into their seventh-grade homework so their teachers would know whom they were up against. She told me about "The Snifflers," a club she formed with friends in junior high school that was dedicated to reading books, writing poems, and smoking cigarettes. She told me about the speakeasies she frequented as a young teenager, about hitchhiking around Philadelphia, and about another friend named June who became a show dancer.

As she told me these stories, Mom scribbled furiously in her notebook. This was a habit she'd acquired as a young girl. Recording her thoughts on paper felt like preparation for her career. From an early age my mother knew what she'd be when she grew up: a famous writer with bohemian tendencies. "I am extremely unconventional," she'd written at thirteen. "I love to flirt and am not averse to necking and kissing a man—if I like him! . . . I am fond of swearing and smoking and I am a 'wet,' but I only like wine and highballs, having never tasted whiskey or champagne."

This thought is scrawled in volume three of the twenty-six notebooks my mother left behind. These journals are filled with philosophical musings and autobiographical notes. In the margins are doodles of women with cigarettes hanging from their lips. Neatly folded inside an early notebook is the typed manifesto of the "Gotta Getta Guy Chapter of the NIGHT CLUB FOR INDEPENDENT SNIFFLERS":

> *Oh, Snifflers are we, are we, are we,*
> *Snifflers till we fall . . .*
> *For goddamn we'd rather be Snifflers*
> *Than anything else at all!*
> ———
> *Seagull, turtle, dove,*
> *What do we love?*
> *Chesterfields, Chesterfields,*
> *Rah, rah, rah!*
> ———
> *What do we always get on a date?*
> *What is it that Snifflers hate, hate, hate?*
> *Luckies!*

Long after the Snifflers took their stand, I watched public relations pioneer Edward Bernays being interviewed on television. Bernays recalled with a chuckle how he fulfilled an early assignment from the American Tobacco Company to make smoking more acceptable for women. A psychiatrist had told him that for many women smoking was both a "sublimation of oral eroticism" and a symbol of freedom. That's why Bernays recruited a group of debutantes to march down Fifth Avenue on Easter Sunday in 1929, waving lit cigarettes. This "parade" was front-page news. Probably my fifteen-year-old mother heard about it. Perhaps she imagined herself marching, too, holding her cigarette high, a walking Statue of Liberty. If so, Edward Bernays certainly won a convert in Charlotte Schachmann. My mother was a dedicated smoker of cigarettes for over half a century, until she died of lung cancer at sixty-six.

Mom and her friend Pat started smoking at twelve. Decades later, Pat told me that one reason they began smoking, drinking, and running around with boys at such an early age was to escape from their homes. Her own parents were divorced, and Mom's should have been. Pat, who became a psychiatric social worker, said my mother's family was dysfunctional long before that concept became a psychological commonplace.

Mom's dentist father was a charming philanderer. One of her notebooks includes a profile of him. "Very handsome," she wrote, "with broad cheekbones, a slender, well-shaped nose with interesting flared nostrils, and beautifully modeled lips." My mother portrayed her father as an old-world gentleman who routinely kissed the hands of women, including her own. "He smoked with great grace," Mom added. "I used to love to watch his curved, graceful fingers holding the cigarette."

In pictures of her taken at Penn State, Mom routinely held a cigarette. These pictures show a voluptuous young woman who liked to strike sultry poses. In one she pulls her skirt up to mid-thigh. In another she laces her finger behind her head and splays both elbows wide. Here Mom throws her chest out like Mae West. There she braces one hand on her hip, Garbo-like. The cigarettes she held were often used as a prop in these poses. Sometimes she held one aloft, like Bette Davis about to say something droll.

Throughout her college career, Mom wrote poems, stories, and essays. Some were published by Penn State's literary magazine. In every story, cigarettes were part of the action or, once, the pipes she and Pat sometimes smoked to save money and shock classmates.

According to Pat, cigarettes were a common medium of exchange at Depression-era Penn State. Many co-eds gave the nod to men who supplied them with cigarettes. My mother wasn't among them. Even though she was surrounded by men thrusting cigarettes at her, and could barely afford to buy her own, Mom ended up with a soft-spoken upperclassman named Scott Keyes who was so poor she sometimes provided them both with cigarettes.

Scott later wrote some notes about a typical evening they spent in his apartment: "I remember you there, pecking away at the typewriter when you were getting out one of your stories for a contest. Sometimes, we would lie on the bed for a while; at other times you would come over to my table, and put your arms around me while I worked. In your lighthearted thoughtfulness you would leave some cigarettes for me from your pack; for I never bought them, always smoking a pipe, except when we were together."

Smoking never had the same resonance for Scott that it did for his wife-to-be. For him it was more of a pastime, something he could take or leave, or give up altogether, as he did in his forties. For Mom smoking was far more than a pastime. For her it was closer to a passion.

I think one reason smoking meant so much to my mother during her forty-two years of marriage to Scott was that it was a last vestige, a single thread tying her to a rambunctious past. Also, in her time writers smoked. Smoking and writing, writing and smoking; to aspiring authors like my mother it might have seemed that one couldn't happen without the other. Mom had more success as a smoker than as an author, however. She left behind a file cabinet full of mostly unpublished literary efforts spanning six decades. They begin with *Two Jolly Friends,* a novella penciled into a composition book, and end with *Peacenik,* an aborted 70s-era novel written longhand on three-hole punched paper. My mother's archives include her journals, lots of poems and stories in manuscript, published biographies of Ralph Waldo Emerson and Herman Melville for young adults, "Four at the Breast," a small magazine piece about breast-feeding her children when few mothers did, a few published poems, and one article in a national publication—*McCall's.*

That wasn't the *oeuvre* Mom had in mind as a young Sniffler. Mom always felt frustrated by not having won the literary recognition she'd felt sure would be hers. Writers usually have ways to explain why they didn't publish more, and my mother was no exception. Mom thought marriage and motherhood had derailed her literary career. She told me this often. My mother felt trapped as a housewife, marooned in a more conventional life than the one she'd dreamed of as a budding Virginia Woolf. Long before Betty Friedan wrote *The Feminine Mystique,* Mom objected vehemently to the lot of housewives and mothers. She enlisted her four children as allies. We grew up with aching sympathy for a mother who hadn't realized her literary potential because she'd been shanghaied into domestic service.

Mom was willing to let Dad be our family's breadwinner. After graduating from Penn State he spent his career working as an economist, planner, and professor. Mom worked intermittently, teaching preschoolers and clerking at a library. But these stints—undertaken when we were strapped for cash—distracted my mother from what she considered her real job: writing. Even worse was the distraction of keeping house.

In the summertime Mom wore shorts and a halter as she swept, mopped, and vacuumed our home in State College, Pennsylvania, a cork-tipped Raleigh cigarette dangling from her lips, or one she paid her kids a penny apiece to make for her in a little roll-your-own machine. Penn State co-eds who roomed with us sometimes followed her about, chatting. They seemed to enjoy my mother's company. So did their boyfriends, who nicknamed Mom "S.W." Years later I discovered that this stood for "Sexy Witch."

Like Mom, I started smoking at twelve. I was "caught" by her after my second cigarette. Probably I wanted Mom to know. Why else would I light up in front of my eight-year-old brother and six-year-old sister? Not that our mother seemed upset when they tattled. Then, as always, she was ambivalent about my smoking. Mom never actually encouraged me to smoke. Nor did she say I couldn't, or shouldn't. I probably wished she had. Why start smoking at all when you're twelve if not to horrify your parents?

I can still recall the flavor of my first cigarettes: a sharp, acrid taste, filled with rebellion and communion. Done as an act of defiance, smoking actually brought me closer to my mother.

Pro forma she counseled me against this habit. But in subtle ways I sensed her approval when I smoked, and disappointment when I stopped seven years later. Dad had long since left the fraternity of smokers. Now Mom had company again. Or so she thought. Despite my mother's invitation to join her—"as long as you're smoking anyway"—holding out her package of Kents, a cigarette for me sticking up from its depths, I always demurred. Who wants to smoke with Mom? Instead I took to sneaking cigarettes in my bedroom or when carousing with pals, as if this activity were just as illicit for me as it was for them. Except it wasn't. Far from increasing the distance from my mother, smoking narrowed it. We didn't just share a love of cigarettes. We also shared a smoker's outlook. Were we timid, respectable people, strait-jacketed by a fear of dying? Hardly. The proof glowed between our fingers.

I think Mom loved the *idea* of smoking cigarettes as much as filling her lungs with smoke. Smokers were bold. They took their life into their own hands. There was magic in the fumes they created. While filling the air with clouds of combustion, my mother may have seen herself as a more imposing figure than five-foot Charlotte Schachmann from West Philadelphia. Surrounded by billowing smoke she had much in common with a circus performer being shot from a cannon. When holding a cigarette delicately between her index and middle fingers, Mom might have imagined she was Greta Garbo, about to be swept into John Gilbert's arms.

Just as my mother once struck Garbo poses, I took to wearing motorcycle boots like Marlon Brando in *The Wild One*, sulking moodily as James Dean did in *Rebel Without a Cause*, and putting a sneer in my smile as if I were Elvis Presley chatting with Ed Sullivan. If smoking couldn't get a rise out of my mother, maybe boots like Brando's would, a hat like his, and a jacket that read THE SATANS, even if The Satans were a mere parody of a gang, one that was threatening only to its members' mothers.

None of it worked. The only item of clothing I ever wore that got a reaction from my mother was a black shirt. That pushed her political buttons—"No son of mine is going to look like a Fascist blackshirt!"—and she forbade me to wear it.

As a one-time hell-raiser herself Mom undoubtedly knew what I was up to. On the surface she didn't seem alarmed when the police called to say they were questioning me about being part of a burglary ring. (I wasn't; my best friend was.) Yet she must have known better than anyone the danger I was courting, and the inner turmoil that pushed me to the brink.

To firm up my bad-boy credentials I added drinking to my smoking, and roaring around late at night in friends' cars. After I became the only one of Mom's four kids to follow in her rowdy footsteps, cigarettes became part of our bond. Or was it our bind?

The knots of this bond-bind grew especially taut during my rocky adolescence. After raising two teenagers of my own,

I came to understand better the grip of love and rage in which Mom and I held each other. As an adolescent I was only aware of how frustrating it was to rebel against a tolerant mother who'd taken risks of her own. As a parent, I can see the ambivalence this must have created in her. How should a mother respond to risky behavior she'd once indulged in herself?

We were too much alike to have an easy relationship. The deeper I got into adolescence, the edgier that relationship grew. Our interaction consisted mainly of pitched battles. One of the few times in my life that I got anything like a spontaneous, heartfelt comment from my mother was when, early in high school, I stood behind her in our kitchen, pressing some demand as she stirred a pot on the stove. Finally Mom dropped her spoon, spun around, and said, "You know, I don't like you." Those words still reverberate in my memory. Did she mean just at that moment? Or while I was being a surly adolescent? Or forever and all time? I never dared to ask.

Even after arguments became our main means of communication, it wasn't our only means. I still discussed any and all subjects with my mother. When girls began to interest me, she became my consultant. Mom said a woman might try to arouse my interest by fluttering her eyelashes down my cheek, then demonstrated how she would do this by brushing her own lashes down my cheek. My mother assured me that I was a good-looking boy but added that even more than good looks something called "sex appeal" was what counted in the mating marketplace. Mom also discussed French kissing with me. That was something she hadn't cared for. Whenever a man tried to stick his tongue in her mouth, Mom said, she pushed it out with her own.

This was one of many ways in which my mother reminded me that she'd once been a woman for men to reckon with. That was hard for me to picture. Mom's face wrinkled early, especially around the lips that had clenched so many cigarettes. Her nose grew more prominent with age, her hair more sparse. She seldom wore makeup. My mother's everyday outfits were whatever she found on sale at J. C. Penney or a Goodwill thrift shop. Her dress-up look was semi-bohemian—hoop earrings in earlobes pierced long before that was common, ruffled peasant blouse, plain skirt, and sensible shoes—as if she'd started out to be fully bohemian but lost interest along the way.

I left for college with some relief on both our parts. Distance lanced the boil of our tension. When I came home on vacation we'd chatter up a storm. What courses are you taking? How do you like your profs? Isn't Vietnam outrageous? Despite our renewed rapport, we continued to argue. During one heated discussion about abortion Mom gave me a knowing look, then said, "Girls in your generation weren't the first ones to get abortions, you know."

The sixties were in full swing and Mom was swinging with them. She demonstrated against the war, took up yoga (or at least read books about it), switched from white bread to whole wheat, and ate the occasional bean sprout. Without irony she began calling herself "a health nut."

There were still the cigarettes, though. Mom smoked as much as ever. She took to carrying a little folding ashtray in her purse so she could smoke politely wherever she happened to be. Changing times put my mother in a bind. For most of her life, smoking was part and parcel of a bohemian lifestyle. A cigarette in one hand and *Das Kapital* in the other made for a dashing figure. During Mom's middle age, however, smoking developed a bad odor among radicals. Dissidents became more concerned with health than dash. As the popularity of Karl Marx waned, that of Andrew Weil soared. This left my mother stranded with a habit she couldn't break and didn't want to break.

Mom considered her lifelong relationship with cigarettes more romance than addiction. This makes better sense to me today than it did then. Smoking, we know now, can be a potent anti-depressant. Undoubtedly, it was for my mother. She called cigarettes "little points of happiness all through the day." I'm sure Mom's exuberance was at least partly nicotine-induced. How could she not love a substance that was her ally in the struggle against depression?

In notes for an essay titled "My Lady Nicotine," my mother defended her lifelong affair with cigarettes:

> I have never joined the ranks of those smokers who admit they don't really enjoy smoking, that it's just a nervous habit (though I'll confess; occasionally I nervously take one & there's no joy at all). But almost every cigarette I smoke is a delight. There's an "ahhhh"to that long inhalation—especially the first one of the morning that accompanies pre-breakfast coffee. But there are also deep breaths of bliss at others during the day—when I pause for a rest and smoke; when I've put off having one for awhile; when I'm doing something I dislike—usually housework—and the smoke & the breathing take the curse off the monotony of the chores. The ever-present fear of cancer does, of course, mar the complete bliss. Where did I read that part of the tremendous condemnation of smoking arises from the puritanism of the United States people which sees all pleasure as sinful? I much prefer the attitude of the Delaware Indians who felt "Tobacco smoke pleases all spirits."

After leaving the ranks of smokers early in college, I urged Mom to join me. Breaking this habit improved my breath, I told her, my stamina, and sense of smell. Food tasted better. My fingers lost their yellowish stain. I didn't miss smoking at all. I did miss the fellowship of smokers, including my mother.

Whether or not one should smoke joined our many subjects of contention:

"Mom, the Surgeon General's report says it could kill you."

"We all have to die sometime."

"But it's such a nasty habit."

"I don't consider it a habit. It's just something I like to do."

"How about its effect on the people around you?"

"Don't be such a Puritan."

During our constant chatter, there were few limits on what Mom and I could discuss. The only taboo topic was how we felt about each other. I don't recall ever saying "I love you" to my mother, or hearing her say those words to me. Not that we didn't love each other. Or not that I didn't love her, anyway. There were just too many footnotes, asterisks, caveats, and qualifying phrases to say those three words outright. Our relationship was chatty, warm, and wary. Only once do I remember hugging my mother in other than a hello or goodbye clench. That was in the kitchen of our home when she was upset about something and I embraced her as I'd learned to do in encounter groups. At first Mom tensed. Then she relaxed and let me hold her. I got the impression that this felt dangerous.

I don't think relationships were easy for my mother. Not that she didn't try. On their thirty-eighth anniversary, Mom wrote to her husband:

The years they are
Thirty-eight
And every one
Has been just great
With my Scott
My love, my mate

Love poems notwithstanding, I doubt that Mom ever resolved her ambivalence about being married, and leading a relatively conventional existence as a wife and mother. But she did her best. Unlike so many unconventional mothers, Charlotte Schachmann Keyes accepted the responsibility of being a wife and parent. She realized that she had to choose between raising hell and raising children. Mom chose.

Dad was not ambivalent, at least about being married. Late in life my father told me often how passionate he was about his wife. On the surface Scott Keyes was a reserved Quaker WASP. Beneath that surface beat the lusty heart of a panting Byron.

On the eve of their fortieth wedding anniversary, Scott wrote this poem for Charlotte:

GOLDEN YEARS
It's so wonderful when
    You're in my arms
And the tip of your cigarette's
    Glowing
And gently you put your
    Lips on mine
And between us the smoke is
    Flowing.
Soon we'll be on the
    Other side, and
Just think—there we'll
    Be able
To light up again in the
    Same old way
And forget what it says on the label.

A few months after he composed this poem my father wrote me a letter, something he seldom did. In his letter Dad said that a "spot" had been found on Mom's lung during a routine checkup. There was no need to get upset. Her doctors were looking into it.

They found a tumor. This tumor was malignant. The half million cigarettes my mother smoked in over half a century's time had finally collected their toll.

After losing part of a lung to the surgeon's knife, my mother finally stopped smoking. She wasn't happy about it. Mom said she enjoyed none of the benefits I'd promised her: better sense of smell, taste, breath, stamina. By then it was probably too late. She just missed her cigarettes. Later I learned that Mom had Dad smuggle some into her hospital room.

Continuing to smoke was part of Mom's fantasy that she was on the mend. This was a fantasy, of course. It lasted only a few weeks. Dad and I were with my mother at the end. I'd been on a book promotion tour. My contribution to the illusion that she wasn't dying was to go on that tour as if her future looked bright. By the time I reached San Diego it was obvious that it didn't. Dad called me there to report that the doctors thought Mom didn't have long to live. After canceling Houston and Atlanta, I went home and spent my mother's last two days in her hospital room.

A hospital is a wretched place to die: cold, barren, sterile. Tubes tie you to your bed. Roommates overhear the grief of your visiting relatives. Doctors summon them into the hallway to ask what plans have been made for the body. Yet—if you're pretending you're not dying—then you're presumably getting better and a hospital is the place to be.

This was our outlook at Carle Hospital, in Champaign, Illinois. We dealt with my mother's impending death by avoiding the subject. That was fine with me. To keep up appearances she, Dad, and I tried to act "normal." We made small talk, cracked jokes, kept things light. On the surface this seemed gutsy; grace under pressure. In retrospect, I think it's a miserable way to die and be with someone who's dying. Because in order to express the important, the felt, the unsaid words you want to say—words like, "I know it hasn't always been easy for us, Mom, but I've always loved you and wouldn't want anyone else to have been my mother"—you must face the fact that the end is near. To maintain an illusion that death can be beat, however, no one can say anything of consequence. Doing so implies that time's running out. What you do instead is try to keep things light and laugh a lot.

All of this is hindsight, however. At the time I was as active as anyone in Keeping Up Appearances. Not long after Mom's second son joined her husband by her bed in Illinois when he was supposed to be on a talk show in Houston, she broke through a morphine haze to say, "We're kidding ourselves, aren't we?"

"About what?" I asked.

"About my getting better," she murmured.

This threw me. I didn't know how to respond. So I said, "What would you rather do?" That's a little technique I learned from psychologist friends: turn a touchy question back on the questioner and play for time.

"Go to sleep," Mom replied. And she did. My tactic worked. I successfully deflected my mother's one attempt to get us to face her death.

All of this took me years to sort out. Today, I wish we'd faced my mother's death more squarely. I wish she'd died at home, in her own bed, without tubes up her nose, technicians doing x-rays, roommates eavesdropping, and doctors whispering nearby. Instead of a hospital I wish she'd died in a comfortable, familiar setting surrounded by as much of her family as possible. What I really wish is that Mom's cancer had never been found. If her tumor had grown at its own pace undetected, I think my mother would have lived longer, died better, and enjoyed more the life she had remaining—surrounded by clouds of smoke.

Critical Thinking

1. How did tobacco companies mainstream smoking among women?
2. What are the health effects related to tobacco usage?

Internet References

Food and Drug Administration
www.fda.gov

National Institute on Drug Abuse
http://www.drugabuse.gov/publications/research-reports/tobacco/letter-director

Unit 6

UNIT

Prepared by: Eileen Daniel, *SUNY College at Brockport*

Sexuality and Relationships

Sexuality is an important part of both self-awareness and intimate relationships. But how important is physical attraction in establishing and maintaining intimate relationships? Researchers in the area of evolutionary psychology have proposed numerous theories that attempt to explain the mutual attraction that occurs between the sexes. The most controversial of these theories postulates that our perception of beauty or physical attractiveness is not subjective but rather a biological component hardwired into our brains. It is generally assumed that perceptions of beauty vary from era to era and culture to culture, but evidence is mounting that suggests that people all over share a common sense of beauty that is based on physical symmetry and scent.

While physical attraction is clearly an important issue when it comes to dating, how important is it in long-term loving relationships? For many Americans, the answer may be very important because we tend to be a "Love Culture" that places a premium on passion in the selection of our mates. Is passion an essential ingredient in love, and can passion serve to sustain a long-term meaningful relationship? Because most people can't imagine marrying someone that they don't love, we must assume that most marriages are based on this feeling we call love. That being the case, why is it that so few marriages survive the rigors of day-to-day living? Perhaps the answer has more to do with our limited definition of love rather than love itself. It appears that married individuals tend to see any unhappiness they experience as a failure of their partner to satisfy their needs. It's common for couples to search for perfection because people believe that they are entitled to the best option there is. Spending time together in challenging activities is suggested to couples to enhance the feelings of closeness and satisfaction with the relationship.

Pornography can be another reason for dissatisfaction in a relationship. The idea that pornography is related to marital infidelity has been a topic of discussion in recent years. With the increase in online options to view pornography, there appears to be a connection to divorce as well.

Two additional topics of interest and controversy in the area of human sexuality are sex education and sex selection. First, although most states mandate some type of school-based sex education, many parents believe that they should be the only source for their children's sex education. Next, should couples have the option of choosing the sex of their baby? Some doctors are willing to accommodate parents' choices, while others question the ethics of choosing gender.

Perhaps no topic in the area of human sexuality has garnered more publicity and public concern than the dangers associated with unprotected sex. Although the concept of "safe sex" is nothing new, the degree of open and public discussion regarding sexual behaviors is. With the emergence of AIDS as a disease of epidemic proportions and the rapid spreading of other sexually transmitted diseases (STDs), the surgeon general of the United States initiated an aggressive educational campaign, based on the assumption that knowledge would change behavior. If STD rates among teens are any indication of the effectiveness of this approach, then we must conclude that our educational efforts are failing. Conservatives believe that while education may play a role in curbing the spread of STDs, the root of the problem is promiscuity and that promiscuity rises when a society is undergoing a moral decline. The solution, according to conservatives, is a joint effort between parents and educators to teach students the importance of values such as respect, responsibility, and integrity. Liberals, on the other hand, think that preventing promiscuity is unrealistic and instead the focus should be on establishing open and frank discussions between the sexes. Their premise is that we are all sexual beings and the best way to combat STDs is to establish open discussions between sexual partners, so that condoms will be used correctly when couples engage in intercourse.

While education undoubtedly has had a positive impact on slowing the spread of STDs, perhaps it is unrealistic to think that education alone is the solution, given the magnitude and the nature of the problem. Most experts agree that for education to succeed in changing personal behaviors, the following conditions must be met: (1) the recipients of the information must first perceive themselves as vulnerable and, thus, be motivated to explore replacement behaviors and (2) the replacement behaviors must satisfy the needs that were the basis of the problem behaviors. To date, most education programs have failed to meet these criteria. Given all the information that we now have on the dangers associated with AIDS and STDs, why is it that people do not perceive themselves at risk? It is not so much the denial of risks as it is the notion of most people that they use good judgment when it comes to choosing sex partners. Unfortunately, most decisions regarding sexual behavior are based on subjective criteria that bear little or no relationship to one's actual risk. Even when individuals do view themselves as vulnerable to AIDS and STDs, there are currently only two viable options for reducing the risk of contracting these diseases. The first is the use of a condom and the second is sexual abstinence, neither of which is an ideal solution to the problem.

Article
Prepared by: Eileen L. Daniel, *SUNY College at Brockport*

My Brother's Secret

Dale always wanted a traditional life with a traditional family. But he found happiness only when he decided to live and love the way he wanted—even if that meant hiding the truth about his sexuality from our parents, right up until his death.

W.K. STRATTON

Learning Outcomes

After reading this article, you will be able to:

• Describe the health effects related to AIDS.

• Understand why many gay men and women hide their sexual orientation from family and friends.

I'd not seen my stepbrother Dale in more than two years when a bitter norther slammed into Texas in December 1989. Schools closed, pipes burst, and sleet-covered highways took on the look of salvage yards. I was sitting alone one blue-gray afternoon, listening to the frozen rain tick on the windows of my house in Belton, when the phone rang.

It was Dale's mother, and she was in a panic. She was at Arlington Memorial Hospital, where her son was in intensive care. "He might not live through the night," she said. "You'll have to tell your mother and stepfather. They'll never believe me if I call them." I knew she was right; ever since her divorce from my stepfather, more than thirty years earlier, he had done little to hide his loathing for her, even after he'd retained custody of their two sons, Elden and Dale, and rebuilt a family with my mother and me. I promised to be at the hospital as soon as I could, then phoned my mother in Oklahoma. "What's wrong with him?" she asked, stunned. I told her I didn't know.

But that was not exactly true. Sitting in the car on my way to the hospital, inching across the ice on Interstate 35, I played news headlines from recent years over and over in my head. AIDS, a disease unknown to Americans just a decade earlier, was filling hospitals and clinics and hospices across the country with patients covered in lesions and fighting for each breath as their lungs were steadily destroyed. And in the late eighties, only one outcome awaited its victims: death.

The disease was not an equal-opportunity killer. True, straight men, children, women, even one nun were among the dead. The disease could take years to develop after initial infection. A blood transfusion during surgery, experimentation with injecting recreational drugs, a one-night heterosexual stand during the wild seventies—even in the early years of the pandemic, people knew that any of these could lead to AIDS. But the overwhelming number of people dying from the disease were gay men who had contracted HIV, the blood-borne virus that causes AIDS, through unprotected anal sex. Some born-again preachers and politicians proclaimed AIDS to be "the gay plague," God's punishment for homosexual perverts.

My family came from a small town in Oklahoma that could hardly be described as open-minded. AIDS was not a topic that my parents discussed. (In fact, I can remember no conversations concerning sex.) My education on the disease had come almost entirely from the book *And the Band Played On,* which I'd read the year before. I'd recognized Dale's life in its pages. Now, thinking of him, I gripped the steering wheel, dreading what awaited me in Arlington.

I arrived at the hospital to find Dale lying unconscious in the ICU. He was connected to a ventilator, and each time it breathed for him, his body jolted. After going bald in his twenties, he'd taken to wearing a toupee, but the dark-brown, almost black bouffant was gone, and his pale head on the pillow struck me as impossibly small. His hospital gown was open, revealing crusty lesions on his chest. I reached down and took his hand. He squeezed, but it seemed like just a reflex.

I asked a nurse what was wrong. When she said she could not comment to anyone unfamiliar with Dale's "underlying physical issue," I lied, saying I knew all about it. She paused. "He has something that's like pneumonia," she said, "but not exactly pneumonia."

"Pneumocystosis?"

"Yes," she said.

I nodded. I knew about pneumocystosis from my reading. Caused by a fungus, it was a devastating lung infection similar to one that had been found only in rats—until, that is, gay men in San Francisco began showing up with it at hospitals in the early eighties. Only one thing could so damage an immune system that someone could contract the infection. My stepbrother, lying before me, was dying of AIDS.

I found a pay phone in the hallway and called my mother. The diagnosis was complicated, I said, and she and my stepfather needed to come to Arlington quickly.

Heading back to the ICU, I ran into my stepbrother's business associate, Tony. We'd met just once before. He and Dale ran a dried-flower store at the massive Grand Prairie marketplace known as Traders Village, where you could seemingly buy everything from used tires to precious stones. It was there, maybe three years earlier, that Dale had given me a promotional vinyl copy of Willie Nelson's *Phases and Stages,* and Tony had shaken his head, muttering, "You like Willie?" He and Dale played LPs like Carly Simon's *Torch.* But Dale knew I was as much shitkicker as aging hippie, and he'd picked up the Willie record for me from a Traders Village dealer.

"I guess you've figured out what's wrong with him," Tony said. I nodded again. "He's so afraid his dad will find out. He's told the doctors and the hospital staff not to discuss anything with anyone unless they know already."

Suddenly, he reached out to embrace me. I hugged him awkwardly. His eyes began to water as he shook his head. "He just can't have his dad find out."

M y mother married my stepfather, Ferdy Waner, a beefy mechanic who'd also worked as a roughneck, three weeks shy of my third birthday. Because my runaway "real" father was out of the picture, I called my stepfather Dad. Elden and Dale were older than me, by five and a half and four years, respectively. Elden was compact, muscular, and outgoing—ready to battle it out with anyone or anything that challenged him. Dale was tall, skinny, and pale; soft-spoken and reserved, he had a stoicism that served him well in the tough environment in which we grew up. Money was hand-to-mouth scarce. Early on, we understood the concept of making do. At home and at school, the rules laid down were strict, and discipline could literally sting. We boys were taught that life was hard, something that only rarely provided much in the way of joy.

Dad governed our world. He was an extraordinary physical and moral force. He had survived the Oklahoma dust bowl and West Texas oil booms. He was the strongest man I've ever known. I once saw him drag a dump truck into his shop using only his massive muscles and a chain wrapped around the truck's bumper. My life eventually brought me into contact with professional rodeo cowboys, football players, and boxers, but none could compare with him in terms of pure toughness. His hands were as hard as a steer horn from decades of brutal work. He left his shop every day scalded, cut, and bruised, yet he accepted the pain as if it were nothing, just part of life. When he said "straighten up and fly right," you listened.

The five of us moved into a trailer house adjacent to the old man's auto repair shop in Guthrie, Oklahoma. We called this five-hundred-square-foot soup can home for five years. Most of that time, Dale and I shared a bed. I remember lying there with him as he did his eye exercise. He suffered from the Waner family curse of amblyopia, or lazy eye. The old man was essentially blind in one eye as a result of it. Dale was at risk of ending up the same way. To save his vision, he'd lie on his back on the bed, his good eye covered, and force his bad eye to track the movements of a ball that was suspended by fishing line above him.

For reasons simply not spoken of, the old man chose not to adopt me, so I bore the last name Stratton while everyone else, Mom included, was a Waner. This bothered Dale, who wanted everything to be consistent, normal. One day we went to get a haircut together, and the barber questioned us about our differences. Why was Dale's hair so dark and thick while mine was so light and fine? Why were his eyes deep blue and mine greenish? I finally told him that we weren't full brothers. That satisfied the barber but made Dale livid. Outside the barbershop, he pushed me around a little and told me to never tell that to anyone, never. He didn't want people to think we came from a weird family.

Dale was a little like the old man that way. Dad had no patience for anything that challenged his sense of order. One evening, as the family watched television coverage of a vintage sixties anti-war protest, he became more and more agitated. "I don't understand," he said, as the gray, fuzzy footage showed demonstrators at a sit-in resisting the police. "Why don't they just bring in machine guns and mow 'em all down?" The old man had flashes of playfulness to be sure, but they were the exception. My stepbrothers and I were careful of what we said, kept our voices low, sat up straight, and did what he said to do, knowing he could turn dangerous in an instant. I was scared shitless of him. My two stepbrothers were scared shitless too—but worshipped him at the same time.

Around age twelve, Dale lost interest in the rough-and-tumble activities that the boys in the neighborhood pursued, preferring to stay with his grandmother, who lived nearby, so he could help her with the greenhouse next to her home. He was obsessively neat and sartorially conscious, so that even in cutoffs, a T-shirt, and sneakers, he looked as flawless as a *GQ* model. In the bedroom we shared, the contents of my drawers were like tossed salad; his, by contrast, were boot-camp tidy. He practiced penmanship endlessly until his everyday handwriting became like calligraphy, impressive enough that friends would remark on it decades later.

Dale was also the only boy I knew who could shimmy. When television dance shows became popular, such as *Shindig!*, he glued himself to our black and white screen, watching every move the dancers made, male or female. Then he'd practice them, with the devotion other boys might have given to learning how to step in on a curve ball. When the shimmy, that old flapper dance move, was resurrected during the age of the frug and the mashed potato, Dale would gyrate his body from ankles to ears, arms held out to his sides. The old man never said anything when he witnessed Dale swaying to music, but disdain registered on his face.

Dad might have been bitter about his first marriage, but he did think it was important that Elden and Dale visit their maternal grandparents, and sometimes we'd make trips to the Fort Worth suburb of Richland Hills. Then, after their mother won visitation rights, Elden and Dale would go on their own, catching the *Santa Fe Texas Chief* and leaving for a couple of weeks at a time. I remember the fabulous red-and-yellow diesel engines at the train station when we dropped them off and how much I envied my stepbrothers for getting to ride the rails. But I felt confused when, a few years later, they decided to move in with their mother permanently, Elden going first, then Dale. I never knew Elden's reasons for leaving. Dale suggested to me that in his case it was because his mother allowed him to smoke in her house, which would never have flown with the old man. (He walloped the hell out of me a few years later when he found out about my own experiments with tobacco.) I don't think I actually said goodbye to either of them when they moved away. I felt neither happy nor sad about their leaving.

Elden returned to Guthrie as often as he could, and after graduating from Richland Hills High School, he moved back, never leaving again except for a stint in the Marines during the Vietnam War. But Dale stayed away, becoming something of a stranger. By the end of his high school years, with hair long enough to risk an ass-whipping from the hometown rednecks, it was clear he'd become a hippie. During one of his rare visits to Oklahoma, we were in the bedroom where he was unpacking when he said to me, "So I hear that you've started smoking grass." It was true, and I told him so. "That's cool," he said. "I've been lighting up for a long time now. Just don't ever let the old man find out. He'll kill you."

I knew Dale was right, and our shared rebellion renewed the bond between us. When he eventually enrolled at Northeastern State University, in Tahlequah, Oklahoma, I loved going to visit him. He had set up house in a well-worn trailer our family owned just a short drive from campus, near the old Cherokee community of Park Hill, outfitting it with a TV and a stereo. While Dale and I lit up, we watched Gailard Sartain's late-night show, *The Uncanny Film Festival and Camp Meeting,* featuring Gary Busey, and listened to John Lennon and the Plastic Ono Band's *Live Peace in Toronto 1969.* My favorite album of his was Dylan's *Nashville Skyline.* The trailer sat a stone's throw from Lake Tenkiller, at the time a remote, emerald-colored reservoir surrounded by thick woods and flint outcroppings, and Dylan's country crooning made the perfect sound track for that landscape.

Dale lasted in college for about a year, then moved to Tulsa, where he found a job with Emery Air Freight. He'd show up in Guthrie from time to time with hippie girls. I remember one with pale skin and dark hair that hung from her head like thin vines. She always seemed to wear the same bellbottoms and flip-flops, with their enormous soles. Then Dale developed a relationship with a young co-worker at Emery. They'd spend hours on the phone, and when he proposed marriage, she accepted.

I was there when he wed her at a chapel in Arlington in the summer of 1976. I *wasn't* there when he gathered afterward with his best man and other buddies for a smoke behind the chapel and announced that he'd just made the biggest mistake of his life; I only heard about that later. Regardless, Dale seemed to want to create a traditional family life. He and his new wife wound up back in Tulsa in a small but neat house that had room enough for his black Lab, Jodi. The only thing their home lacked was air-conditioning.

But some part of Dale also required a life contrary to tradition, and within days, his bride discovered he was heavily into drugs—not just the weed and uppers I'd known him to use but also windowpane LSD and mescaline. It was too much for the young couple, and their marriage collapsed after only a few months. Dale, who couldn't tell his family why things had gone awry, said the breakup had happened because she'd run away. When he attempted suicide a few weeks later, my parents told me that he was in the hospital because of bleeding ulcers. By that time I was so busy with college, I didn't make the drive to Tulsa to visit him.

I met his next wife just once. Not long after his recovery, Dale returned to Texas and his air freight job. His new girlfriend, who wore her hair styled like my mother's, seemed a strange choice for Dale, far removed from anything hippie and with a peculiar demeanor, but Dale willingly exchanged vows with her in 1979. The marriage lasted a year on the books; in actuality it survived a much shorter time. I later heard that it began falling apart on their wedding night. Whatever happened, Dale retreated to Tulsa for a short time. He then went back to Texas a changed man.

Meanwhile, in Guthrie, my parents' life was undergoing substantial change. They scraped and saved and eventually were able to build their dream house. The old man expanded his business to include wrecker service. Elden worked for him after he was honorably discharged from the military. They made a good team, and I assumed Elden would take over the family business at some point. But he was unsettled after the Marines. He left the business after a few short years to become a cop. Later he would become, at various times, a heavy-equipment operator, long-haul trucker, and firefighter. I know Elden's departure from the business at first upset the old man. Yet he and his oldest son energized each other, and they remained close, even though they sometimes engaged in screaming arguments. My stepfather and my mother ran the auto repair shop and wrecker service, occasionally hiring guys I'd gone to high school with as helpers. The hours were long and draining. Mom set many of her enthusiasms aside (oil painting, working at the local museum) to work in the cramped, dusty shop office. She often spent nights alone in the new house while the old man was off untangling multi-vehicle pileups on the interstate. She never seemed to resent it, though. She and the old man were inseparable as a couple.

I was the only one of the boys to live in that house. I graduated high school in 1974 at the top of my class and scored high on the college entrance exams. But no money was available for me to go to any of the universities I wanted to attend. I took a job as a reporter at my hometown newspaper and enrolled in classes at the state college fifteen miles down the highway. My parents allowed me to stay in the new house while I was in school, but the old man and I had little to say to each other. He couldn't understand my interest in movies or why I majored in something as foolish as English. He sure as hell couldn't appreciate my zest for the Pigpen-era Grateful Dead or even a long-haired Waylon Jennings. There wasn't much for us to share. Besides, he thought I lacked strength, physical and otherwise.

I'm sure he understood even less about what was going on with Dale. As was the custom of their generation at that time and in that place, my parents hardly spoke of Dale's failed marriages. Some things you just don't talk about. Yet whatever misgivings he might have held, the old man seemed happy to see Dale when he visited at Thanksgiving and Christmas. After his second marriage crumbled, he always arrived alone except for his Lab. Sometimes Dale would drive a pickup he had bought and overhaul it in the old man's shop. They enjoyed each other's company. Elden seemed to distance himself from his brother. Dale put on a good face around the family, nodding at the litanies delivered about lazy workers, corrupt local politicians, and worthless businessmen. But when Dale and I were alone,

he lampooned the small-town fashions, way of speaking, and coarse manners. And he let me know he loathed Guthrie.

Dale told me he was the happiest he'd ever been living in the Dallas–Fort Worth suburbs. After his second divorce, it was as if he'd made a calculation—a decision to let go of the life he'd been tied to, or thought he was tied to. He quit his air freight job and opened a dried-flower business, catering to Dallas and Fort Worth homeowners and designers looking to save money. He began working out at health clubs. And except for the toupee he'd started wearing, he looked better than he ever had—smiling a lot, laughing frequently. He was at ease.

But the more intimate details of his private life are a mystery to me. I can't say if he frequented gay bars or anything like that. I know he had two relationships with men, both younger than him. The first one lasted for a year, maybe longer. Now, nearly three decades later, I can't even remember that boyfriend's name, let alone any details about him. Then Tony became part of his life, both as a romantic partner and a business associate. Tony looked strikingly like Dale, with matching dark-brown mustache and eyebrows. He was shorter than Dale, but thin like him. Tony was about my age. I knew he'd made his way from North Carolina to Texas, but that was about all. I wish I could say how they met, what attracted them to each other, when they realized they were in love. But I can't. I was around Dale from time to time, a couple of times staying at his house in Arlington, yet it never occurred to me to ask about those things.

Still, we eventually addressed it in our own way. One December, after a family Christmas get-together, Dale had a plane to catch in Oklahoma City, and I offered to give him a ride to Will Rogers International Airport. As soon as we were on the road, he confessed how painful he found these visits. He talked about how difficult it was to return to the old hometown, how completely out of place he felt there, how he could no longer understand the relatives and friends he'd thought he knew. And he said something about how he feared what the old man must think about him. In the middle of our conversation, he stopped and looked over at me. "You know how I am?" he said.

After a pause, I replied, "Sure."

And that was it: Dale's admission that he was gay. Though we never actually discussed it beyond those six words, I hoped he knew he wouldn't have to pretend anymore around me. But he would pretend around the rest of the family. Already, news about the disease called AIDS ravaging gay communities in the U.S. was familiar. Beyond that, just being gay was still taboo in many, maybe most, quarters. There was also the family dynamic. Some things you just don't talk about. I knew a part of Dale was still that little boy who didn't want anyone to know that ours was a weird family, the little boy who kept his socks and underwear so neatly arranged in his drawers. Appearances mattered.

I was the only one in the family who knew his secret.

It was Tony who told me, that first night at Arlington Memorial, when Dale had found out he'd contracted HIV. Two years earlier, in 1987, the two had applied for life insurance to secure a bank loan for their business. To get the insurance, they'd had to take physicals. Both had tested positive for the disease. The insurance policy was canceled, as was the loan. Not too long after that, Dale developed a cough that would not go away. For months, that was it—just a cough. Then, suddenly, his health went into a tailspin. He quickly lost his strength, to the point that he could not walk or stand. He and Tony gave up their house and moved to an apartment. Once, while Dale was home alone, in bed, a toilet began leaking and he could do nothing except lie helpless as water crept across the floors. Yet he refused to see a doctor.

Now, here he was, at death's door. He was not the only one. In 1989 Texas had 6,312 confirmed cases of AIDS; nearly 4,000 Texans had already died from the disease. The American medical establishment offered no hope to the afflicted. People were so desperate for any chance of survival that they were willing to take drugs that had been smuggled in from Mexico; the drugs weren't approved by the FDA and their effectiveness was doubtful, but it was something. Still, even an option like that was too little, too late for Dale. He remained at Arlington Memorial for another couple of weeks, until, because of his lack of health insurance, he was sent to the county hospital in Fort Worth. The hospital staff respected his order not to discuss his condition with anyone. My parents' questions about what was wrong with him were dodged. They were left to speculate on their own. They ignored the obvious.

The frigid bluster never let up that holiday season, and my memories of that time are of driving and driving, slowly on the ice, between Belton, Arlington, Fort Worth, and Guthrie. At my folks' house, the artificial Christmas tree stood in the corner, Dale's gifts in a cluster behind everyone else's. I don't know what became of them, because Dale never had a chance to open them. He died on January 18, 1990, at the age of 38.

His funeral was in Guthrie a few days later. It fell to me to take Dale's burial clothes to the funeral home. When I saw the mortician, an old family friend, I asked him what the death certificate said. "I'm so glad you said something," he replied, pulling it out to show me. "Your folks were down here, and I don't think they have a clue."

There were the letters: HIV/AIDS. "He'll have to sign this," the mortician said, referring to the old man. "He's next of kin. I don't know how he'll react when he sees it."

At my parents' house, I helped my mother prep beds for guests staying over for the funeral, including Tony, whom my parents at that point considered to be Dale's business associate and roommate but nothing more. As she spread out a sheet still warm from the dryer, she began reciting what had become the narrative for her and the old man as to the cause of death: Dale had gone to Mexico to purchase bulk goods for his dried-flower business, and while there, he'd picked up some sort of pathogen borne by blowing sand that had settled in his lungs.

"Mom," I said, "Dale died of AIDS." I told her about the death certificate. She stuttered a bit and asked how he'd contracted the disease.

"Mom," I said again, "Dale was gay." It was eighteen hours before he was to be buried in our hometown's red clay, and it was the first time any of us had ever talked about Dale's sexuality. She protested that he had been married—not once but twice. I told her it made no difference.

"Don't tell Dad," she said after a pause. "Let me do it."

I don't know how exactly she told him, but I remember his sitting at the counter that separated the kitchen and the dining room, staring into nothingness and saying, "If he'd just told me, I think I could have helped him." He'd trailed off. "If he'd just told me …"

I remember the awkwardness between the old man and Dale's mother. I remember Tony, who spoke achingly to me about his love for my stepbrother, and whom I would never see again. I remember Dale's new grave in the winter-dead cemetery.

The old man himself died this summer. His exit was not easy, concluding with miserable weeks in a nursing home. One morning he told Mom that Dale had come to see him during the night and was still standing in the corner of his room. Mom did not disavow him of that notion. In the days to come, she'd ask him if Dale had come to visit. But he never said more about it.

Over the quarter of a century that had passed since his death, Dale had not been spoken of often at family get-togethers, and certainly no one ever brought up his sexuality or how he had died. Even in private moments, I never heard the old man open up about Dale's gayness or his AIDS death. I suspect it troubled him until his dying breath. Mom, on the other hand, began to talk to me about it eventually. She accepts that he was gay and is nonjudgmental about it. And one day a woman who had been a schoolmate of mine told Mom about her own gay son, who had been stricken with AIDS. Mom gave her a sympathetic ear, saying she knew what she was going through, she'd been there herself.

My schoolmate's son has survived because of drug therapy that was unavailable 25 years ago. AIDS seldom makes headlines these days, though it remains a significant health issue. Today's news is more likely to concern gay marriage, a concept that was hardly conceivable in early 1990. The military has progressed beyond "Don't ask, don't tell." Politicians, entertainers, and other public figures not only are out of the closet but openly celebrate their gayness. It's a shame Dale didn't live to experience the changes that American society has undergone.

It's even more unfortunate that he didn't have a chance to make peace with his father. I thought about that the day of Dad's funeral. As he aged, my stepfather was more accepting of things he would not have tolerated decades earlier. An openly gay son might have been too much, but maybe not. I'll never know. We buried the old man up the hill from Dale's grave, separated by half a mile of tombstones.

Critical Thinking

1. Why do many gay men and women hide their sexual orientation from friends and family?

2. What are some of the health effects of HIV?

Internet References

Welcome to AIDS.gov
https://www.aids.gov/

International lesbian, gay, bisexual, trans and intersex association
http://ilga.org/

The Marriage Paradox

Love, Lies, and the Power of Self-Deception

CLANCY MARTIN

Learning Outcomes

After reading this article, you will be able to:

- Explain why political, educational, and labor equality for women has changed marriage.

- Understand why the author considers marriage to be a "leap of faith."

- Describe why Martin calls marriage a kind of self-deception.

Last thanksgiving, at the turn-of-the-century house Amie and I just bought in old Kansas City: Amie, my third wife; Rebecca, my second; Alicia, my first; Amie's mom, Pat; and my three daughters sat around the harvest table. My first wife, Alicia, who has a large, ambitious heart, had proposed this act of holiday lunacy. My second wife, Rebecca, had suggested we just have fun without her, but then came anyway. Amie had felt powerless to say no, and now it was taking place.

Once the guests arrived, Amie hid in the kitchen until dinner. She spent most of her time there, making eggnog cappuccinos, roasting sweet potatoes, and baking pumpkin pies. I was afraid of the dinner table but took the head, my daughters flanking me on either side. Amie's mother was at the other end. The four women and three girls all seemed to have a good time. My first wife and my third wife discussed cleaning supplies and ghosts. Three of the four women—everyone but Amie—were single mothers, I realized. They'd all been married; they were all presently single.

Coming out of the kitchen with a roasted chicken on a platter, I listened nervously to the conversation:

"I know the wood needs oil," Amie said, gesturing to the mahogany paneling in the dining room. "But you can't really do it before company comes."

My eldest daughter was musing aloud about what she would do if she accidentally killed someone. She thought it would be best to hide the body.

"No," her mother, my first wife, said. "You would call me."

"I'd call my attorney!" my daughter said, and she pointed to my second wife (a divorce lawyer), who laughed.

Two ex-wives and my present wife all together: my divorce mediator had warned against it. I stood at the end of the table, amateurishly carved the chicken—these were the first I'd roasted in a few years—and talked with my daughters.

Dinner and dessert went well. Every time I looked up to check on Amie, she was smiling and chatting. When they all left, the hugs were natural. They all took pumpkin pies home with them.

Good luck always makes me anxious. That night I woke at 3 A.M. in a sweat. Why had those once-married women stayed single? Did they understand something I didn't? Did Amie and I get married too quickly? Was it because I need someone to love me? Did she love me? But if not, why marry a twice-divorced man with three children? I couldn't get back to sleep.

I went downstairs to the study, sat at our new desk, and made a list of all the reasons I'd married for a third time. I decided to be as rough on myself as I could. The first reason I wrote was: "I fell madly in love with Amie. She's the one." Wait, that's a cop-out. That was what I would say in a Nora Ephron play. I started a new list. Tougher.

"Reason No. 1: I don't like to be alone. Reason No. 2: Life seems mostly sane when I am with the person who is my best friend." The list had 11 reasons. I could have kept going.

After my second divorce, a friend and mentor said to me, "Give me this much: You'll wait as long as I did before trying it again." This friend had an interval of about 15 years between his two marriages. I reassured him that there was no chance I was getting married again. Then, a few months after my promise, less than two weeks after the signing of my divorce decree, at the beginning of the monsoon season in a Tibetan colony in the Himalayas, I married for the third time. "For Christ's sake, why?" my married male friends asked me. My single male friends were quiet. My female friends laughed or shook their heads. My brothers were relieved. My ex-wives were emphatic: "Promise you won't have any more children." My mother said: "Listen to me. There's only one way to make a marriage work, Clancy. You simply refuse to let it fail."

"Marriage is like a cage," Montaigne wrote. "One sees the birds outside desperate to get in, and those inside equally desperate to get out." The metaphor is hardly value-neutral; there is something noble if frightening about living outside the cage, secure but slavish within. (My father, himself twice married, used to quote Groucho Marx: "Marriage is a wonderful institution, but who wants to live in an institution?") For better or worse, Montaigne was right to point out that so many people who are married confess, after half a bottle of wine, that they would rather not be; catch a single person in a weak moment and he will often admit his longing for a lover who is more than temporary.

Divorce and the fortunate trend toward political, educational, and labor equality for women have changed the way we understand and practice marriage (in the West, anyway), but most of us continue to value the ideal of dedicating one's erotic and affectionate attention to another human being for a lifetime. The story of Odysseus striving to get back to Penelope, of Penelope weaving and unweaving her tapestry to delay her suitors while she hopes for the return of her husband, is no less compelling today than it was more than 3,000 years ago.

In the first months of our marriage, when Amie told me she loved me, she often added, "I've never loved anyone like this since my best friend in the third grade." Best friendship in childhood is something like marriage. Kierkegaard had the idea that, in every life, there was both a first and a second "immediacy." The first is the kind you enjoy when you are encountering the world for the first time: the smell of snow in your first few winters (even as a teenager, I could smell the snow in a way I no longer can), the first times you swim, what food tasted like. Then life proceeds: familiarity and habit creep in, and the world loses its newness, its ease, and its golden quality. For many of us, perhaps, we never recapture that immediacy of youth. But there can be a second immediacy, experienced perhaps through love, perhaps only through faith (the Danish word, *tro,* or faith, also means "belief").

This second immediacy sometimes sounds like a mystical state in Kierkegaard's writing, but sometimes like the very ordinary, though uncommon, experience of rediscovering the newness of something you've experienced before—as when you reread a favorite book or swim in the ocean after you haven't done so for a few years. Most simply, I think, it's re-experiencing what it's like to feel fully alive. In this state, we do not forget what the world was like before, when we were satiated with it; rather, we rediscover its wonder, and appreciate it more because of all that we've been through. The world is, as Max Weber (writing under Kierkegaard's influence) put it, "re-enchanted."

Having a best friend as a kid, or falling in love: these are good examples of first immediacy. The world is an enchanted place. Then the disappointments of love disenchant us. But marriage might offer the possibility of re-enchantment. The idea is that in first immediacy, you don't know how lucky you are. In the second immediacy, you bring both the knowledge that you have chosen this situation and your understanding of the past to your new way of looking at the world, your new appreciation of love.

For this reason, a good remarriage might be a particularly powerful case of re-enchantment. I bring to my new marriage everything I learned from my previous two: the immediacy I once had in those marriages; the knowledge of how I lost that freshness and what it is like to lose that; and, consequently, a deeper appreciation of the preciousness of that kind of love when you experience it again. Clearly I'm a slow learner. But I think that, in my third marriage, for the first time, I am starting to understand gratitude.

One of my philosopher friends would argue: how about a fourth marriage, then? Better still! And a fifth! Well, there's a practical limit to human resilience. You love a second child as much as the first; a new career revives you, and so does exotic travel; but most of us don't pursue those goods endlessly. And most long-term love relationships go through phases of enchantment, disenchantment, and re-enchantment: it's not required and probably not recommended that one change partners to appreciate what I'm trying to describe.

The truth is, there's not just one best mate out there waiting for us. If we allow that love relies not just on luck but also on our own ability to choose our partners and creatively apply our minds to romantically loving well, then there might be many potential lifelong mates who can fulfill us. And so we might need to search for re-enchantment following a disenchantment in love. The term "codependent" has gone out of style, and it is not fashionable to suggest that I am "more me" when I am with someone else. But what if it's simply true that—to quote from my list (No. 4)—"I am at my best when I am sharing my life with someone with whom I am deeply in love?"

The contemporary American philosopher Eric Schwitzgebel has identified what he calls a paradox in the marriage vow: to promise to love for a lifetime, while recognizing that both life and love are unpredictable, seems like a risky move. But as Schwitzgebel correctly argues, to promise to love a partner for a lifetime is both to acknowledge the future's unpredictability ("for better, for worse, for richer, for poorer, in sickness, and in health") and to insist that one part of life won't change: one's commitment to one's partner. Which is not to say that the feelings of both partners won't change along the way.

If this vow is paradoxical the first time it's made, think how much more so it is a second time and, in my case, a third. But belief in the meaning of that vow, despite its inherent paradox, despite the evidence that many of us don't live up to it, adds to the passion that one brings to it. Kierkegaard observed that if we knew that God existed, we wouldn't need to believe in him; it's precisely the irrationality of faith that gives its punch.

Marriage as a slightly crazy promise—even, perhaps, a special kind of self-deception: to believe a proposition and at the same time not to believe it. Psychologically, self-deception is even more paradoxical than the marriage vow; it ought to be impossible, and yet we do it with fluency from a young age.

One side of the self-deception allows us to get ourselves into the kinds of love-destroying situations that I created when I ended my first two marriages. Like lying to others, lying to yourself can lead to a whole lot of trouble—as in, for example, sliding into bed with someone while telling yourself (and even telling your new lover), "No, this needn't be the first step toward destroying my happy marriage." Self-deception may also keep people in certain marriages long after they should have left them. The difference between bad self-deception and good, I think, is that in the latter kind you know that you're doing it and you know why you're doing it. The benevolent power of self-deception is, in fact, what makes long, happy marriages—and all successful relationships—possible.

Shakespeare's "Sonnet 138" shows how this works:

> When my love swears that she is made of truth
> I do believe her, though I know she lies,
> That she might think me some untutor'd youth,
> Unlearned in the world's false subtleties.
> Thus vainly thinking that she thinks me young,
> Although she knows my days are past the best,
> Simply I credit her false speaking tongue:
> On both sides thus is simple truth suppress'd.
> But wherefore says she not she is unjust?
> And wherefore say not I that I am old?
> O, love's best habit is in seeming trust,
> And age in love loves not to have years told:
>> Therefore I lie with her and she with me,
>> And in our faults by lies we flatter'd be.

The first two lines are a terrific double paradox: he believes her, though he knows she's lying—but for him to believe her, he can't know she's lying. Given our facility with the pretzel logic that enables us to believe the lies we tell ourselves, how do we believe a lie someone else is telling us, while knowing it's a lie? The poet admits that he lets his lover believe that he believes her lies so that she will think he is young, which is also the lie she is telling him, and he uses his performance in the same way he believes her lie—to convince himself of the lie she is telling him ("thus vainly thinking that she thinks me young"). This is subtle, convoluted, hilarious, and yet entirely true to the phenomenology of love.

My favorite line: "O, love's best habit is in seeming trust." Real trust in love comes in trusting even when we know there may be reason for distrust, when we recognize that complete trust is an illusion and should not even be a goal. To truly trust is to *seem* to trust, to trust with the acceptance of doubt, to be willing to extend the feigning of trust while hoping, even expecting, that the feint will be returned.

As Nietzsche observed, the wisdom of the ancient Greeks was in the fact that, at least before Socrates, they preferred seeming to being. They understood that "the naked truth" was not what good lovers seek: "It is necessary to keep bravely to the surface, the fold and the skin; to worship appearance, to believe in forms, tones, and words, in the whole Olympus of appearance! Those Greeks were superficial—from profundity!"

Do we really want to know the truth about our lovers? We don't even know that about ourselves—it's simply too elusive, too protean, too complex.

Do we really want to know the truth about our lovers? We don't even know that about ourselves—it's simply too elusive, too protean, and too complex—and we don't want to know it, we don't need to know it. Would I love my wife more, would our marriage be stronger, if we knew every detail of each other's past lovers and love affairs? Even writing this essay about marriage is scary. I am wildly in love; my marriage, though it has its ups and downs, is splendid: Do I really want to put it under a microscope? Will my commitment be stronger because of a 3 A.M. dissection?

In love we are artists, not scientists. Who among us hasn't had the feeling, when first falling in love, of "wait, but aren't I making this all up?" That can be a bad thing, as when the young narrator, at the close of James Joyce's story "Araby," concludes that all of love is a kind of vain trick one plays on oneself. Yet deceptions and self-deceptions are a desirable, vital part of falling and staying in love. The make-believe of first love (and first heartbreak) is just warm-up for the game to come. We have to creatively participate in the romantic appreciation of our beloved—just as we creatively participate in the romantic enhancement of ourselves (both consciously and unconsciously).

Hans Vaihinger called that kind of instrumentally false belief a "necessary fiction"; Coleridge called it "the willing suspension of disbelief." Kids call it playing (although it crucially excludes the illusion-killing cynicism of the "player"). In Shakespeare's sonnet, healthy illusions are being championed, not ironized away.

This is what being married three times has taught me: engaging in this kind of playful, open-eyed deception and self-deception is how love is fostered, nurtured, and maintained. It is necessary to learn how to do it. "Couples last longer if they tend to overrate each other compared to the other's self-evaluation," the evolutionary biologist Robert Trivers teaches us. (That sounds awfully similar to No. 9 on my 3 A.M. Thanksgiving list: "I have doubts about myself and even tend to fail when I don't have a partner who believes in me. When I have a partner who believes in me, I tend to be a better person.")

In his 1996 book, Monogamy, the psychotherapist Adam Phillips succinctly views the same idea in a more negative light: "The point about trust is that it is impossible to establish. It is a risk masquerading as a promise." But we can take blind risks, foolish risks, ill-advised risks; we can also take practiced risks; we can enjoy risk; we can risk because to risk is to live.

A friend of mine, the philosopher R.J. Hankinson, who is a scholar of the ancient skeptic Sextus Empiricus, once raised the argument that being a skeptic might not be all that attractive a way to live, because skepticism—despite or because of the tranquilizing benefits that *ataraxia* ("freedom from disturbance") might have—threatens to take the fun out of life. If you aren't willing to be swayed by appearances, if you aren't stimulated and even scared once in a while, what's the point of it all?

Yes, to get married is a leap of faith. But really, who would want to be marriage because "it makes sense"?

Yes, to get married is a leap of faith: Hell, it's not a rational thing to do, but how much of life is rational? Is it rational to have kids, to chase a career, to write books, to believe that tomorrow will be better than yesterday? If it is all a dream, is a

nightmare more honest? And really, who would want to be in a marriage because "it makes sense"?

The Buddhist lama Dzongsar Khyentse Rinpoche (also known as Khyentse Norbu) gave a famous lecture on love and relationships in 2010, in Bir, in northern India. With romantic relationships, he said, "We don't really have a choice. When it comes, it comes. What is important about relationships is not to have expectations. If you are a couple, your attitude should be that you have checked into a hotel for a few days together. I might never see her again tomorrow. This might be our last goodbye, our last kiss, together. Maybe it will help; it will bring out the preciousness of the relationship. When the relationship comes, you should not be afraid."

Or, as Mark Twain wrote in a letter, sounding very Buddhist himself: "Marriage—yes, it is the supreme felicity of life. I concede it. And it is also the supreme tragedy of life. The deeper the love, the surer the tragedy."

When Khyentse Rinpoche married my wife and me, he warned us: "You know, Buddhism doesn't have a marriage ceremony. We don't really believe in marriage." To married couples, he says: "The best thing you can do is live in the world. I would tell you from the day you are married, your practice is, let's forget about giving freedom to the sentient beings"—a fundamental Buddhist motivation—"but start with giving freedom to your husband, and husband to the wife."

In this view, marriage is not supposed to constrain but to liberate. What does that mean, practically speaking? I think it means that I am supposed to help Amie pursue the things that matter most to her—many of which will also, with luck, turn out to be the things that matter most to me.

The lama goes on to say that marrying can be good practice for freeing oneself from the selfish cravings that we all suffer from. In the ideal marriage, which is understood as a goal, Amie's well-being will matter to me more than my own. We do love our children this way, and sometimes one or two friends. Of course we should acknowledge that, if life is impermanent (as indeed it is), marriage may be much more so—but here we are, stuck in the world, so why not risk it? Part of the risk is honestly acknowledging that the other human being, your spouse, is free: there's no telling what he or she might do. You're free, too, and sometimes there's no telling what you might do.

Of course all of this is just a philosopher stumbling awkwardly around the real story, which is that Amie called one afternoon to do a tarot-card reading on me for a column she eventually wrote for a magazine (the cards said I should work and avoid romance). I Google-imaged her and, single at the time, flirted with her. Facebook led to emails led to texts and then long phone calls. I flew Amie to Kansas City, and one morning, coming upstairs from the basement of my apartment with laundry in my arms, I caught sight of her in the eastern sunlight making coffee, smiling with that half-frown she makes when she's working, her long, dark brown hair in her face and on her shoulders. I flew back with her to Seattle, and walking through the jewelry department of Barney's, I saw a ring. That afternoon I proposed. That's the truth of it. We met; we fell in love; I asked her to spend the rest of her life with me; she said yes.

Yes, you might have your heart broken; yes, the whole thing might be an impossible joke, a game with outrageous odds; yes, you might have failed at it twice before, and there's no guarantee—just the opposite, really—that the third time's the charm. Life is risky; love, riskier still; marriage might be riskiest of all. But to choose to be married is, *contra* Montaigne, a paradoxical expression of one's freedom. It's not the only game in town, but it's one helluva good game.

Critical Thinking

1. Why does the author believe that divorce has changed the way we practice marriage?

2. Why does the author believe that there's not just one best mate out there waiting for us?

Create Central

www.mhhe.com/createcentral

Internet References

American Psychological Association
   http://www.apa.org/topics/divorce

Psychology Today
   http://www.psychologytoday.com/basics/marriage

CLANCY MARTIN is a professor of philosophy at the University of Missouri at Kansas City and the author of the novel *How to Sell* (2009) and the forthcoming nonfiction book *Love, Lies, and Marriage* (both Farrar, Straus and Giroux).

Clancy Martin, "The Marriage Paradox: Loves, Lies, and the Power of Self Deception" from *The Chronicle Review* (February 28, 2014): 7–10.

Article   Prepared by: Eileen L. Daniel, *SUNY College at Brockport*

Sexual Paranoia

How Campus Rules Make Students More Vulnerable

Laura Kipnis

Learning Outcomes

After reading this article, you will be able to:

- Understand the basic premise of Title IX.

- Understand how campus rules may make students more vulnerable to charges of sexual misconduct.

You have to feel a little sorry these days for professors married to their former students. They used to be respectable citizens—leaders in their fields, department chairs, maybe even a dean or two—and now they're abusers of power avant la lettre. I suspect you can barely throw a stone on most campuses around the country without hitting a few of these neo-miscreants. Who knows what coercions they deployed back in the day to corral those students into submission; at least that's the fear evinced by today's new campus dating policies. And think how their kids must feel! A friend of mine is the offspring of such a coupling—does she look at her father a little differently now, I wonder.

It's been barely a year since the Great Prohibition took effect in my own workplace. Before that, students and professors could date whomever we wanted; the next day we were off-limits to one another—verboten, traife, dangerous (and perhaps, therefore, all the more alluring).

Of course, the residues of the wild old days are everywhere. On my campus, several such "mixed" couples leap to mind, including female professors wed to former students. Not to mention the legions who've dated a graduate student or two in their day—plenty of female professors in that category, too—in fact, I'm one of them. Don't ask for details. It's one of those things it now behooves one to be reticent about, lest you be branded a predator.

Forgive my slightly mocking tone. I suppose I'm out of step with the new realities because I came of age in a different time, and under a different version of feminism, minus the layers of prohibition and sexual terror surrounding the unequal-power dilemmas of today.

When I was in college, hooking up with professors was more or less part of the curriculum. Admittedly, I went to an art school, and mine was the lucky generation that came of age in that too-brief interregnum after the sexual revolution and before AIDS turned sex into a crime scene replete with perpetrators and victims—back when sex, even when not so great or when people got their feelings hurt, fell under the category of life experience. It's not that I didn't make my share of mistakes, or act stupidly and inchoately, but it was embarrassing, not traumatizing.

As Jane Gallop recalls in *Feminist Accused of Sexual Harassment* (1997), her own generational cri de coeur, sleeping with professors made her feel cocky, not taken advantage of. She admits to seducing more than one of them as a grad student—she wanted to see them naked, she says, as like other men. Lots of smart, ambitious women were doing the same thing, according to her, because it was a way to experience your own power.

But somehow power seemed a lot less powerful back then. The gulf between students and faculty wasn't a shark-filled moat; a misstep wasn't fatal. We partied together, drank and got high together, slept together. The teachers may have been older and more accomplished, but you didn't feel they could take advantage of you because of it. How would they?

Which isn't to say that teacher-student relations were guaranteed to turn out well, but then what percentage of romances do? No doubt there were jealousies, sometimes things didn't go the way you wanted—which was probably good training for the rest of life. It was also an excellent education in not taking power too seriously, and I suspect the less seriously you take it, the more strategies you have for contending with it.

It's the fiction of the all-powerful professor embedded in the new campus codes that appalls me. And the kowtowing to the fiction—kowtowing wrapped in a vaguely feminist air of rectitude. If this is feminism, it's feminism hijacked by melodrama. The melodramatic imagination's obsession with helpless victims and powerful predators is what's shaping the conversation of the moment, to the detriment of those whose interests are supposedly being protected, namely students. The result? Students' sense of vulnerability is skyrocketing.

I've done what I can to adapt myself to the new paradigm. Around a decade ago, as colleges began instituting new "offensive environment" guidelines, I appointed myself the task of actually reading my university's sexual-harassment handbook, which I'd thus far avoided doing. I was pleased to learn that our guidelines were less prohibitive than those of the more draconian new codes. You were permitted to date students; you just weren't supposed to harass them into it. I could live with that.

However, we were warned in two separate places that inappropriate humor violates university policy. I'd always thought inappropriateness was pretty much the definition of humor— I believe Freud would agree. Why all this delicacy? Students were being encouraged to regard themselves as such exquisitely sensitive creatures that an errant classroom remark could impede their education, as such hothouse flowers that an unfunny joke was likely to create lasting trauma.

Knowing my own propensity for unfunny jokes, and given that telling one could now land you, the unfunny prof, on the carpet or even the national news, I decided to put my name down for one of the voluntary harassment workshops on my campus, hoping that my good citizenship might be noticed and applauded by the relevant university powers.

At the appointed hour, things kicked off with a "sexual-harassment pretest." This was administered by an earnest mid-50s psychologist I'll call David, and an earnest young woman with a master's in social work I'll call Beth. The pretest consisted of a long list of true false questions such as: "If I make sexual comments to someone and that person doesn't ask me to stop, then I guess that my behavior is probably welcome."

Despite the painful dumbness of these questions and the fading of afternoon into evening, a roomful of people with advanced degrees seemed grimly determined to shut up and play along, probably aided by a collective wish to be sprung by cocktail hour. That is, until we were handed a printed list of "guidelines." No. 1 on the list was: "Do not make unwanted sexual advances."

Someone demanded querulously from the back, "But how do you know they're unwanted until you try?" (OK, it was me.) David seemed oddly flustered by the question and began frantically jangling the change in his pants pocket.

"Do you really want me to answer that?" he finally responded, trying to make a joke out of it. I did want him to answer, because it's something I'd been wondering—how are you supposed to know in advance? Do people wear their desires emblazoned on their foreheads?—but I didn't want to be seen by my colleagues as a troublemaker. There was an awkward pause while David stared me down. Another person piped up helpfully, "What about smoldering glances?" Everyone laughed, but David's coin-jangling was becoming more pronounced.

A theater professor spoke up, guiltily admitting to having complimented a student on her hairstyle that very afternoon (one of the "Do Nots" involved not commenting on students' appearance) but, as a gay male, wondered whether not to have complimented her would have been grounds for offense. He mimicked the female student, tossing her mane around in a "Notice my hair" manner, and people began shouting suggestions about other dumb pretest scenarios for him to perform, like sexual-harassment charades. Rebellion was in the air. The man sitting next to me, an ethnographer who studied street gangs, whispered, "They've lost control of the room." David was jangling his change so frantically that it was hard to keep your eyes off his groin.

I recalled a long-forgotten pop-psychology guide to body language that identified change-jangling as an unconscious masturbation substitute. If the leader of our sexual-harassment workshop was engaging in public masturbatory-like behavior, seizing his private pleasure in the midst of the very institutional mechanism designed to clamp such delinquent urges, what hope for the rest of us?

Let's face it: Other people's sexuality is often just weird and creepy. Sex is leaky and anxiety-ridden; intelligent people can be oblivious about it. Of course the gulf between desire and knowledge has long been a tragicomic staple. Consider some notable treatments of the student-professor hookup theme—J.M. Coetzee's *Disgrace;* Francine Prose's *Blue Angel;* Jonathan Franzen's *The Corrections*—in which learning has an inverse relation to self-knowledge, professors are emblems of sexual stupidity, and such disasters ensue that it's hard not to read them as cautionary tales about the disastrous effects of intellect on practical intelligence.

The implementers of the new campus codes seemed awfully optimistic about rectifying the condition, I thought to myself.

The optimism continues, outpaced only by all the new prohibitions and behavior codes required to sustain it. According to the latest version of our campus policy, "differences in institutional power and the inherent risk of coercion are so great" between teachers and students that no romance, dating, or sexual relationships will be permitted, even between students and professors from different departments. (Relations between graduate students and professors aren't outright banned, but are "problematic" and must be reported if you're in the same department.) Yale and other places had already instituted similar policies; Harvard jumped on board last month, though it's a sign of the incoherence surrounding these issues that the second sentence of *The New York Times* story on Harvard reads: "The move comes as the Obama administration investigates the handling of accusations of sexual assault at dozens of colleges, including Harvard." As everyone knows, the accusations in the news have been about students assaulting other students, not students dating professors.

Of course, the codes themselves also shape the narratives and emotional climate of professor-student interactions. An undergraduate sued my own university, alleging that a philosophy professor had engaged in "unwelcome and inappropriate sexual advances" and that the university punished him insufficiently for it. The details that emerged in news reports and legal papers were murky and contested, and the suit was eventually thrown out of court.

In brief: The two had gone to an art exhibit together—an outing initiated by the student—and then to some other exhibits and bars. She says he bought her alcohol and forced her to drink, so much that by the end of the evening she was going in and out of consciousness. He says she drank of her own volition. (She was under legal drinking age; he says he thought she was 22.) She says he made various sexual insinuations, and that she wanted him to drive her home (they'd driven in his car); he says she insisted on sleeping over at his place. She says she woke up in his bed with his arms around her, and that he groped her. He denies making advances and says she made advances, which he deflected. He says they slept on top of the covers, clothed. Neither says they had sex. He says she sent friendly texts in the days after and wanted to meet. She says she attempted suicide two days later, now has PTSD, and has had to take medical leave.

The aftermath has been a score of back-and-forth lawsuits. After trying to get a financial settlement from the professor, the student filed a Title IX suit against the university: She wants her tuition reimbursed, compensation for emotional distress, and other damages. Because the professor wasn't terminated, when she runs into him it triggers her PTSD, she says. (The university claims that it appropriately sanctioned the professor, denying him a raise and a named chair.) She's also suing the professor for gender violence. He sued the university for gender discrimination (he says he wasn't allowed to present evidence disproving the student's allegations)—this suit was thrown out; so were several brought by the student. The professor sued various colleagues, administrators, and a former grad student he previously dated, for defamation; a judge dismissed those suits last month. He sued local media outlets for using the word "rape" as a synonym for sexual assault—a complaint thrown out by a different judge who said rape was an accurate enough

summary of the charges, even though the assault was confined to fondling, which the professor denies occurred. (This professor isn't someone I know or have met, by the way.)

What a mess. And what a slippery slope, from alleged fondler to rapist. But here's the real problem with these charges: This is melodrama. I'm quite sure that professors can be sleazebags. I'm less sure that any professor can force an unwilling student to drink, especially to the point of passing out. With what power? What sorts of repercussions can there possibly be if the student refuses?

Indeed, these are precisely the sorts of situations already covered by existing sexual-harassment codes, so if students think that professors have such unlimited powers that they can compel someone to drink or retaliate if she doesn't, then these students have been very badly educated about the nature and limits of institutional power.

In fact, it's just as likely that a student can derail a professor's career these days as the other way around, which is pretty much what happened in the case of the accused philosophy professor.

To a cultural critic, the representation of emotion in all these documents plays to the gallery. The student charges that she "suffered and will continue to suffer humiliation, mental and emotional anguish, anxiety, and distress." As I read through the complaint, it struck me that the lawsuit and our new consensual-relations code share a common set of tropes, and a certain narrative inevitability. In both, students and professors are stock characters in a predetermined story. According to the code, students are putty in the hands of all-powerful professors. According to the lawsuit, the student was virtually a rag doll, taken advantage of by a skillful predator who scripted a drunken evening of galleries and bars, all for the opportunity of some groping.

Everywhere on campuses today you find scholars whose work elaborates sophisticated models of power and agency. It would be hard to overstate the influence, across disciplines, of Michel Foucault, whose signature idea was that power has no permanent address or valence. Yet our workplaces themselves are promulgating the crudest version of top-down power imaginable, recasting the professoriate as Snidely Whiplashes twirling our mustaches and students as helpless damsels tied to railroad tracks. Students lack volition and independent desires of their own; professors are would-be coercers with dastardly plans to corrupt the innocent.

Even the language these policies come packaged in seems designed for maximum stupefaction, with students eager to add their voices to the din. Shortly after the new policy went into effect on my campus, we all received a long email from the Title IX Coordinating Committee. This was in the midst of student protests about the continued employment of the accused philosophy professor: 100 or so students, mouths taped shut (by themselves), had marched on the dean's office (a planned sit-in of the professor's class went awry when he pre-emptively canceled it). The committee was responding to a student-government petition demanding that "survivors" be informed about the outcomes of sexual-harassment investigations. The petition also demanded that the new policies be amended to include possible termination of faculty members who violate its provisions.

There was more, but my eye was struck by the word "survivor," which was repeated several times. Wouldn't the proper term be "accuser"? How can someone be referred to as a survivor before a finding on the accusation—assuming we don't want to predetermine the guilt of the accused, that is. At the risk of sounding like some bow-tied neocon columnist, this is also a horrifying perversion of the language by people who should know better. Are you seriously telling me, I wanted to ask the Title IX Committee, that the same term now encompasses both someone allegedly groped by a professor and my great-aunt, who lived through the Nazi death camps? I emailed an inquiry to this effect to the university's general counsel, one of the email's signatories, but got no reply.

For the record, I strongly believe that bona fide harassers should be chemically castrated, stripped of their property, and hung up by their thumbs in the nearest public square. Let no one think I'm soft on harassment. But I also believe that the myths and fantasies about power perpetuated in these new codes are leaving our students disabled when it comes to the ordinary interpersonal tangles and erotic confusions that pretty much everyone has to deal with at some point in life, because that's simply part of the human condition.

In the post-Title IX landscape, sexual panic rules. Slippery slopes abound. Gropers become rapists and accusers become survivors, opening the door for another panicky conflation: teacher-student sex and incest. Recall that it was incest victims who earlier popularized the use of the term "survivor," previously reserved for those who'd survived the Holocaust. The migration of the term itself is telling, exposing the core anxiety about teacher-student romances: that there's a whiff of perversity about such couples, notwithstanding all the venerable married ones.

These are anxious times for officialdom, and students, too, are increasingly afflicted with the condition—after all, anxiety is contagious. Around the time the "survivor" email arrived, something happened that I'd never experienced in many decades of teaching, which was that two students—one male, one female—in two classes informed me, separately, that they were unable to watch assigned films because they "triggered" something for them. I was baffled by the congruence until the following week, when the *Times* ran a story titled "Trauma Warnings Move From the Internet to the Ivory Tower," and the word "trigger" was suddenly all over the news.

I didn't press the two students on the nature of these triggers. I knew them both pretty well from previous classes, and they'd always seemed well-adjusted enough, so I couldn't help wondering. One of the films dealt with fascism and bigotry: The triggeree was a minority student, though not the minority targeted in the film. Still, I could see what might be upsetting. In the other case, the connection between the student and the film was obscure: no overlapping identity categories, and though there was some sexual content in the film, it wasn't particularly explicit. We exchanged emails about whether she should sit out the discussion, too; I proposed that she attend and leave if it got uncomfortable. I was trying to be empathetic, though I was also convinced that I was impeding her education rather than contributing to it.

I teach in a film program. We're supposed to be instilling critical skills in our students (at least that's how I see it), even those who aspire to churn out formulaic dreck for Hollywood. Which is how I framed it to my student: If she hoped for a career in the industry, getting more critical distance on material she found upsetting would seem advisable, given the nature of even mainstream media. I had an image of her in a meeting with a bunch of execs, telling them that she couldn't watch one of the company's films because it was a trigger for her. She agreed this could be a problem, and sat in on the discussion with no discernable ill effects.

But what do we expect will become of students, successfully cocooned from uncomfortable feelings, once they leave the sanctuary of academe for the boorish badlands of real life? What becomes of students so committed to their own vulnerability, conditioned to imagine they have no agency, and protected from unequal power arrangements in romantic life? I can't help asking, because there's a distressing little fact about the discomfort of vulnerability, which is that it's pretty much a daily experience in the world, and every sentient being has to learn how to somehow negotiate the consequences and fallout, or go through life flummoxed at every turn.

Here's a story that brought the point home for me. I was talking to a woman who'd just published her first book. She was around 30, a friend of a friend. The book had started at a major trade press, then ended up published by a different press, and I was curious why. She alluded to problems with her first editor. I pressed for details, and out they came in a rush.

Her editor had developed a sort of obsession with her, constantly calling, taking her out for fancy meals, and eventually confessing his love. Meanwhile, he wasn't reading the chapters she gave him; in fact, he was doing barely any work on the manuscript at all. She wasn't really into him, though she admitted that if she'd been more attracted to him, it might have been another story. But for him, it was escalating. He wanted to leave his wife for her! There were kids, too, a bunch of them. Still no feedback on the chapters.

Meanwhile he was Skyping her in his underwear from hotel rooms and complaining about his marriage, and she was letting it go on because she felt that her fate was in his hands. Nothing really happened between them—well, maybe a bit of fumbling, but she kept him at a distance. The thing was that she didn't want to rebuff him too bluntly because she was worried about the fate of her book—worried he'd reject the manuscript, she'd have to pay back the advance, and she'd never get it published anywhere else.

I'd actually once met this guy—he'd edited a friend's book (badly). He was sort of a nebbish, hard to see as threatening. "Did you talk to your agent?" I asked the woman. I was playing the situation out in my mind, wondering what I'd do. No, she hadn't talked to her agent, for various reasons, including fears that she'd led the would-be paramour on and that her book wasn't any good.

Suddenly the editor left for a job at another press, and the publisher called the contract, demanding a final manuscript, which was overdue and nowhere near finished. In despair, the author finally confessed the situation to our mutual friend, another writer, who employed the backbone-stiffening phrase "sexual harassment" and insisted that the woman get her agent involved. Which she did, and the agent negotiated an exit deal with the publisher by explaining what had taken place. The author was let out of the contract and got to take the book to another press.

What struck me most, hearing the story, was how incapacitated this woman had felt, despite her advanced degree and accomplishments. The reason, I think, was that she imagined she was the only vulnerable one in the situation. But look at the editor: He was married, with a midlevel job in the scandal-averse world of corporate publishing. It simply wasn't the case that he had all the power in the situation or nothing to lose. He may have been an occluded jerk, but he was also a fairly human-sized one.

So that's an example of a real-world situation, postgraduation. Somehow I don't see the publishing industry instituting codes banning unhappily married editors from going goopy over authors, though even with such a ban, will any set of regulations ever prevent affective misunderstandings and erotic crossed signals, compounded by power differentials, compounded further by subjective levels of vulnerability?

The question, then, is what kind of education prepares people to deal with the inevitably messy gray areas of life? Personally I'd start by promoting a less vulnerable sense of self than the one our new campus codes are peddling. Maybe I see it this way because I wasn't educated to think that holders of institutional power were quite so fearsome, nor did the institutions themselves seem so mighty. Of course they didn't aspire to reach quite as deeply into our lives back then. What no one's much saying about the efflorescence of these new policies is the degree to which they expand the power of the institutions

themselves. As for those of us employed by them, what power we have is fairly contingent, especially lately. Get real: What's more powerful—a professor who crosses the line, or the shaming capabilities of social media?

For myself, I don't much want to date students these days, but it's not like I don't understand the appeal. Recently I was at a book party, and a much younger man, an assistant professor, started a conversation. He reminded me that we'd met a decade or so ago, when he was a grad student—we'd been at some sort of event and sat next to each other. He said he thought we'd been flirting. In fact, he was sure we'd been flirting. I searched my memory. He wasn't in it, though I didn't doubt his recollection; I've been known to flirt. He couldn't believe I didn't remember him. I apologized. He pretended to be miffed. I pretended to be regretful. I asked him about his work. He told me about it, in a charming way. Wait a second, I thought, was he flirting with me now? As an aging biological female, and all too aware of what that means in our culture, I was skeptical. On the heels of doubt came a surge of joy: "Still got it," crowed some perverse inner imp in silent congratulation, jackbooting the reality principle into assent. My psyche broke out the champagne, and all of us were in a far better mood for the rest of the evening.

Intergenerational desire has always been a dilemma as well as an occasion for mutual fascination. Whether or not it's a brilliant move, plenty of professors I know, male and female, have hooked up with students, though informal evidence suggests that female professors do it less, and rarely with undergraduates. (The gender asymmetries here would require a dozen more articles to explicate.) Some of these professors act well, some are jerks, and it would benefit students to learn the identifying marks of the latter breed early on, because postcollegiate life is full of them. I propose a round of mandatory workshops on this useful topic for all students, beginning immediately.

But here's another way to look at it: the longue durée. Societies keep reformulating the kinds of cautionary stories they tell about intergenerational erotics and the catastrophes that result, starting with Oedipus. The details vary; so do the kinds of catastrophes prophesied—once it was plagues and crop failure, these days it's psychological trauma. Even over the past half-century, the story keeps getting reconfigured. In the preceding era, the Freudian version reigned: Children universally desire their parents, such desires meet up with social prohibitions—the incest taboo—and become repressed. Neurosis ensues.

These days the desire persists, but what's shifted is the direction of the arrows. Now it's parents—or their surrogates, teachers—who do all the desiring; children are conveniently returned to innocence. So long to childhood sexuality, the most irksome part of the Freudian story. So too with the new campus dating codes, which also excise student desire from the story, extending the presumption of the innocent child well into his or her collegiate career. Except that students aren't children.

Among the problems with treating students like children is that they become increasingly childlike in response. *The New York Times Magazine* recently reported on the tangled story of a 21-year-old former Stanford undergraduate suing a 29-year-old tech entrepreneur she'd dated for a year. He'd been a mentor in a business class she was enrolled in, though they'd met long before. They traveled together and spent time with each other's families. Marriage was discussed. After they broke up, she charged that their consensual relationship had actually been psychological kidnapping, and that she'd been raped every time they'd had sex. She seems to regard herself as a helpless child in a woman's body. She demanded that Stanford investigate and is bringing a civil suit against the guy—this despite the fact that her own mother had introduced the couple, approved the relationship every step of the way, and been in more or less constant contact with the suitor.

No doubt some 21-year-olds are fragile and emotionally immature (helicopter parenting probably plays a role), but is this now to be our normative conception of personhood? A 21-year-old incapable of consent? A certain brand of radical feminist—the late Andrea Dworkin, for one—held that women's consent was meaningless in the context of patriarchy, but Dworkin was generally considered an extremist. She'd have been gratified to hear that her convictions had finally gone mainstream, not merely driving campus policy but also shaping the basic social narratives of love and romance in our time.

It used to be said of many enclaves in academe that they were old-boys clubs and testosterone-fueled, no doubt still true of certain disciplines. Thanks to institutional feminism's successes, some tides have turned, meaning that menopausal women now occupy more positions of administrative power, edging out at least some of the old boys and bringing a different hormonal style—a more delibidinalized one, perhaps—to bear on policy decisions. And so the pendulum swings, overshooting the middle ground by a hundred miles or so.

The feminism I identified with as a student stressed independence and resilience. In the intervening years, the climate of sanctimony about student vulnerability has grown too thick to penetrate; no one dares question it lest you're labeled antifeminist. Or worse, a sex criminal. I asked someone on our Faculty Senate if there'd been any pushback when the administration presented the new consensual-relations policy (though by then it was a fait accompli—the senate's role was "advisory").

"I don't quite know how to characterize the willingness of my supposed feminist colleagues to hand over the rights of faculty—women as well as men—to administrators and attorneys in the name of protection from unwanted sexual advances," he said. "I suppose the word would be 'zeal.'" His own view was that the existing sexual-harassment policy already protected students from coercion and a hostile environment; the new rules infantilized students and presumed the guilt of professors. When I asked if I could quote him, he begged for anonymity, fearing vilification from his colleagues.

These are things you're not supposed to say on campuses now. But let's be frank. To begin with, if colleges and universities around the country were in any way serious about policies to prevent sexual assaults, the path is obvious: Don't ban teacher-student romance, ban fraternities. And if we want to limit the potential for sexual favoritism—another rationale often proffered for the new policies—then let's include the institutionalized sexual favoritism of spousal hiring, with trailing spouses getting ranks and perks based on whom they're sleeping with rather than CVs alone, and brought in at salaries often dwarfing those of senior and more accomplished colleagues who didn't have the foresight to couple more advantageously.

Lastly: The new codes sweeping American campuses aren't just a striking abridgment of everyone's freedom, they're also intellectually embarrassing. Sexual paranoia reigns; students are trauma cases waiting to happen. If you wanted to produce a pacified, cowering citizenry, this would be the method. And in that sense, we're all the victims.

Critical Thinking

1. How can campus rules make students feel more vulnerable to charges of sexual misconduct?

2. What role does Title IX play on campuses?

Internet References

American Association of University Women
  www.aauw.org

Title IX
  http://www.titleix.info/

LAURA KIPNIS is a professor in the department of radio, television, and film at Northwestern University and the author, most recently, of *Men: Notes From an Ongoing Investigation* (Metropolitan Books).

Article

Prepared by: Eileen L. Daniel, *SUNY College at Brockport*

Swipe and Burn

Dating apps that connect people in the here and now are being linked to a surge in sexually transmitted infections.

SHAONI BHATTACHARYA

Learning Outcomes

After reading this article, you will be able to:

- Understand the link between location-based dating apps and sexually transmitted infections.

- Understand why the number of syphilis cases has risen in the United States.

S ome people do it in bed. Others slope off to the bathrooms at work. Look carefully and you'll probably spot someone at it on the train. You might even be one of them.

Whether or not you have joined the millions regularly logging on to hook-up apps such as Tinder and Grindr, it is clear that over the past few years they have become an accepted part of today's dating scene. With touchscreen interfaces that allow users to swipe through profiles of available matches, they make finding a date as quick and easy as flicking through the pages of a magazine.

Tinder, used by men and women, generates 15 million mutual matches a day. Grindr, a similar app for men seeking men, has 6 million users, with 10,000 joining daily. And because these apps rely on GPS to recommend potential matches within a given radius, they make meeting people in the flesh easier than ever.

But for all the fun and spontaneity, a darker side is emerging. The rise of such apps has coincided with a surge in outbreaks of sexually transmitted infections (STIs) that had long been under control, and an increase in other rare diseases. Public health officials are now pointing the finger of blame at a combination of relaxed attitudes toward safe sex and the easy access to partners provided by these apps.

"What it comes down to is mobile convenience leading to more efficient STI transmission," says epidemiologist Matthew Beymer at the Los Angeles LGBT Center. That's not all. Research is starting to explore the idea that this technology makes you more likely to change your behaviour, causing you to leave your common sense at the bedroom door.

Syphilis was once one of the most feared STIs but was almost confined to the history books after it became treatable with penicillin in the 1940s. By 2000, it was on the brink of elimination in both the US and the UK.

But cases of syphilis have rocketed over the past few years in many Western countries, including the US, Canada, UK, Germany, Sweden, and Australia. Now the UK sees more than 3000 cases a year and the US more than 16,500. Australia had its highest-ever recorded levels last September.

It's not just syphilis. Infection rates for other STIs that had plummeted during the AIDS epidemic in the 1980s are also on the rise. In Australia, gonorrhoea cases rose by 70 per cent between 2009 and 2013. Chlamydia and multidrug-resistant gonorrhoea are on the increase in numerous countries.

In their public responses to these outbreaks, health officials have repeatedly blamed hook-up apps. "You've suddenly invented a way of discovering where the nearest sexually available person is to the nearest metre—it's not difficult for you to get with them," says Peter Greenhouse at the British Association for Sexual Health and HIV.

Rash Behaviour

Research into the cause of the STI increase is still in the early stages, but evidence is starting to stack up in support of this idea.

An investigation of six regional outbreaks of syphilis across the UK since 2012 found that location-based networking apps played an important part in how patients had met their sexual partners, especially for men who have sex with men.

The team behind the research, led by Ian Simms at Public Health England in Colindale, UK, says that as well as making it quicker and easier to find new partners, the technology joins together isolated sexual networks in which disease would previously have been contained. This results in "hyper-efficient transmission" of infections, Simms says, so epidemics spread faster and further.

Further evidence that links app use with STIs comes from a small study of men who have sex with men. This found that those who met up through smartphone apps had significantly more past sexual partners and were more likely to have ever been diagnosed with an STI than those who didn't use the apps (PLoS One, DOI: 10.1371/journal.pone.0086603).

That finding was backed up by Beymer and his colleagues, who conducted the first major study to compare STI rates in people who use apps and those who don't. The clinic had noticed that increasingly, men who came in for testing were using apps such as Grindr, Jack'd, Recon, and Scruff.

The team looked at disease incidence in 7000 men who came in for screening and found that those who used phone apps to meet sexual partners were 40 per cent more likely to test positive for gonorrhoea than those who met sexual partners online. They were 25 per cent more likely to have the disease than men who had met partners socially.

What was "startling", Beymer says, is that even when they controlled for other factors that are known to influence STI risk, such as age, ethnicity and drug use, the link to phone app use remained.

STIs are the core concern, but in the past two years, Simms and others have been surprised to find that infections that weren't traditionally thought to spread through sexual contact also now seem to be spreading this way. Two infections that had hitherto been known as travel-related stomach bugs, the gastroenteric bacterium Shigella flexneri and the rare verocytotoxin-producing Escherichia coli (VTEC), were reported in clusters of gay and bisexual men in the UK. Many cases weren't linked to travel to countries where the disease is endemic, and later interviews with the men revealed factors such as the use of the internet and apps to meet partners.

"Essentially we are saying all these overlapping epidemics are all sides of the same dice," Simms says. "They are sustained by very closely related sexual networks facilitated by geospatial networking apps which allow all these previously un-joined networks to be linked up."

These studies suggest a link, but it could be that the results aren't about the apps but the users, says Ian Holloway at the Luskin School of Public Affairs at the University of California, Los Angeles. "We don't yet know if there's something inherent about these apps or the individuals choosing to use them," he says.

Anecdotally, the spontaneity involved seems to make people more relaxed. "You are more likely to throw caution to the wind," says Kate (not her real name), who started using Tinder after a breakup. She didn't originally sign up to Tinder for casual sex but ended up sleeping with three of the five men she met. "Sometimes we'd been chatting for ages so you feel more advanced in your flirtation when you meet them for the first time than with someone you meet in a bar, so it's more likely that things will happen," she says.

But what's the evidence? Working out why and how people behave the way they do when it comes to sex is delicate and complicated. Yet studies suggest that the way people meet their sexual partners might influence what happens when they end up in bed—translating into health consequences.

"We have done work to show that the actual process of interaction online can increase risk-taking," says John de Wit at the University of New South Wales, Australia. With colleague Philippe Adam, he conducted a survey of 2000 men who have sex with men to see if their online experiences affected their actions.

"We found out that 70 per cent of gay men who use these online chat sites or apps fantasise around unprotected sex with their partner as a way of getting aroused—without the intention to actually do that. But in fact all these fantasies modify their sexual script," says Adam, and some men act on them regardless of their initial intentions.

Safer Swiping

Much of the research has so far focused on men having sex with men, but the surge of STIs is far from confined to this community, with outbreaks also occurring in heterosexual adults. Similar research on Tinder would be interesting, says Holloway.

One of the reasons some officials believe that apps are helping to drive the problem is a result of contact tracing, one of the first things they do when trying to address an outbreak. Those who test positive in the clinic are asked for the contact details of recent sexual partners so that they can be alerted of the risk. And it's this process, they say, which often reveals the role of hook-up apps: in the Canadian city of Winnipeg, for example, 50 per cent of people being treated for syphilis said they had met sexual partners through them.

Apps may also make contact tracing harder than if people meet through social connections as there is no need for users to reveal their real name or contact details, making halting an outbreak more difficult.

But although apps have been implicated in the STI surge, they are far from the only factor. Cases of syphilis have been rising for around a decade, and this coincides with a reduction in sexual health campaigns and a change in attitudes toward HIV.

As the perception of AIDS has changed from it being seen as a death sentence to a chronic condition that can be managed with drugs, a so-called "safe-sex fatigue" has ensued. The same generation that is now connecting more easily using mobile devices is also less concerned about safe sex than the generation before.

The success of preventative pre- and post-exposure pills for HIV, which protect against HIV but don't stop other STIs, may add to the issue, officials say, as well as the popularity of "sero-sorting" websites. These connect people on the basis of their HIV status. Without the HIV risk, people may be less likely to practice safe sex.

With such a complex issue, Holloway cautions against vilifying networking apps. Instead, he thinks they could be harnessed as valuable prevention tools.

That's why he and his colleagues have teamed up with Online Buddies, which owns internet sites and mobile apps such as Manhunt and Jack'd, to conduct a study into how HIV prevention advice through mobile apps might be received by at-risk groups.

Online Buddies has a research arm, OLB Research Institute in Cambridge, Massachusetts, which is focused on gathering evidence on the best way to get sexual health messages across on their platforms. It also acts as a consultancy to health agencies to help them design mobile campaigns that users are more likely to engage with. The institute is headed by David Novak, who was previously National Syphilis Elimination Coordinator at the US Centers for Disease Control but felt that he could do more by working in the industry.

The approach can work. During a deadly meningitis outbreak in New York City in 2012, Novak says they worked with local public health authorities and directed one-third of local Manhunt users to get vaccinated using an advert on the site.

Other app companies are also getting on board. In October last year, Grindr and six other app makers formed a collaboration with the San Francisco AIDS Foundation and the Foundation for AIDS Research with the aim of finding new ways to encourage testing, raise awareness and reduce stigma.

Getting the message right is crucial, however. "Once you make a change to a site of millions of users, if you don't do it properly it can have a bad health outcome," says Novak.

Online Buddies will turn down paid public health advertising or campaigns it feels aren't right for their mobile platforms. For example, it recently refused a syphilis campaign that it felt stigmatised people who had the disease.

And a barrage of criticism fell on the public health department of San Mateo County in northern California recently for its use of fake Grindr accounts to send users sexual health advice. The accounts use stock photos as avatars and are operated by trained STI counsellors, says Darryl Lampkin, Community Program Supervisor at the department. Once they get chatting to users, the counsellors find the first opportune moment to reveal that they are actually healthcare providers and use the chat to supply health information. But critics have slammed this as patronising and unethical and have likened it to entrapment.

"We recognise how this strategy can be perceived as being deceptive," says Lampkin. But he says it works, with 80 per cent of men remaining online after the counsellors they are chatting to have come clean. They have also seen a rise in the number of men coming in to be tested.

Encouraging testing is crucial, but sending people their results quickly and in a shareable, electronic format can also help to increase dialogue about STIs, says Ramin Bastani, CEO of health platform Healthvana, which works with public health bodies in the US to develop electronic test results. Bastani envisages a day when app users will expect to see some kind of verified sexual health tick or "badge" on people's profiles noting that many men in the gay community already post their HIV status on their online profiles.

Quite how this technology will evolve remains to be seen. Holloway points out that the possible resharing of test results raises privacy issues that have yet to be resolved.

But what is clear is that there is a real drive to change the way sexual health messages are presented. "Young people don't want boring messages about public health," says Adam. "They want to know about relationships. Sexual health messages need to be embedded in this." As Basani puts it, "the healthcare of the 21st century will not look like healthcare—it will look like your iPhone, your computer. The things you use every day."

Critical Thinking

1. How does the use of dating apps relate to sexually transmitted diseases?
2. Why are some sexually transmitted diseases such as syphilis increasing in the United States, Britain, and Australia?

Internet References

Centers for Disease Control and Prevention
www.cdc.gov

Mayo Clinic
http://www.mayoclinic.org/diseases-conditions/sexually-transmitted-diseases-stds/in-depth/std-symptoms/art-20047081

Unit 7

UNIT

Prepared by: Eileen Daniel, *SUNY College at Brockport*

Preventing and Fighting Disease

Cardiovascular disease and cancer are the leading killers in this country. This is not altogether surprising given that the American population is growing increasingly older, and one's risk of developing both of these diseases is directly proportional to one's age. Another major risk factor, which has received considerable attention over the past 30 years, is one's genetic predisposition or family history. Historically, the significance of this risk factor has been emphasized as a basis for encouraging at-risk individuals to make prudent lifestyle choices, but this may be about to change as recent advances in genetic research, including mapping the human genome, may significantly improve the efficacy of both diagnostic and therapeutic procedures.

Just as cutting-edge genetic research is transforming the practice of medicine, startling new research findings in the health profession are transforming our views concerning adult health. This new research suggests that the primary determinants of our health as adults are the environmental conditions we experienced during our life in the womb. According to Dr. Peter Nathanielsz of Cornell University, conditions during gestation, ranging from hormones that flow from the mother to how well the placenta delivers nutrients to the tiny limbs and organs, program how our liver, heart, kidneys, and especially our brains function as adults. While it is too early to draw any firm conclusions regarding the significance of the "life in the womb factor," it appears that this avenue of research may yield important clues as to how we may best prevent or forestall chronic illness.

Of all the diseases in America, coronary heart disease is this nation's number one killer. Frequently, the first and only symptom of this disease is a sudden heart attack. Epidemiological studies have revealed a number of risk factors that increase one's likelihood of developing this disease. These include hypertension, a high serum cholesterol level, diabetes, cigarette smoking, obesity, a sedentary lifestyle, a family history of heart disease, age, sex, race, and stress. In addition to these well-established risk factors, scientists think they may have discovered several additional risk factors. These include the following: low birth weight, cytomegalovirus, *Chlamydia pneumoniae,* porphyromonasgingivalis, and c-reactive protein (CRP). CRP is a measure of inflammation somewhere in the body. In theory, a high CRP reading may be a good indicator of an impending heart attack.

One of the most startling and ominous health stories was the recent announcement by the Centers for Disease Control and Prevention (CDC) that the incidence of Type 2 adult onset diabetes increased significantly over the past 15 years. This sudden rise appears to cross all races and age groups, with the sharpest increase occurring among people ages 30 to 39 (about 70 percent). Health experts at the CDC believe that this startling rise in diabetes among 30 to 39 year olds is linked to the rise in obesity observed among young adults (obesity rates rose from 12 to 20 percent nationally during this same time period). Experts at the CDC believe that there is a time lag of about 10–15 years between the deposition of body fat and the manifestation of Type 2 diabetes. This time lag could explain why individuals in their 30s are experiencing the greatest increase in developing Type 2 diabetes today. Current estimates suggest that 16 million Americans have diabetes, and it kills approximately 180,000 Americans each year. Many experts now believe that our couch potato culture is fueling the rising rates of both obesity and diabetes. Given what we know about the relationship between obesity and Type 2 diabetes, the only practical solution is for Americans to watch their total calorie intake and exercise regularly. Currently, there has been a rise in the incidence of Type 2 diabetes among our youth and young adults, and the term *adult onset diabetes* may be a misnomer, given the growing number of young adults and teens with this form of diabetes.

Cardiovascular disease is America's number one killer, but cancer takes top billing in terms of the "fear factor." This fear of cancer stems from an awareness of the degenerative and disfiguring nature of the disease. Today, cancer specialists are employing a variety of complex agents and technologies, such as monoclonal antibodies, interferon, and immunotherapy, in their attempt to fight the disease. Progress has been slow, however, and the results, while promising, suggest that a cure may be several years away. A very disturbing aspect of this country's battle against cancer is the fact that millions of dollars are spent each year trying to advance the treatment of cancer, while the funding for the technologies used to detect cancer in its early stages is quite limited. A reallocation of funds would seem appropriate, given the medical community posits that early detection and treatment are the key elements in the successful cure of cancer. An interesting issue related to early detection has arisen. A government task force recently announced that women in their 40s do not need annual mammograms, a long-held belief. Until we have more effective methods for detecting cancer in the early stages, our best hope for managing cancer is to prevent it through our lifestyle choices. The same lifestyle choices that may help prevent cancer can also help reduce the incidence of heart disease and diabetes.

Refusing Vaccination Puts Others at Risk

Ronald Bailey

Learning Outcomes

After reading this article, you will be able to:

- Explain why vaccine refusal puts others at risk.

- Understand why defenseless people such as infants who are too young to be vaccinated and individuals whose immune systems are compromised are at particular risk for disease prevented by vaccination.

- Understand the concept of herd immunity.

Millions of Americans believe it is perfectly all right to put other people at risk of death and misery. These people are your friends, neighbors, and fellow citizens who refuse to have themselves or their children vaccinated against preventable infectious diseases.

Aside from the issue of child neglect, there would be no argument against allowing people to refuse government-required vaccination if they and their families were the only ones who suffered the consequences of their fool-hardiness. But that is not the case in the real world. Let's first take a look at how vaccines have improved health, then consider the role of the state in promoting immunization.

Vaccines are among the most effective health care innovations ever devised. A November 2013 New England Journal of Medicine article, drawing on the University of Pittsburgh's Project Tycho database of infectious disease statistics since 1888, concluded that vaccinations since 1924 have prevented 103 million cases of polio, measles, rubella, mumps, hepatitis A, diphtheria, and pertussis. They have played a substantial role in greatly reducing death and hospitalization rates, as well as the sheer unpleasantness of being hobbled by disease.

A 2007 article in the Journal of the American Medical Association compared the annual average number of cases and resulting deaths of various diseases before the advent of vaccines to those occurring in 2006. Before an effective diphtheria vaccine was developed in the 1930s, for example, the disease infected about 21,000 people in the United States each year, killing 1,800. By 2006, both numbers were zero. Polio, too, went from deadly (16,000 cases, 1,900 deaths) to nonexistent after vaccines were rolled out in the 1950s and 1960s. Chickenpox used to infect 4 million kids a year, hospitalize 11,000, and kill 105; within a decade of a vaccine being rolled out in the mid-1990s, infections had dropped to 600,000, resulting in 1,276 hospitalizations and 19 deaths. Similar dramatic results can be found with whooping cough, measles, rubella, and more.

And deaths don't tell the whole story. In the case of rubella, which went from infecting 48,000 people and killing 17 per year, to infecting just 17 and killing zero, there were damaging pass-on effects that no longer exist. Some 2,160 infants born to mothers infected by others were afflicted with congenital rubella syndrome-causing deafness, cloudy corneas, damaged hearts, and stunted intellects—as late as 1965. In 2006 that number was one.

It is certainly true that much of the decline in infectious disease mortality has occurred as a result of improved sanitation and water chlorination. A 2004 study by the Harvard University economist David Cutler and the National Bureau of Economic Research economist Grant Miller estimated that the provision of clean water "was responsible for nearly half of the total mortality reduction in major cities, three-quarters of the infant mortality reduction, and nearly two-thirds of the child mortality reduction." Providing clean water and pasteurized milk resulted in a steep decline in deadly waterborne infectious diseases. Improved nutrition also reduced mortality rates, enabling infants, children, and adults to fight off diseases that would have more likely killed their malnourished ancestors. But it is a simple fact that vaccines are the most effective tool yet devised for preventing contagious airborne diseases.

Vaccines do not always produce immunity, so a percentage of those who took the responsibility to be vaccinated remain vulnerable. Other defenseless people include infants who are too young to be vaccinated and individuals whose immune systems are compromised. In America today, it is estimated that about 10 million people are immunocompromised through no fault of their own.

This brings us to the important issue of "herd immunity." Herd immunity works when most people in a community are immunized against an illness, greatly reducing the chances that an infected person can pass his microbes along to other susceptible people.

People who refuse vaccination for themselves and their children are free riding off of herd immunity. Even while receiving this benefit, the unvaccinated inflict the negative externality of being possible vectors of disease, threatening those 10 million most vulnerable to contagion.

Vaccines are like fences. Fences keep your neighbor's livestock out of your pastures and yours out of his. Similarly, vaccines separate people's microbes. Anti-vaccination folks are taking advantage of the fact that most people around them have chosen differently, thus acting as a firewall protecting them from disease. But if enough people refuse, that firewall comes down, and innocent people get hurt.

Oliver Wendell Holmes articulated a good libertarian principle when he said, "The right to swing my fist ends where the other man's nose begins." Holmes' observation is particularly salient in the case of whooping cough shots.

Infants cannot be vaccinated against whooping cough (pertussis), so their protection against this dangerous disease depends upon the fact that most of the rest of us are immunized. Unfortunately, as immunization refusals have increased in recent years, so have whooping cough infections. The annual number of pertussis cases fell from 200,000 pre-vaccine to a low of 1,010 in 1976. Last year, the number of reported cases rose to 48,277, the highest since 1955. Eighteen infants died of the disease in 2012, up from just four in 1976.

The trend is affecting other diseases as well. In 2005, an intentionally unvaccinated 17-year-old Indiana girl brought measles back with her from a visit to Romania and ended up infecting 34 people. Most of them were also intentionally unvaccinated, but a medical technician who had been vaccinated caught the disease as well, and was hospitalized.

Another intentionally unvaccinated 7-year-old boy in San Diego sparked an outbreak of measles in 2008. The kid, who caught the disease in Switzerland, ended up spreading his illness to 11 other children, all of whom were also unvaccinated, putting one infant in the hospital. Forty-eight other children younger than vaccination age had to be quarantined.

Some people object to applying Holmes' aphorism by arguing that aggression can only occur when someone intends to hit someone else; microbes just happen. However, being intentionally unvaccinated against highly contagious airborne diseases is, to extend the metaphor, like walking down a street randomly swinging your fists without warning. You may not hit an innocent bystander, but you've substantially increased the chances. Those harmed by the irresponsibility of the unvaccinated are not being accorded the inherent equal dignity and rights every individual possesses. The autonomy of the unvaccinated is trumping the autonomy of those they put at risk.

As central to libertarian thinking as the non-aggression principle is, there are other tenets that also inform the philosophy. One such is the harm principle, as outlined by John Stuart Mill. In On Liberty, Mill argued that "the only purpose for which power can be rightfully exercised over any member of a civilized community, against his will, is to prevent harm to others." Vaccination clearly prevents harm to others.

So what are the best methods for increasing vaccination? Education and the incentives of the market have encouraged many Americans to get themselves and their children immunized, and surely those avenues of persuasion can and should be used more. Perhaps schools and daycare centers and pediatric clinics could attract clients by advertising their refusal to admit unvaccinated kids. Or social pressure might be exercised by parents who insist on assurances from other parents that their children are vaccinated before agreeing to playdates.

But it would be naive not to acknowledge the central role of government mandates in spreading immunization. By requiring that children entering school be vaccinated against many highly contagious diseases, states have greatly benefited the vast majority of Americans.

For the sake of social peace, vaccine opt-out loopholes based on religious and philosophical objections should be maintained. States should, however, amend their vaccine exemption laws to require that people who take advantage of them acknowledge in writing that they know their actions are considered by the medical community to be putting others at risk. This could potentially expose vaccine objectors to legal liability, should their decisions lead to infections that could have been prevented.

In terms of net human freedom, the trade-off is clear: in exchange for punishment-free government requirements that contain opt-out loopholes, humans have freed themselves from hundreds of millions of infections from diseases that maimed and often killed people in recent memory. People who refuse vaccination are asserting that they have a right to "swing" their microbes at other people. That is wrong.

Being intentionally unvaccinated against highly contagious airborne diseases is like walking down a street randomly swinging your fists without warning.

Critical Thinking

1. Why don't vaccines always produce immunity and who is most at risk?
2. What are some of the best ways to increase the vaccination rates?

Create Central

www.mhhe.com/createcentral

Internet References

Centers for Disease Control and Prevention
http://www.cdc.gov/vaccines

National Vaccine Information Center
http://www.nvic.org

Article   Prepared by: Eileen L. Daniel, *SUNY Brockport*

The High Cost of "Hooking Up"

KURT WILLIAMSEN

Learning Outcomes

After reading this article, you will be able to:

- Explain the health risks associated with promiscuous sex.

- Describe the types of pathogenic organisms that can be transmitted sexually.

- Describe why there is such a high rate of sexually transmitted diseases among teenagers.

Hydeia Broadbent became somewhat of a mini-celebrity 20 years ago as a seven-year-old when she appeared on a Nickelodeon AIDS special. She appeared on the show with basketball great and HIV-positive athlete Magic Johnson—she had been diagnosed with AIDS, basically believed at the time to be a death sentence. She is still alive, and is a public-speaking dynamo. As an early recipient of anti-viral treatments that made AIDS a livable disease, one might expect her to be one of the many who reiterate their positive experiences having the disease, also inadvertently pooh-poohing the seriousness of the disease.

Not her. She does the opposite. She lays bare the consequences of having the disease, in order to encourage people to abstain from behaviors that might lead them to acquire it. She explained in a story for CNN: "If you're HIV-negative, I would say 'Stay that way.' If you're positive, I would say, 'There's life after a positive test, but it is a hassle.'"

As she told CNN last year, what she accomplishes in a day depends on how she feels:

There are days when Hydeia can't get out of bed. Sometimes she is so sick her mornings are spent with her head hung over the toilet.

Every morning, she must take her cocktail of five pills. Her tiny frame is partly a result of medicine stunting her growth.

If it's a good day, she goes to the gym to exercise. Staying fit is key to living with AIDS, she says. She eats healthy too, because a person with HIV/AIDS is more prone to cancer and heart disease. . . .

"There's so much misinformation. People think there's a cure . . .," she said. "There is no cure." . . .

Although a positive test result is no longer a death sentence, Hydeia says, "it's a life sentence."

"It's always there. You're always going to have HIV or AIDS. You're always going to be taking medicine. You're always going to be going to the doctor's office. You're always going to be getting your blood drawn."

Her medicine costs $3,500 to $5,000 a month.

The story soberly added that "16,000 Americans will die this year from AIDS."

Yet despite the very harsh realities of HIV/AIDS, according to the National Center for Health Statistics, in 2010, in the United States, "for all races combined in the age group 15–24 years, HIV disease moved from the 12th leading cause of death in 2009 to the 11th leading cause of death in 2010." It is the "7th leading cause of death in 2010 for the age group 25–44 years."

Moreover, there are, according to the Centers for Disease Control's "2010 Sexually Transmitted Diseases Surveillance," about 47,000 new diagnoses of HIV made each year, with a lifetime cost for each person conservatively estimated at $379,668—that's $17,844,396,000 of medical costs added to an already overwhelmed and over-budgeted U.S. medical system yearly. (Note: Many people catch HIV by sharing intravenous needles, not via sex.)

There are also 19 million new infections of sexually transmitted gonorrhea, chlamydia, and syphilis yearly, which cost $17 billion to treat each year. Then there are the costs to treat all of the other STDs—human papillomavirus, herpes, genital warts, hepatitis, trichomoniasis, scabies, etc. The World Health Organization says that there "are more than 30 different sexually transmissible bacteria, viruses and parasites." Treatment for those in the United States is also in the billions of dollars per year—when they're treatable and not drug resistant.

Whooping It Up over Whooppee

Though it's likely that literally everyone who is having sex is aware of STDs, such as herpes and HIV, and that STDs have consequences that include death, casual sex in our country is practically revered by youths and leftists. Sex on a whim, to them, is the be-all and end-all of life.

Accordingly, public schools, Hollywood celebs, and teen magazines often teach youths that no one should be allowed to tell them that they should not have sex until they are married, that every type and manner of sex is OK, and that having sex is just another bodily function and should be considered only with the same level of care as eating: Be careful about what you put in your body; try to prevent the transmission of pathogens via hygienic practices and barriers to disease transmission, such as latex products; and then dig in.

As well, even network TV tantalizes viewers with titillation and works to convince viewers that bed hopping is no big deal—everyone does it, with ones they love or ones they merely like. The term "friends with benefits"—friends who have sex with each other when no one better is available—is now such common slang that Hollywood used it as the basis for a movie.

Human nature being what it is, it's really no surprise to learn that there's not much difference between the percentage of youths who latch on to the "safe sex" message and the percentage of those who heed the appeals to participate in "uninhibited sex." A CDC survey showed that about 60 percent of high-school students who have had sex used a condom the last time they had sex, and 50 percent of them say they've had sex at least once. That's a lot of young people, with a lot of exposure to STDs. (Of course, in both cases there's probably some false data: In the case of the number of youths having sex, many youths don't consider oral sex to be sex at all, and so don't count it.)

In 2008, according to an AP article entitled "1 in 4 teen girls has sexually transmitted disease," not only did 25 percent of teenage girls have an STD, "among those who admitted to having sex, the rate was even more disturbing—40 percent had an STD." Black girls suffered worst: 48 percent of them had an STD, though blacks as a group are the most likely to use condoms, using them between 65 and 70 percent of the time.

Lest one believe the oft-cited refrain that such high rates of venereal disease in the United States demonstrate, as stated by Cecile Richards, the head of Planned Parenthood, that "the national policy of promoting abstinence-only programs is a . . . failure," know that "abstinence-only" is far from national policy—with only 34 percent of school principals in a Kaiser study saying that their school's "main message was abstinence-only" and with two-thirds of U.S. teens having had school lessons about condom usage. More importantly, it should be clear to all by studying France that sex-ed programs are a proven failure at eliminating such problems.

In France, sex education has been part of the school curricula since 1973, and students are given condoms in eighth and ninth grades. Moreover, in that country there can be no claims of hidden sexual repression influencing findings: Sex is not only part of the national dialogue, it's part of the country's national pride—alongside French cuisine—and public sex is not uncommon. Yet according to the World Health Organization, nearly 45 percent of French women tested under 25 years of age had sexually transmitted human papillomavirus (HPV). When women of all ages are considered, the evidence is equally damning: 12.8 percent of French women had HPV versus 7.3 percent for women of Western Europe as a whole. The worldwide HPV rate is 11.4 percent.

One Disease, Then Another

But sex-related diseases and costs go far beyond those directly associated with STDs. The National Cancer Institute at the

National Institutes of Health stated that the human papillomavirus, which is "spread through direct skin-to-skin contact during vaginal, anal, and oral sex," causes "virtually all cervical cancers" and "most anal cancers and some vaginal, vulvar, penile, and oropharyngeal cancers [cancers in the middle part of the throat]." And the risk isn't limited to women. The title of a 2011 NBCNews.com article adequately sums up the situation: "Cancer spike, mainly in men, tied to HPV from oral sex." The article added that "we can expect some 10,000 to 15,000 patients with (the [oropharyngeal] cancers) per year in the United States, with the great majority having HPV-positive (cancers)." All told, "High risk HPV infections account for approximately 5 percent of cancers worldwide."

With the total cost of treating cancer in the United States in excess of $124.6 billion in 2010, the cost of treating cancer caused by HPV infections is likely upward of $6.23 billion per year—five percent of $124.6 billion. (This total is based on average costs from 2001 to 2006, before many expensive treatments were introduced, so costs now are likely higher.)

Also, according to the CDC, "Chlamydia and gonorrhea are important preventable causes of infertility," even though "most women infected with chlamydia or gonorrhea have no symptoms." There are "an estimated 2.8 million cases of chlamydia and 718,000 cases of gonorrhea [that] occur annually in the United States." "Each year untreated STDs cause 24,000 women in the United States to become infertile." STDs cause approximately one-fourth of all infertility in women, and treatment to rectify infertility can be very costly.

STDs also cause ectopic pregnancy, wherein a woman's egg gets fertilized in her fallopian tubes, instead of her uterus, again causing a life-threatening situation.

And the effects of STDs travel further than between the couple having sex: The effects can get passed on to newborns. The CDC commented:

STDs can be passed from a pregnant woman to the baby before, during, or after the baby's birth. Some STDs (like syphilis) cross the placenta and infect the baby while it is in the uterus (womb). Other STDs (like gonorrhea, chlamydia, hepatitis B, and genital herpes) can be transmitted from the mother to the baby during delivery as the baby passes through the birth canal. . . .

A pregnant woman with an STD may also have early onset of labor, premature rupture of the membranes surrounding the baby in the uterus, and uterine infection after delivery.

The harmful effects of STDs in babies may include stillbirth (a baby that is born dead), low birth weight (less than five pounds), conjunctivitis (eye infection), pneumonia, neonatal sepsis (infection in the baby's blood stream), neurologic damage, blindness, deafness, acute hepatitis, meningitis, chronic liver disease, and cirrhosis.

STDs truly are the gifts that keep on giving.

Too, taking "the pill" to avoid begetting any infants increases the risk of getting blood clots, strokes, and heart attacks.

A study published in the June *New England Journal of Medicine* determined that some types of pill double the risk of heart attack and stroke. (Much of this extra risk is borne by smokers.) For every 10,000 pill users, there is approximately one extra heart attack and one extra stroke. Combined with the fact that the pill can cause high blood pressure, possibly damaging organs; more than double the increase in risk of blood clots in veins, called deep venous thrombosis; and cause pulmonary embolism, which is when blood clots break loose from a vein and go into the lungs—potentially causing death—taking the pill is akin to playing bingo in a very large room and waiting for your chance to "win" an ailment.

Taking the pill also frequently results in increased headaches and, rarely, in liver tumors.

And the pill isn't the birth-control choice only of women in long-term monogamous relationships. A May report released by the CDC said that 60 percent of teen girls who have sex use the pill.

Though this is admittedly already a horrific list of physical consequences of sexual promiscuity—accompanied with a tab of many billions of dollars—it is far from an all-encompassing list. It really only covers some of the obvious "biggies." It ignores such things as the blisters, lesions, sores, and pain that come with STDs and their complications, such as pelvic inflammatory disease.

Moreover, to fully account for costs of the free-sex ethic, we must add emotional trauma and its consequences and treatment to the list of physical ailments.

Ouch, My Head/Heart Hurts

The emotional trauma that often comes with promiscuity includes, but is definitely not limited to, the embarrassment of having to tell someone with whom you want to become intimate that you have incurable herpes or HIV, telling your family that you're dying of AIDS, or grieving over the knowledge that your herpes caused your newborn to be blind or brain damaged.

The online article "Life With Herpes: One Woman's Story" recounts a woman named Angela's experience with contracting herpes:

In the summer of 1995, Angela, who was 25 at the time, felt like she had the flu and found it difficult and painful to urinate. She saw a doctor and, after being treated with several different medications for a possible bladder infection, felt worse than ever. "At the end of the three weeks I was miserable, couldn't walk and the pain was beyond description," she said.

Angela finally insisted on a vaginal examination and was diagnosed with genital herpes. . . .

She later realized she had contracted the virus from a sexual contact two weeks earlier. She was angry that her partner hadn't informed her he had herpes. . . . Shocked, terrified and alone, she struggled to find support and information about her disease.

Her physician wasn't helpful. "He basically handed me a box of tissues and told me my life would never be the same and sent me on my way." . . .

The emotional effects of having genital herpes have been as painful for Angela as the physical effects. "The first year I was ashamed, got flare ups all the time and didn't have anybody I trusted to talk to about what was happening in my life," she said. Frustrated by the lack of support systems where she lived, Angela started her own support group . . .

The HELP group meets monthly and offers a confidential environment where people can relate to others experiencing similar difficulties. . . . Herpes support groups allow attendees to vent their feelings, which can range from denial, depression, isolation and intense anger.

The CDC states that "nationwide, 16.2% [of], or about one out of six, people aged 14 to 49 years have genital HSV-2 infection"—one of two types of genital herpes. Women are more apt to catch it than men. Insidiously, the disease can move to different areas of the body: "If a person with genital herpes touches their sores or the fluids from the sores, they may transfer herpes to another part of the body. This is particularly problematic if it is a sensitive location such as the eyes."

Then there's the litany of findings that were released in 2003 by the Heritage Foundation, compiled from the U.S. Department of Health and Human Services' National Survey of Family Growth, in which 10,000 sexually active women between the ages of 15 and 44 were interviewed about both their sex lives and their lives in general.

The study, which asked women about how early in their lives they initiated voluntary sexual encounters, found that the younger a girl is when she becomes sexually active, the more likely she is to give birth out of wedlock. (At the time of the study, "nearly 40 percent of girls who commence sexual activity at ages 13 or 14 will give birth outside of marriage [versus] . . . 9 percent of women who begin sexual activity at ages 21 or 22.") Starting sex earlier also correlated to higher levels of child and maternal poverty, increased single motherhood, more abortions, more unstable marriages (once they did get married), decreased personal happiness, and increased depression.

Servings of sex came with heaping helpings of emotional pain, mental pain, and stress.

Please, Sir, May I Have Some More

Here again, the negative effects snowball. It's clearly evident in a Heritage Foundation study entitled "Marriage: America's Greatest Weapon Against Child Poverty" that over the years as the free-sex ideology has increasingly found acceptance, single motherhood has jumped dramatically—"in 2010 nearly 60 percent of all births in the U.S. were to single mothers," while "in 1964, 93 percent of children born in the United States were born to married parents." Moreover, as "free sex" and single motherhood took hold, poverty has prospered.

As the report says,

According to the U.S. Census, the poverty rate for single parents with children in the United States in 2009 was 37.1 percent. The rate for married couples with children was 6.8 percent. Being raised in a married family reduced a child's probability of living in poverty by about 82 percent.

And single motherhood costs this country dearly. In terms of dollars, the Heritage report stated:

In fiscal year 2011, federal and state governments spent over $450 billion on means-tested welfare for low-income families with children. Roughly three-quarters of this welfare assistance, or $330 billion, went to single-parent families. Most nonmarital births are currently paid for by the taxpayers through the Medicaid system, and a wide variety of welfare assistance will continue to be given to the mother and child for nearly two decades after the child is born. On average, the means-tested welfare costs for single parents with children amount to around $30,000 per household per year.

And that's just a part of the "economic costs." There are other heavy costs.

Studies have shown that 63 percent of youth suicides are from fatherless homes, as are 90 percent of all homeless and runaway children, 85 percent of all children that exhibit behavioral disorders, 80 percent of rapists motivated with displaced anger, and 85 percent of youths in prison. As well, single parenting results in a lower likelihood of graduating from high school for kids.

And women, who are already more inclined to abuse their children than are men, become more likely to abuse their children when they have a heavier "parenting and housework load." Even when the children of single-mother homes do have a man in the picture, it's not all good. According to the U.S. Department of Health and Human Services' Administration for Children and Families, "Unrelated male figures and stepfathers in households tend to be more abusive than biological, married fathers." The report specifically says:

Children who live in father-absent homes often face higher risks of physical abuse, sexual abuse, and neglect than children who live with their fathers. A 1997 Federal study indicated that the overall rate of child maltreatment among single-parent families was almost double that of the rate among two-parent families: 27.4 children per thousand were maltreated in single-parent families, compared to 15.5 per thousand in two-parent families. One national study found that 7 percent of children who had lived with one parent had ever been sexually abused, compared to 4 percent of children who lived with both biological parents.

And the wounds from maltreatment run deep. Remuda Ranch, which bills itself as "the nation's leading eating disorder treatment center," said that "more than 50 percent of its patients have experienced trauma in their lives. The trauma is usually sexual, physical and emotional abuse." It added: "Forty-nine percent of our patients have experienced childhood sexual abuse."

Remuda gave a brief explanation of how eating disorders may be generated from abuse:

Research has shown that childhood sexual abuse increases binge-eating, purging, restricting calories, body shame and body dissatisfaction. Eating disorders become a way of helping victims cope with shame. They feel they may need to modify their body in ways that reduce shame or distress. For example, a woman suffering from trauma and an eating disorder may wish to reduce her breast size in order to appear less feminine and therefore, less appealing to men because of her past history of abuse.

A girl named Kacy at Pandora's Project, a resource for victims of rape and sexual abuse, related the story of her abuse:

About twice a year my family would fly out to where my grandparents lived. Thats how my young life started, being violently raped and abused over and over again [by my grandfather]. And thats how the sexual abuse continued throughout my entire childhood.

When I reached 9th grade, I was sent away to an all girls boarding school. I had been in and out of schools every year of high school and when I was in 11th grade (in yet again, a new school) thats where I met perp #2. She was my teacher, and I confided in her, the secret that I had been holding in all those years. She responded with kindness and compassion. But soon after, she went on to take advantage of my vulnerability, and continued the horrid pattern that my life had claimed. She would crawl into my bed at night and exploit and shatter whatever human part of me my grandfather had left behind. She stole any innocence that had been forgotten, she tore me apart once again—leaving me more broken than I had ever been.

The next two years went by, filled with numbness and unbearable pain. Filled with emotions I had never known existed. Filled with an emptiness that was so hollow, I was a walking dead person. The endless amount of sleepless nights became a ritual in my twisted schedule. The daily confusion and absolute loss that consumed me is indescribable. This torturous hell was my life as I had come to know it.

Porn's Part

Sadly, according to Dr. Laura Berman, "up to one-third of the sexual abuse in this country is committed by minors. (It is worth noting that while a small percentage of those who are sexually abused become abusers, almost all child abusers—adult or otherwise—are victims of sexual abuse)." And for this, pornography—another segment of the "sexual freedom" mantra—can be partially blamed.

An article entitled "Children as Victims," about the effect of porn on children, reported the following statistic: "A Los Angeles Police Department study of every child molestation case referred to them over a ten-year period, found that in 60% of the cases adult or child pornography was used to lower the inhibitions of the children molested and/or to excite and sexually arouse the pedophile." Also, "87% of convicted molesters of girls and 77% of convicted molesters of boys admit to using pornography, most often in the commission of their crimes." Let's not forget that, as Massachusetts U.S. Attorney Carmen Diaz said in an AP article, demand for child porn—images and videos of children being "raped by adults"—is increasing rapidly, and increasing numbers of children are abused to satisfy the demand: "This demand leads to the abuse of children, yet there is this misconception that somehow, viewing child pornography is a victimless crime." Diaz prosecuted one member of a global child porn ring, a ring in which the members had hundreds of thousands of images on their computers of children being abused.

Many users of porn would likely dismiss its use as innocuous, but the preponderance of evidence shows that it has a cost far beyond its huge—but unknowable—dollar costs. (The most popular "adult website" on the Web gets "32 million visitors a month, or almost 2.5% of all Internet users!" according to a *Forbes* interview of scientists who crunched the numbers.) Not only do children act out things they see during porn viewing, even committing rape, but, according to psychologist Steve

Livingston, porn may similarly affect "vulnerable" adults by "strengthen[ing] existing violent proclivities." Moreover, he added, experts haven't yet investigated whether there are ties between jurors using porn and the likelihood they'll convict rapists.

Additionally, porn has the same addicting physiological effects as gambling; it causes men to desire more and more graphic sexual imagery to remain stimulated; it causes men to objectify women and see them merely as sperm receptacles; and it causes men and women to have problems with emotional intimacy. According to a news release entitled "Internet Porn Ruining Male-Female Relationships, Studies Show" for Jim Wysong, the author of *The Neutering of the American Male,* "In a 20,000-person study recently conducted by TED.com [a website containing "remarkable" speeches], porn is the most prevalently cited obstacle for romantic relationships between men and women in their teens and 20s. Women say guys are emotionally unavailable, and men say porn makes them less interested in pursuing a relationship."

One woman told about her porn experience with the man in her life:

My ex told me that he knew porn was an "addiction" for him. He used that term, and he said he wanted to stop and that because he couldn't porn had "ruined his life." He also showed me a scar from [performing a sex act] to the point of bleeding because he was unable to stop.

He said porn made him want to cheat all the time, and made him constantly fantasize about "nasty" sex with strangers, and young (teen) girls. . . . He would become agitated, irritable and mean when he could not look at porn because I was home, and he would become so angry and abusive due to frustration that I would unwittingly give him what he wanted by leaving. He would also abandon me places and run home and get online.

And porn has other, even more dramatic, effects: It causes men both to instigate sex that is actually physically painful to the woman and to even completely lose the ability to have sex with an actual woman. Sex, for a heavy porn user, often becomes reduced to self-stimulation while watching pornographic videos.

And that's what some people call sexual freedom.

Sex and Security

The problems with porn and a lack of sexual restraint are societal and, believe it or not, actually even have a negative effect on U.S. national defense and crime-fighting. During the Cold War with Russia, it was common to hear of diplomats and military personnel turning traitor through a "honeytrap"—an intelligence operative using sex. Even now weak willpower and sex could easily lead to secrets being leaked. In recent months, nine Secret Service agents responsible for protecting the president were forced out of their positions after they engaged in liaisons with prostitutes while doing advanced work for the president's trip to Colombia; four-star general and director of the CIA David Petreaus admitted to having an extramarital affair with a woman named Paula Broadwell and resigned; presidential candidates Newt Gingrich, John Edwards, and Herman Cain were involved in trysts with women who were not their wives; and Bill Clinton had a sexual encounter with Monica Lewinsky in the White House. Who knows what deals these men were willing to make—or did make—to protect their prestige and not get exposed diddling around. Meanwhile, last July the Pentagon's Missile Defense Agency had to warn its staff not to watch porn on U.S. government computers. (Gee, I wonder if computer viruses embedded in porn videos could allow hackers to gain access to government computers?)

Dangers and crimes that threaten U.S. citizens have been allowed to slide because of sexual obsessions: Dozens of members of the Securities and Exchange Commission, tasked with monitoring the country's financial system, watched porn at work—for up to eight hours a day—instead of responding to credible, repeated accusations against Bernie Madoff, who was eventually caught running a $50 billion Ponzi scheme.

The list of problems and costs associated with the free-sex mantra go on and on. Not covered here are its implications for abortion, sex trafficking, and drug and alcohol use, among others.

In response to the weighty evidence aligned against them, the best libertines could do in the way of defense of their ideology—the best defense I could find—came from a young woman writing for Salon.com in an article entitled "In defense of casual sex." She claims that numerous sexual exploits "lead to better adult relationships." She believes that it's good to try "on different men to see how they fit." Women are "romantically vetting—and being vetted. . . . Hopefully, by taking several test-drives before buying, we'll be happier with our final investment." (And as a feminist she likes "empowerment," "respect," and "choice"—meaning she wants to do what she feels, whenever she feels.)

Of course, studies don't back her up (and it *is* possible to vet possible spouses without having sex), but there it is.

U.S. Representative Joe Pitts (R-Pa.) makes a good point about the propensity of schools—and others—to promote sexual freedom:

How would it look if the federal government took the same approach to reducing teenage drinking that it takes to reducing teenage pregnancies? . . . School programs would teach teens how to drink, but also encourage them to use good judgment through messages like: "Wait until you know you are ready before you have your first drink." . . . They would be told: "The only one who can decide when you are ready to drink is you."

Knowing what we know about teenagers and their ability to assess risk and act accordingly, this sort of approach sounds ludicrous. Nevertheless, that's precisely the approach we've been taking to sex ed for decades. . . . We do it right in other areas. Teens are simply told "no" when it comes to other risky activities like smoking, drinking, and driving below a certain age.

He added that a government report entitled "A Better Approach to Teenage Pregnancy Prevention: Sexual Risk Avoidance" gave the science fortifying his claims.

Moreover, it seems as if liberals subconsciously acknowledge the damage that's done by their teachings, even as they promulgate their views: In so-called sex-ed classes, students learn little about STDs (except perhaps HIV/AIDS), according to a study reported on by ScienceDaily, even though additional details go a long way toward keeping youth abstinent.

In a sense liberals are correct: Sex *is* just another physical activity that people do—such as eating, sleeping, and exercising—but it is also much more than that. It changes behavior, moods, attitudes, views of self-worth, moral constraints, and more, and so-called free sex is nowhere near being "free." It imposes heavy costs on both individuals and society, and the chance that anyone who participates in the free-sex lifestyle—or their children—will remain unscathed is low.

Since this information is not hard to find, any individual or organization that takes a public position pushing a free-sex ideology goes far beyond the point of being simply ignorant to being brainwashed, stupid, depraved, or in serious denial. Where do you stand on the issue?

Critical Thinking

1. What are the health and social risks associated with promiscuous sex?

2. What types of organisms can cause sexually transmitted diseases?

Create Central

www.mhhe.com/createcentral

Internet References

National Institute of Allergy and Infectious Diseases (NIAID)
www3.niaid.nih.gov

Planned Parenthood
www.plannedparenthood.org

Sexuality Information and Education Council of the United States (SIECUS)
www.siecus.org

Article   Prepared by: Eileen Daniel, *SUNY College at Brockport*

The Secret Life of Dirt

At the Finnish-Russian Border, Scientists Investigate a Medical Mystery

ANDREW CURRY

Learning Outcomes

After reading this article, you will be able to:

- Understand why exposure to dirt in childhood may lead to lower rates of certain diseases.

- Describe why allergies are less common in areas that resemble a "pre-hygiene" past.

- Explain the relationship between exposure to dirt and the risk of childhood diabetes.

After eight hours in an overheated Soviet-era sleeper car, we pull into the Petrozavodsk train station just after 1 A.M. The streets are silent, the night air chilly. Our taxi shudders and swerves along roads pitted with axle-gulping potholes. Identical concrete apartment blocks built in the 1960s flash by in a blur. Winter temperatures here, some 250 miles northeast of St. Petersburg, sometimes plunge to minus 40 degrees Fahrenheit. A traffic circle in the middle of town boasts what locals claim is Russia's only statue of Lenin holding a fur hat.

I'm traveling with Mikael Knip, a short, energetic Finnish physician and University of Helsinki researcher with a perpetual smile under his bushy mustache. He has come to Petrozavodsk—an impoverished Russian city of 270,000 on the shores of Lake Onega and the capital of the Republic of Karelia—to solve a medical mystery, and perhaps help explain a scourge increasingly afflicting the developed world, the United States included.

For reasons that no one has been able to identify, Finland has the world's highest rate of Type 1 diabetes among children.

Out of every 100,000 Finnish kids, 64 are diagnosed annually with the disease, in which the body's immune system declares war on the cells that produce insulin. Type 1 diabetes is usually diagnosed in children, adolescents, and young adults.

The disease rate wasn't always so high. In the 1950s, Finland had less than a quarter of the Type 1 diabetes it has today. Over the past half-century, much of the industrialized world has also seen a proliferation of the once rare disease, along with other autoimmune disorders such as rheumatoid arthritis and celiac disease. Meanwhile, such afflictions remain relatively rare in poorer, less-developed nations.

Why?

Petrozavodsk, only about 175 miles from the Finland border, may be the perfect place to investigate the question: The rate of childhood Type 1 diabetes in Russian Karelia is one-sixth that of Finland. That stark difference intrigues Knip and others because the two populations for the most part are genetically similar, even sharing risk factors for Type 1 diabetes. They also live in the same subarctic environment of pine forests and pristine lakes, dark, bitter winters, and long summer days. Still, the 500-mile boundary between Finland and this Russian republic marks one of the steepest standard-of-living gradients in the world: Finns are seven times richer than their neighbors across the border. "The difference is even greater than between Mexico and the U.S.," Knip tells me.

Since 2008, Knip and his colleagues have collected tens of thousands of tissue samples from babies and young children in Russia and Finland, as well as in nearby Estonia. In his spotless lab on the fourth floor of a modern research complex in Helsinki, nearly two dozen freezers are filled with bar-coded vials of, among other things, umbilical cord blood, stool samples, and nasal swabs. The freezers also hold tap water and dust collected at the different locations. By comparing the samples, Knip hopes to isolate what's driving Finland's diabetes rate up—or what's keeping Russian Karelia's low.

For all the sophisticated analysis involved, the theory that Knip is testing couldn't be more basic. He thinks the key difference between the two populations is . . . dirt. In a sense, he wonders if kids in Finland, and in the United States and other developed nations as well, are too clean for their own good.

The idea that dirt, or the lack of it, might play a role in autoimmune disease and allergy gained support along another border. In the late 1980s, Erika von Mutius was studying asthma in and around Munich. At the time, researchers thought air pollution was the cause. But after years of work, the young German researcher couldn't clearly link Munich's pollution and respiratory disease.

On November 9, 1989, an unusual opportunity came along: The Berlin Wall fell. For the first time since the 1940s, West Germans could conduct research in the East. Von Mutius, of Ludwig-Maximilians University Munich, seized the opportunity, expanding her study to include Leipzig, a city of 520,000 deep in East Germany.

The countryside around Leipzig was home to polluting chemical plants and was pocked with open-pit coal mines; many residents heated their apartments with coal-burning ovens. It was a perfect experiment: two groups of children with similar genetic backgrounds, divided by the Iron Curtain into dramatically different environments. If air pollution caused asthma, Leipzig's kids should be off the charts.

Working with local doctors, von Mutius studied hundreds of East German schoolchildren. "The results were a complete surprise," von Mutius says. "In fact, at first we thought we should re-enter the data." Young Leipzigers had slightly lower rates of asthma than their Bavarian counterparts—and dramatically less hay fever, a pollen allergy.

Puzzling over her results, von Mutius came across a paper by David Strachan, a British physician who had examined the medical records of 17,000 British children for clues to what caused allergies later in life. Strachan found that kids with a lot of older brothers and sisters had lower rates of hay fever and eczema, probably because the siblings brought home colds, flus, and other germs.

After learning of Strachan's study, von Mutius wondered whether air pollution might somehow protect East Germans from respiratory allergies.

Soon, studies from around the world showed similarly surprising results. But it was germ-laden dirt that seemed to matter, not air pollution. The children of full-time farmers in rural Switzerland and Bavaria, for example, had far fewer allergies than their non-farming peers. And a study following more than 1,000 babies in Arizona showed that, unless parents also had asthma, living in houses with dogs reduced the chances of wheezing and allergies later in life. Researchers proposed that the more microbial agents that children are exposed to early in life, the less likely they are to develop allergies and autoimmune diseases later on. Studies also showed that baby mice kept in sterile environments were more likely to face autoimmune disease, seeming to back what came to be called the "hygiene hypothesis."

"It was so unexpected," says von Mutius, who now believes air pollution was a red herring. Instead, East German children may have benefited from time spent in daycare.

Think about it this way: At birth, our immune cells make up an aggressive army with no sense of who its enemies are. But the more bad guys the immune system is exposed to during life's early years, the more discerning it gets. "The immune system is programmed within the first two years of life," says Knip. "With less early infection, the immune system has too little to do, so it starts looking for other targets."

Sometimes the immune system overreacts to things it should simply ignore, like cat dander, eggs, peanuts, or pollen. Those are allergies. And sometimes the immune system turns on the body itself, attacking the cells we need to produce insulin (Type 1 diabetes) or hair follicles (alopecia) or even targeting the central nervous system (multiple sclerosis). Those are autoimmune disorders.

Both appear to be mostly modern phenomena. A century ago, more people lived on farms or in the countryside. Antibiotics hadn't been invented yet. Families were larger, and children spent more time outside. Water came straight from wells, lakes, and rivers. Kids running barefoot picked up parasites like hookworms. All these circumstances gave young immune systems a workout, keeping allergy and autoimmune diseases at bay.

In places where living conditions resemble this "pre-hygiene" past-rural parts of Africa, South America, and Asia—the disorders remain uncommon. It can be tempting to dismiss the differences as genetic. But disease rates in the industrialized world have risen too fast, up to 3 or 4 percent a year in recent decades, to be explained by evolutionary changes in DNA "You can see quite clearly in a pre-hygiene situation you don't see allergic disease," says Thomas Platts-Mills, an allergy specialist at the University of Virginia. "Move to a hygiene society, and it does not matter your race or ethnicity—allergy rises."

These findings don't mean that people should eschew basic hygiene. Its benefits are clear: In the past 60 years or so, our overall life expectancy has continued to rise. The trick for scientists is to determine exactly which early life exposures to germs might matter and identify the biology behind their potentially protective effect.

That's one big way Knip's research on the Finland-Russia border can contribute. The accident of geography and history playing out there offers a chance to work in what Knip calls a "living laboratory."

"It's really an exciting opportunity," says Richard Insel, chief scientific officer for the New York City-based Juvenile Diabetes Research Foundation.

Just a few hours after we arrive in Petrozavodsk, I follow Knip and his team to a morning meeting at the Karelian Ministry of Health. Russian officials on the other side of a long conference table explain through an interpreter that they haven't recruited as many study participants as their Finnish and Estonian colleagues. Parents in Petrozavodsk are unfamiliar with the practice of conducting medical studies, reluctant to submit their babies to what they see as painful blood tests and too stressed to fill out long surveys on diet and family history.

If Knip is frustrated, he hides it well. The recruitment phase of the study was supposed to end in 2012. He's trying to buy his Russian colleagues another year to conduct their work, he says, smiling and shaking hands before heading to a taxi waiting outside. "It's turned out to be a lot more complicated than we expected," Knip tells me later. "Cultural differences have been a big learning process for us."

The next stop is Petrozavodsk Children's Hospital, a building on the city's outskirts surrounded by concrete apartments. While Knip gives a pep talk to pediatricians charged with gathering study samples, I sit down with Tatyana Varlamova, a young doctor in a thigh-length white lab coat and black pumps. Varlamova's drab exam room is a world away from Knip's gleaming lab in Helsinki. It's equipped with a plug-in space heater and particleboard desk. Wilted potted plants sit next to an open window. In a long corridor outside are wood benches filled with exhausted-looking parents and children edging toward tears.

Varlamova is clear-eyed about the differences between Russian Karelia and Finland. "Karelia is poorer," she says, "there's no hysterical cleaning of apartments and a lot more physical activity."

Conducting the study in Russia has been a struggle, she says. While extra attention from doctors encourages Finnish and Estonian parents to participate, that's not the case in Russia. Babies here are already required to visit a pediatrician once a month in the first year of life, more often than in Finland. Enrolling young children has also been challenging. Since 2008, doctors have seen 1,575 children in Es-poo, a suburb of Helsinki; 1,681 have been sampled in Estonia, where the diabetes rate falls between that of Finland and of Russian Karelia. But after three years, researchers had recruited only 320 Russian children.

"People don't need more time with the doctor," Varlamova tells me softly in Russian. "They're not as motivated to take part in scientific investigations. They have more important problems in their life."

Then there's the Russian bureaucracy. All the samples taken for the study have to be analyzed in the same Finnish lab for consistency. But just as Knip's study was taking shape, Russian legislators passed a law requiring special permission to export human tissue

samples. (Some lawmakers argued that foreigners might use the samples to develop biological weapons targeting Russians.) As a result, Varlamova explains, thousands of study samples from Petrozavodsk had to be individually reviewed by three ministries, including the dauntingly named Federal Agency for the Legal Protection of Military, Special, and Dual-Use Intellectual Property, before being exported. Finally, though, samples going all the way back to 2008 and filling two industrial freezers crossed the border into Finland last December, along with a 30-pound stack of paperwork.

Early results are pointing to different immune system challenges during infancy in the study regions. Russian children, Knip says, spend the first years of their lives fighting off a host of infections virtually unknown in Finland. The Russian kids, as other studies have shown, have signs of regular exposure to hepatitis A, the parasite Toxoplasma gondii and the stomach bug Helicobacter pylori. "Helicobacter pylori antibodies are 15 times more common in children in Russian Karelia than in Finland," says Knip. "We did expect more microbial infections. But we didn't expect such a huge difference."

Identifying important differences may lead to a Type 1 diabetes prevention strategy, for kids in Finland and the rest of the developed world. "If one could identify specific microbes, you'd have to consider whether you could expose children—in a safe way—to those microbes," Knip says.

Such an intervention could prime the immune system much like a vaccine but might use a collection of bacteria rather than a specific microbe.

Knip's in a hurry to find out: Living laboratories don't last forever. Von Mutius, for her part, says she might have missed her chance to prove her hypothesis that crowded daycare centers, not pollution, protected kids in East Germany. Leipzig's coal pits have been flooded and turned into lakes ringed with beaches and bike paths. "We cannot go back—the East and West German phenomenon will remain an enigma," von Mutius says.

In Russia, Karelia's living standards, though they lag behind those in the most developed nations, have been rising slowly—alongside cases of Type 1 diabetes, celiac disease, hay fever, and asthma.

If Knip and his team can identify the culprits soon enough, perhaps Karelia, and other developing regions, can enjoy the upsides of modernity without some of the disorders that have accompanied economic advancement elsewhere in the world.

Kids with a lot of older brothers and sisters had lower rates of hay fever and eczema, probably because the siblings brought home colds, flus, and other germs.

Sometimes, the immune system overreacts to things that it should simply ignore, like cat dander, eggs, peanuts, or pollen. And sometimes the immune system turns on the body itself.

"People don't need more time with the doctor. They're not as motivated to take part in scientific investigations. They have more important problems in their life."

A poorly trained immune system may overreact to allergens such as pollen.

Critical Thinking

1. Because better hygiene has improved health overall, why should we consider increasing exposure to dirt?

2. In what ways does the immune system respond to dirt and microbes in childhood?

Create Central

www.mhhe.com/createcentral

Internet References

American Academy of Allergy, Asthma, and Immunology
http://www.aaaai.org/conditions-and-treatments/allergies.aspx

National Institutes of Health
http://www.ncbi.nlm.nih.gov/pubmed/15167035

Andrew Curry, "The Secret Life of Dirt: At the Finnish-Russian Border, Scientists Investigate a Medical Mystery" from *Smithsonian* (April 2013): 40–45.

Article   Prepared by: Eileen L. Daniel, *SUNY Brockport*

The Broken Vaccine

Whooping cough is on the rise, exposing a worrisome trend: The vaccine that holds it in check is losing its potency, and nobody is sure why.

MELINDA WENNER MOYER

Learning Outcomes

After reading this article, you will be able to:

- Explain why the pertussis vaccine is losing its effectiveness.

- Describe how the Centers for Disease Control and Prevention tracks outbreaks and epidemics.

- Discuss why there is an increase in the number of pertussis cases in the United States since the 1990s.

Seth Fikkert had a head cold. The 30-year-old worked in a hospital and had two kids, so he didn't think much of it. But after three weeks, he still felt short of breath, and his 2-year-old son was coughing a little, too.

Fikkert, who resembles Jim from the NBC television show *The Office* in both his boyish good looks and his sharp sense of humor (he jokes about the mispronunciations his last name inspires), lived in Everett, Washington, which last summer was in the midst of one of the country's most serious whooping cough epidemics. So he thought it best to get tested.

"I just wanted to rule it out," Fikkert says. He had gotten his adult booster for pertussis, the bacterium that causes whooping cough, only a year before, so it was highly unlikely that he had the infection. On the morning of Thursday, June 28, he walked into the employee health clinic at Providence Regional Medical Center, where he worked, and asked for a test.

The clinic did not take his concern lightly. Fikkert recalls that afterward, "they masked me up, sent me down for a Z-Pak [the antibiotic Zithromax] at the pharmacy, and sent me directly home."

And for good reason: Four days later, Fikkert learned he had tested positive. "It was a huge surprise," he says. His daughter also tested positive; his son tested negative, though if a test is administered more than two weeks after symptoms arise, it may yield a false negative. To keep the infection from spreading, the hospital and the local health department in Snohomish County gave antibiotics to 35 hospital patients and 77 employees that Fikkert had been in close contact with over the 28 days before his diagnosis, despite the fact that almost all of the staff had had boosters.

Before pertussis vaccines came into use in the 1930s, the infection killed about 4,000 Americans (mostly infants) a year—10 times as many as the number of people who died annually from measles and 12 times more than died from smallpox.

Although infection rates dropped dramatically with the vaccine, pertussis has recently returned with dangerous fervor: 2012 was the country's worst year for pertussis since 1959, with more than 38,000 cases reported nationally, 16 deaths of infants and children, and large spikes in every state except California. Most health officials believe that because many cases go undetected, the actual infection numbers are far higher. Pertussis is now considered the most poorly controlled vaccine-preventable bacterial disease in the developed world.

The resurgence is not the fault of parents who haven't immunized their kids. "We don't think those exemptors are driving this current wave," Anne Schuchat, director of the National Center for Immunization and Respiratory Diseases at the Centers for Disease Control and Prevention (CDC), told reporters at a July press briefing.

Indeed, 73 percent of kids aged 7 to 10 who caught pertussis last year in Washington State—where the infection hit particularly hard—had been fully vaccinated. And 81 percent of adolescents had not only had full childhood vaccinations, but also a booster shot.

The problem is the pertussis vaccine itself. In 1992, U.S. doctors began switching to a new formulation with fewer side effects. But the CDC, which monitors infectious disease outbreaks, is learning the hard way that it just doesn't work very well. "It wanes, and it wanes more quickly than we expected," says CDC epidemiologist Stacey Martin. Scientists are trying hard to find out why.

In the meantime, more than 228 million Americans—some kids and teens, as well as most adults—think that they are protected from whooping cough, but they are not.

Pertussis is caused by *bordetella pertussis,* a bacterium that has been around for at least 400 years. The microbes attach to tiny, hairlike structures in the lungs and release toxins that cause a terrible and persistent cough. Every outburst projects live bacteria into the air, and anyone within three feet can breathe them in and become infected.

Often the relentless hacking causes people to throw up, or to have so much trouble catching their breath that they make a "whooping" sound while inhaling. Antibiotics stop a person from being contagious but do not always ease symptoms.

Babies younger than 3 months are particularly vulnerable. They can suffocate because of the cough, and since their immune systems are undeveloped, their white blood cells can spike so high that they literally clog the veins, obstructing blood flow and causing cardiovascular problems. Babies get their first pertussis vaccine at 2 months, but it provides only a small amount of protection.

Prior to 1992, children in the United States were inoculated with whole-cell pertussis vaccines, which were made using whole killed bacteria. These were quite effective but often caused side effects like local swelling, fevers, and, in rare instances, neurological problems.

That year, the CDC began recommending a new vaccine that contained two to five proteins isolated from *B. pertussis* rather than the entire bacterium. While these acellular vaccines, as they are called, cause fewer side effects, they do not seem to last very long.

In 2010 California experienced a particularly devastating pertussis outbreak that sickened 9,000 people and killed 10 babies. At the time, David Witt, an infectious disease specialist at Kaiser Permanente Medical Center in San Rafael, assumed that most of the infected kids were unvaccinated; the very first patient he treated, for instance, was from a non-vaccinating family.

To confirm his suspicions, Witt assigned a project to his son, a University of California, Berkeley, public health major who was home for the Christmas holiday: Check the vaccination records of all of the kids the medical center had treated so far that year.

"The original impetus was just to show how virulent an effect not being vaccinated has," Witt explains. Instead, Witt's son found that whooping cough rates were not significantly different in vaccinated, unvaccinated and undervaccinated children between the ages of 8 and 12.

Kids typically finish their initial vaccine series between ages 4 and 6, and the results suggested that protection starts to wane three years later—a big problem, considering that they don't get another shot until they're 11 or 12. "It's awfully worrisome," Witt says.

In November 2012, the CDC announced the results of its own analysis of the California outbreak. The agency found that the vaccine's effectiveness begins to drop after one year, and that five years after the final dose, it provides only 70 percent protection. An Australian study recently reported that kids who were given the acellular vaccine as infants were more than three times as likely to get pertussis between 2009 and 2011 than were those who received the whole-cell version.

No one knows why the acellular vaccine is so ineffective. It exposes the immune system to only a handful of bacterial proteins, and it may be that exposure to more—as occurred when people were inoculated with the whole-cell vaccine—is more powerful. But the CDC's Martin notes that the United States will probably never use the whole cell vaccine again because of concerns about its possible side effects.

Frits Mooi, a molecular microbiologist at the Centre for Infectious Disease Control in the Netherlands, has a controversial theory about the acellular version: The pertussis bacteria may have adapted to it, much like bacteria become resistant to antibiotics.

Mooi sequenced the genomes of today's *B. pertussis* strains and found they have acquired mutations in each of the proteins used to make the acellular vaccines. This means, he says, that our immune systems are being primed to fight an attacker that is slightly different from what they actually encounter. While Martin agrees that the vaccine does not precisely match today's circulating strains, she says it is unclear whether this mismatch is actually causing the observed vaccine failure.

Jean Zahalka, a soft-spoken public health nurse with shortly cropped gray hair, sat in a small office at the headquarters of the Snohomish Health District, conducting a phone interview with the mother of a 7-month-old baby who had just been diagnosed with whooping cough.

Luckily, the little boy didn't attend daycare, which meant that he hadn't had many opportunities to infect others. And despite his persistent cough, he was holding up well, possibly because he'd already had two doses of DTaP, the childhood vaccine for diphtheria, tetanus, and pertussis.

But then the mom told Zahalka that the boy's 3-year-old sister was also coughing. Zahalka winced. Next, it came to light that the mother's 14-year-old niece had spent three days with the family earlier that week, which meant she was probably infected as well. The niece's mother had just lost her job and could not afford to buy antibiotics, so the health department was going to have to cover the cost of her treatment in order to curb the spread of the infection.

As health departments across the country are coming to learn, it is extremely difficult to monitor and control pertussis outbreaks. For one thing, many cases go undetected. "We're reporting just the tip of the iceberg," says Sandi Paciotti, communicable disease manager at the Skagit County Health Department, which tallied the most pertussis cases in Washington State in 2012. Paciotti estimates that three to five times more people have been infected than are reflected in her official numbers.

One reason is that 15 percent of the Skagit County population is uninsured and unwilling to pay for the $300 test. Teens are another overlooked pertussis reservoir; the director of the Skagit County Health Department, Peter Browning, says his 13-year-old son caught pertussis early in the outbreak, but since he had been immunized, Browning didn't suspect it. "We don't stop loving our kids after age 13, but we don't rush them to the doctor, either," he says.

The vaccine's effectiveness begins to drop after one year. Five years after the final dose, it provides only 70 percent protection.

There are probably also thousands of adults who have suffered through the infection without seeking treatment. Adults who have been vaccinated, like Fikkert, often have milder symptoms, but they are still contagious. Some do go to the doctor but only after they have been sick for several weeks, at which point the test can come back negative even if they had the infection. And some doctors do not even consider pertussis when adults come in complaining of a persistent cough. "They don't think adults can get it," the CDC's Martin says.

With an infection so difficult to control, the best hope is prevention. But a better vaccine may be years, if not decades, away. "We just don't know what we should be targeting," says Martin, pointing out that no one knows what parts of the bacterium should be included in the vaccine to make it more effective.

Scott Halperin, the director of the Canadian Center for Vaccinology in Halifax, believes that changing the immune-boosting chemicals, called adjuvants, in the vaccine could make a difference. Camille Locht, a microbiologist at Inserm and Institut Pasteur de Lille in France, is developing a live vaccine for newborns; he says it could give infants enough protection to survive until they get their childhood series, but so far he has tested the vaccine only in adults.

The CDC began recommending a tetanus, diphtheria, and pertussis (Tdap) booster shot for most people over age 11, including adults up to age 64, in 2005. But as of 2010, only 8 percent of the adult population had actually received one. Moreover, an ongoing CDC investigation suggests that, like the childhood vaccine, the adult Tdap booster lasts only a few years at most.

Yet with the exception of childbearing women, who are advised to get the booster during every pregnancy, Tdap is licensed only for one-time use in adults. "That probably isn't enough," says Amie Tidrington, the immunization clinic manager for the Skagit County Health Department.

Still, it is crucial to vaccinate as many people as possible, says Gary Goldbaum, the health officer of the Snohomish Health District in Everett. Unprotected people are much less likely to encounter the infection if most of the population is protected. Despite a slew of recent funding cuts, Goldbaum's district has held 20 vaccination clinics since the outbreaks started.

Last spring the American Congress of Obstetricians and Gynecologists sent pertussis information packets to more than 33,000 of its members to increase awareness among doctors, and a joint program between the AmeriCares charity and pharmaceutical company Sanofi-Pasteur has given more than 117,000 free Tdap booster shots to health clinics around the country to immunize uninsured, low-income families. "If we are serious about trying to protect the most vulnerable," Goldbaum says, "the rest of us have to be fully protected too."

Critical Thinking

1. Why is the number of cases of pertussis increasing?
2. How does the Centers for Disease Control and Prevention track disease outbreaks and epidemics?

Create Central

www.mhhe.com/createcentral

Internet References

Centers for Disease Control and Prevention
cdc.gov

National Institute of Allergy and Infectious Diseases (NIAID)
www3.niaid.nih.gov

Article Prepared by: Eileen L. Daniel, *SUNY College at Brockport*

No Exit

50 Percent of people will develop some form of dementia by their eighty-fifth birthday. 76 Million people by 2030. It is the illness that will define our times. How are we going to get through this?

KENT RUSSELL

Learning Outcomes

After reading this article, you will be able to:

- Explain the societal costs related to Alzheimer's disease.

- Describe the symptoms of Alzheimer's disease.

- Understand the difficulties faced by those who care for Alzheimer's patients.

Try as we do, us Americans still croak. One and all, somehow, even today. We are done in by ten likely suspects: heart disease, cancer, stroke, diabetes, nephritis, and suicide. Yet we can and do fight these things. We have working cures, preventive regimens, ways to halt the damage for all of these commonest causes of death. All of them, that is, save one.

Alzheimer's disease is practically unheard of in adults younger than 40, and very rare (one in 2,500) for those under 60. It affects 1 percent of 65-year-olds, 2 percent of 68-year-olds, and 3 percent of 70-year-olds. After that, the odds start multiplying. The likelihood of your developing Alzheimer's more or less doubles every five years past 65. Should you make it to 85, you will have, roughly, a fifty-fifty shot at remaining sane.

Eighty-five, though! That's infinity-and-a-day away. Except that, by 2030, the population of Americans aged 65 and over also will have doubled. At that point, the number of people suffering from Alzheimer's or related dementias around the world is expected to hit 76 million. Twenty years after that, in 2050, the number will be 135 million, including new cases in rapidly modernizing places like China and sub-Saharan Africa. The cost of their care in this country alone is projected to hit $1 trillion per annum, inflation not included.

There's nothing new about aging. But Alzheimer's is not simply a by-product of old age. It is a degenerative brain disease, a fatal one. A degenerative brain disease that almost exclusively targets people who, prior to the twentieth century, were demographic anomalies.

In 1900, about 4 percent of the U.S. population was older than 65. Today, 90 percent of all babies born in the developed world will live past that age. Barring a miracle cure, or some kind of *Stand*-esque superfluenza, dementia will become *the public health crisis of our* time. A late interpolation into the shared story of human existence.

So far in the future, my guy! you might say. Who knows what medical science will cook up in the meantime? Anyway, I've seen the movies; I remember the dad from The Corrections. I know how this story plays out.

To the former bit of rhetoric, about the future: very true. A breakthrough *may* come. To the latter statements, about artistic representation—that all is great! It is great that the specter of Alzheimer's disease (in particular) and dementia (in general) is beginning to ghost around our culture.

But this trickle of Alzheimer's narratives will one day be an inundation. And, already, it's ossifying into a genre. We know what to expect in a dementia tale: The devastated spouse, say, whose husband of 60 years flinches fearfully whenever she wipes at his mouth. Or else the pampered (if not little loved) child who comes of age while overseeing what age has ravaged.

I could tell you any number of such true stories. I could tell you about one or another patient at Isabella Geriatric Center in north Manhattan, which I frequented when I lived a few blocks up the street. I could tell you about the mute, smiling seniors I met on a reporting trip to Hogewey, the pioneering dementia facility just outside of Amsterdam. I could tell you my own story, about the three family members who metamorphosed into jabbering Lears before my eyes.

The thing about these stories—compelling as they can be—is that they tend to work against themselves. They have a dampening effect. Emerging from one, you feel a little stupefied, and bone-tired, as though you yourself have just swum through six feet of cemetery dirt. The reading or viewing experience is not only harrowing, grievous—truly *scary*—but also inconsequential, in a way.

Scary because dementia creates what should not be: mindless persons. Mindless, selfless, unreasonable creatures, somehow still looking like human beings. We see a metaphysical incompatibility in them, and it is deeply unsettling. They might as well be headless bodies, up and shambling around.

Inconsequential because, for all their pathos, each dementia story comes across as an individual tragedy. You read it or watch it or hear about it, and you might fear something similar happening to you, but you can't really *imagine* such a thing ever happening to you. Literally—dementia is unimaginable. We can't put ourselves in the place of the demented; we can't wrap our minds around what it must be like to lose your mind. Instead, you and me, storytelling animals that we are—we invent confident memories of our future.

And then, of course, it happens to us.

There is no cure, preventive regimen, or way to halt the damage of Alzheimer's. Right now, the only means for change lie within *us:* how we conceive of the illness, how we think of the afflicted. So many people are going to have to live with this dehumanizing disease! How do we make sure that they are able to do so with dignity, compassion? The importance of this question cannot be overstated. How are we going to accommodate the least of us—and those tasked with their care—once they become so many?

Well. Here I will humbly suggest that, before we put down this magazine to blanch the kale, swallow the softgel fish oil (mercury-free), and retreat further into the crenelated abbeys of our hotyoga bodies—we entertain a thought experiment.

Your correspondent in this story is a youngish guy, not terribly old, maybe your same age. He, too, lives in the city and bounces around creative industries doing real au courant, new-economy-type stuff. Freelance graphic design, Web development, and all manner of "content creation." A guy who, once upon a time, preferred not to work a full-time job. Who is now getting his demented old man ready for a journey.

Come on, he's saying. He's using two fingers to stretch the folds of his old man's skin. With his other hand, he's running a razor down his neck. The abrasive sibilance calls to mind shuffleboard pucks, or skateboards on sidewalks.

Remember when you finally bought me that short board? he asks his old man. *And I cracked my tailbone within the hour?*

The old man's isn't a thousand-yard stare; it stretches past that, barren and edgeless. Searching it makes your correspondent's own eyes desperate.

He can no longer rely on his old man to change clothes, much less shave. Hygiene is too overwhelming for him. It involves too many steps: shed the garments, turn the tap, spread the lather, blot the blood, open the drawer, match the socks, and tie the tie. The last time he was left to his own devices, the old man slept in his same outfit far days, overripening.

The shaving finished, your correspondent steers his old man into one of the apartment's bedrooms, where clothes have been laid on a bed. He picks up a pair of looser-fitting jeans and says, *OK, sit at the foot for me.* [Misting through the old man's head is a lingual vapor that cannot condense into the phrase, *I don't know how to act—I've never been here before.*]

Do you want to wear your flannel shirt? your correspondent wonders. *Or maybe the vintage Starter jacket you thought was so cool?*

Cool, the old man manages. *Too cool.* Your correspondent dusts off a little smile for him, then turns away. Out the window, he sees snow sifting in wet, neuronal clumps. He hears his super scraping the front steps. You're right, he says. *We'll put you in something heavier.*

The old man scoots to the lip of the mattress, but when the jeans start sliding up his legs, he paws languidly at your correspondent's head. *Frankly,* he says, buffeting the younger man with crepey palms. *Frankly. I took my eyes off of you, and a steep street. You went down.*

Some days he'd be so normal that your correspondent was guilty of thinking, *Could it be that he really isn't...?* But then he'd come home and find the old man attempting to repair the toaster oven, which wasn't broken but *was* plugged in, saying, *Call her and tell her to bring home salami for hot sandwiches,* his eyes flickering like bulbs half screwed in. The truth was that whenever your correspondent became the slightest bit comfortable with the condition, his old man took the next stumble along the downhill progression of his disease.

For his sake, your correspondent has: blocked the radiators; removed the knobs from the oven, stove, and front door; hidden a baby monitor in the spare bedroom; and remodeled the bathroom in blue and yellow. (His old man's vision has deteriorated to the point where he has trouble differentiating between objects that don't contrast. When the toilet, sink, and tub were all white … mistakes were made.) Rock bottom was when your correspondent hastily painted his bedroom door-handle, hinges, and all-the same cream color as the surrounding wall, so that, should he need a moment to himself, he could drop out.

Your correspondent isn't one to complain. But honestly, this was some horseshit. He had been robbed of his leisure time (*hard to find a pro-bono sitter*), his peace of mind (*turn your head, and he's off on another obscure mission*), his savings (*Medicare doesn't cover this*), nearly all of his rest (*old man naps in the day and then rises at night, reanimated*), and any visitors or well-wishers (*they're too politely embarrassed*). He has ordered a cable package for the first time in 15 years, for a periscope's view of the outside world. He reaches for words like *millstone* while making too much eye contact with delivery guys. He feels himself devolving into a cipher, a nonentity, by the day, hour, minute.

Buttoning his old man up, turning down his collar, your correspondent sees something scintillate in his face. [*What did I do that this guy's so pissed at me?*] Maybe cognizance, he thinks, though probably not. [*Kill 'em with kindness,* his old man recalls, and so decides to beam.] At this smile, your correspondent very nearly loses it.

A fiancé, some kids, a blossoming creative life—dreams deferred. Would that this grinning life-leach perceived *anything* about the money and man-hours and future he was bleeding dry. Your correspondent wasn't even free enough to fear that he was missing out.

OK, stand up, he says. *We've got a plane to catch.*

S now is falling fast, lending the narrow street a confettied depth. Your correspondent made sure to leave five hours before their flight, plenty of time. The Internet said the precipitation will have stopped by then. Right now, though, it is a velvet crunch underfoot. Leading his old man carefully by the hip, your correspondent grasps just how much thinner he has become. Were he to give him a squeeze, his old man might keen like bagpipes.

As they come to the broad avenue, the old man points to the brown, tire-treaded snow that has been churned atop the pure white. [*Crumb cake,* he envisages. An associative flipbook of memories flitters past: *Entenmann's. Dad allowed one piece after dinner. The last dinner party. Friends gestured to shake, but their palms were lost in space. Blankness where names should be. Faces, too. As blank as clocks without hands.*]

Where is everyone? the old man asks as harried pedestrians flow around them in the crosswalk. *Where's dad? Did he get out?*

Your correspondent sighs deeply, applying a bellows to his spirit. He has learned not to correct him. *Reality orientation,* the literature calls it. It was one of the more popular care strategies, up until the 1990s. *No, Mr. Jones, it's not 1984. See the calendar? Your father couldn't have just visited; he's been dead for years.* Gradually, it dawned on oft-bitten caretakers that this practice

was quite upsetting to the demented—and more than a little sadistic. Getting the rug pulled out from under you á la Charlton Heston at the end of *Planet of the Apes?* With all the attendant anguish and disbelief? Imagine. Also, imagine forgetting that it ever happened, and then experiencing it anew, day in and out.

Instead, your correspondent says, *They're in Amsterdam, waiting for us. It's supposed to be in the mid-fifties there! Not bad, eh?*

[The old man offers a response—and thinks it came out OK—but sees on the face of the other guy that not one word was understood. This other guy, he resembles the old man—the old man of a few years ago, at least—and is speaking to him now, but the old man is not sure which language he's using.] *Take the steps slow,* your correspondent is telling him as they duck into the subway station. *Real widow-makers, these.* [The old man looks up at him with lamblike credulity in his eyes. He has no choice but to believe he is being led somewhere in good faith.]

They stand far from the platform edge. As a train approaches, the old man squints into the false gale. He looks like none of a father, husband, or son; rather, a boy standing at the edge of a nighttime forest, listening.

Corroded brakes screech. Doors thump open.

T he floor of the crowded train is wet and whorled with shoeprints. Seated between two strangers, the old man holds his ears while dragging a foot through the muck.

Your correspondent is hanging from a bar across the aisle, watching. Perhaps he could be forgiven for failing to identify the beginning. That was what unnerved him most about Alzheimer's: Its onset was as insidious as a haunting's.

Whenever he had visited his old man at *his* apartment (long since sold to fund the visiting nurse, occupational therapist, medication, moisture-proof pads, petroleum jelly…) in the years before diagnosis, your correspondent had found that, although a little softer and browner at the edges, his old man appeared fresh enough. Sometimes he couldn't find his glasses, or the linen closet, but so what—who wasn't seized by fleeting moments of confusion every now and then? When he spent whole afternoons trying to recall just which word he wished to say, your correspondent chalked it up to advanced age, "senior moments." Even as the slipups became more egregious—a coffee can full of urine, the stereo remote hidden and half-melted in the oven—your correspondent ascribed them to flu, or a bad night's sleep, or the general way in which the world spins faster and faster until those who used to be a part of it got separated, like sediment in a centrifuge.

All that time, the old man volunteered nothing about his loosening grip on reality. He was the kind of guy who prided himself on control—over himself, his emotions—and the incremental loss of it had been a continual shock to him. More and more frequently, he was confounded by what had been routine.

The subway, for instance. One day, he rode past his stop on the F train. When he couldn't remember which he'd gotten on at, or what the announced names meant, or even why he was there to begin with, he rode the train end to end for many hours, a complete stranger to himself. A station manager noticed him wandering at one terminus; all the old man could manage by way of explanation was, *I fear I am not in my right mind.*

After that, he would sometimes go months without incident or outage. Until—very suddenly—he would feel as if he'd woken from another in a long string of concussions. He was conscious but dumbstruck then, trapped in the space between words. He wouldn't know whom he was talking to, or he couldn't follow their line of questioning. He groped his way through social situations by relying on inference, body language. Amazing, what he was able to read from the lines in a forehead or the corners of a mouth. But the walls closed in. Scared of outing himself, he became quiet, still.

And he never dared think "Alzheimer's," much less say it out loud. Saying its name might make it real.

When the evidence of his old man's altered state finally became irrefutable, your correspondent booked a long trip to a cabin in the woods, just the two of them. He hoped maybe to stir up the residue of happier times: rocks skipped, talks had, and skillets scrubbed with sand. But during one squally night, your correspondent looked through a window and proclaimed, *Raining cats and dogs outside.* His old man—who had been sitting in cobwebbed silence throughout the preceding afternoon—jumped from his armchair as if electrically jolted. He rushed your correspondent, nodded into his face, and stormed out of the cabin's front door, the wind spitting leaves and rain behind him. Your correspondent had never been so spooked. It was as though, this entire time, he'd been vacationing not with his old man, but a doppelgänger.

It took him weeks to realize: His old man hadn't heard a *sentence.* He'd heard a string of individual *words* and had taken his cue from the last one.

Dementia itself is not a disease but a set of symptoms; a syndrome, like Down or Asperger's. It is a spectrum of traits and behaviors that together suggest the presence of some underlying malady. There are more than 70 known triggers, but Alzheimer's disease accounts for about 70 percent of all cases.

Despite their many working hypotheses, scientists have yet to confirm a single theory that proves where Alzheimer's comes from, or why. The disease seems to have sprung itself from deep within the human architecture, a curse written over the door to our last, hitherto unexplored chamber.

Some advocate for the cholinergic hypothesis, which supposes that Alzheimer's is caused by the reduced synthesis of a neurotransmitter called acetylcholine. Alternatively, there's the tau hypothesis, which posits that abnormalities in the brain's tau protein end up dismantling neurons' transport systems, loosing Alzheimer's in the process. Some say Herpes simplex plays a role; others, an age-related breakdown of myelin, the brain's electric insulation. Some researchers are taking a closer look at what air pollution might be doing to trigger the disease. Silver dental fillings, the crackpots say. If not flu shots. Or aspartame. Or aluminum cookware.

Long before the old man's forgetting had begun, Alzheimer's disease was there in his brain, lying in wait. Specifically, it was in his hippocampus, where it had sprouted. There, it germinated for who knows how long—years, maybe decades. Slowly, imperceptibly, it began to slither its way through and around his neurons and synapses, this ooze of dense, extracellular material. It coiled across his gray matter like kudzu, the invasive vine that kills as it spreads, obscuring the sun.

The farther that Alzheimer's disease advanced into the old man's hippocampus, the more his memory formation began to falter. There came relatively stable periods in his decline—plateaus—but Alzheimer's disease is relentless and irreversible. In time, he was locked into the burning library of his existing memories.

The disease wreathed his limbic system, then wormed its way into the temporal, parietal, and frontal lobes of his cerebral cortex. From his temporal lobes—just inside his ears on either side of his brain—the disease took away his ability to fully process sensory input. Now, he sometimes heard or saw… *things.* Hallucinations.

He also began to ask your correspondent, *Who are you? What are you doing in my house?* This wasn't a problem of memory. He hadn't forgotten. But when he beheld your correspondent, the image he saw did not match the contours of the image he knew. Agnosia is the term.

From the parietal lobes on the top of his brain, the kudzu wrecked his ability to comprehend physical contact. Touch, pain, and spatial awareness lost what meaning they used to have. The old man had never been a particularly affectionate person—he treated his body like a fish tank, no tapping on the glass—but as the disease stole over him, he began to act as though he'd ingested an empathogenic drug, Ecstasy or some such. He sought out rough, pebbled surfaces to run his hands over. He sometimes allowed your correspondent's touch to linger and would shift his body into it, like a cat. He seemed to be looking for friction.

When the kudzu crept into his amygdala, he began to lose control over his baser emotions—fear, anger, and yearning. There came new, startling outbursts in response to non-events. Occasional crying jags. These, from the man who used to sigh neutrally when he hammered a thumbnail black, were more than alarming. [*You think I'm goddamn nuts,* he wished to say then. *But if you were getting what I'm getting here, you'd be doing likewise.*]

The disease has reached as far as his frontal lobes, which house the brain's system of retrieval. Previously, when he ran memories through this system, they were made clearer and more concrete by the reproductions. The paradox was that remembering reinforced the memories; remembering created copies that *gained* detail. As things are now, though, the old man can't replicate his remaining memories. He can't even rake through the deep ash of those already consumed by the disease.

The frontal lobes are also where his brain compares and contrasts the continuous flow of *what's happening now with what's happened before.* Because his frontal lobes have very little left to check against, the old man's will—his very sense of himself—is vanishing. His crutches and quick fixes have already come to naught. He can't program reminders into his phone anymore. He isn't sure what a phone *is.* And the explanatory Post-its your correspondent slapped on every household item—they frighten him. He doesn't see letters; he sees squiggles writhing across yellow.

Soon, the present will simply pass through him, unencumbered, like wind through a bare tree.

But that doesn't mean the disease will stop. Once the plaques and tangles have reached the depths of his brain that control gross motor function, he will be susceptible to *retrogenesis,* a return to infancy observed in many late-stage Alzheimer's patients. The physical capabilities he picked up over the course of his life will be undone in the reverse order in which they were acquired. He will lose the ability to walk, to stand, to even straighten his legs to the ground. His eyes will no longer focus, and his newborn reflexes will reemerge. At this point, if someone were to tickle the soles of his feet, he'd raise his big toes and spread the others outward, a phenomenon known as the Babinski sign, common only to infants younger than six months and the terminally demented.

Finally, his body will begin to shut down. The last in his long series of deaths. The old man's extremities will leach heat and grow unresponsive. Complete incontinence will set in. His skin will lose all elasticity and become like wax paper wrapped around butcher bones. He will experience no hunger, thirst, or apparent consciousness as he drifts off in the third person. At his bedside, your correspondent will watch for more infrequent spouts of breath. The immediate cause of death might be a complicating condition like pneumonia, dehydration, or infection. But it's Alzheimer's that will kill him.

In booking this trip, your correspondent discovered that direct fares from New York City to Amsterdam are indefensibly expensive. The most reasonable ticket would see them travel first to Moscow before continuing on to the Netherlands. There, they would visit Hogewey, the Oz-like dementia facility that is pined after in chain e-mail after chain e-mail exchanged by caregivers the world over.

It was all irresponsible and ill-advised, traveling with his old man. Your correspondent understood that. But he also understood the last-ditch logic that compels one to thrust a baby through an embassy gate, or onto a lap in a whirring helicopter—the logic that prefers uncertainty to the end that's encroaching.

[*Calm. Remaining calm is the thing to do here,* the old man concludes, glancing around the jetliner's cabin. *Hurtling. That is the word for what this thingy is doing.*] *I'll try not to stop in the middle and …* He tries again. *Sometimes I stop right in the middle. And I get … can't get on … what you need to tell me … big hand … the thingy?* [*How long will this hurtling last, young man?* he wants to know.]

I told you, we're going to a special place, your correspondent answers. He hadn't mentioned this trip to anyone else. He didn't know what he would've said if he had. That he was hoping these Dutch miracle workers would take pity on him and his old man? That they would lower the bridge, grant sanctuary? All he knew was the two of them didn't have a lot of time left. What else was he supposed to do? Hide his old man in the apartment until he hit his expiration date? *We'll be there soon enough,* he adds.

When … to home? the old man asks, stiffening in his seat. [*I want to go home.*]

Unconsciously, your correspondent runs through the conditionals of his caregiver's if/then programming:

If out of nowhere his old man whimpers, "I don't want to die!" *Then he* probably means, "I feel sick, though I don't feel pain. I feel this way all the time, so I must be dying."

If he ransacks the apartment one day before dawn, accusing: "You! You stole my money, you son of a bitch!" *Then* he most likely wants to say, "I used to carry a wallet. I used to be able to support myself. I've become shamefully dependent, and I don't understand how."

If he grows as taut as a string before it snaps, and mentions "home," *then* he might be thinking, "I wish I could return to the time when I had a past, and an identity, and a purpose, and a place."

Your correspondent pats his old man's hand before settling in his seat and dinging the ding for a mini Glenlivet. A dour Russian stewardess arrives, spinning down foil trays of carp and taking no drink orders. Your correspondent spends the next ten minutes plucking wee bones from the filet, paring it into bite-sized wedges. It has been a while since his old man ate his last solid meal. If there's more than one texture in his mouth, he doesn't know whether to chew or swallow.

Elbows tucked in, wrists bent, utensils prodding *ever so delicately* around the tray, he pictures a Tyrannosaurus trying to defuse a bomb.

Your correspondent had packed a couple Alzheimer's memoirs for the flight, but he couldn't bring himself to read them. What bothered him about these tales—almost always written from the point of view of the caregiver—was how invariably they turned into horror stories. The memoirist loves someone deeply, thinks of that person as unbreakably bound to him … until, one day, he discovers that this person might not be who he thought.

Usually, what follows is a painstaking reconstruction of the psychological gauntlet endured by the memoirist. The inversion of his life; the day-by-day descent into a personal hell. Meanwhile, the mask of his formerly loved one slips little by little until the big reveal: wife/mom/bubby is no more. In her place is a pod person, a boogieman who doesn't care about the memoirist, may even mean him harm.

What's taken for granted in these stories is the conclusion that a demented person is *dead,* or at least the *living dead.* So the main drama then—as in any zombie flick—centers on the living, how they're managing to survive. The *real* victims here are the caregivers.

Rather than one of those, your correspondent cracks a new care guide, something with a beach-ready title like *The Misery of Inertia.* It, like all the literature, begs the reader to please, *please* look into nursing homes before the real bad dementia symptoms emerge. Like, the moment you begin to suspect that your loved one might have Alzheimer's? Look into a goddamned nursing home. Good facilities require you to get on a waiting list years in advance. If you don't—if you wait until you have to find a place for your loved one *right now*—you'll have to take what's available.

Some months back, your correspondent decided to do just that, check out the closest eldercare facility in the city.

When the elevator doors opened onto the eighth floor dementia ward, the funk that greeted him and his old man was not exactly offensive; it had the zoological tang of a petting farm. The ward was shaped like a serif T, with two wings of rooms branching off of a hallway that led to an activity center. Only the ambulatory demented were allowed here. As soon as a patient stopped moving, he or she was hustled off the ward, which was euphemized as "the neighborhood."

Your correspondent had to drag his old man off the elevator. Black mats had been placed in front of its doors, and to his (and any potential defectors') compromised sensory system, the mats appeared to be bottomless pits.

The care strategy here—as at most U.S. nursing homes—was originally modeled after that of hospitals, in part because that's what reimbursement and regulatory policies supported. In a hospital, a patient arrives, waives his autonomy, gets put into an assless gown, gets treated, goes home. It's a short-term medical model with an emphasis on hierarchy, routine, and efficient but depersonalized care. Not all U.S. nursing homes retain this operational structure—just the more affordable ones. It is at odds with the needs of the demented.

On the eighth floor, almost every one of the three dozen patients was seated around a long table in the activity center. They arranged themselves like kids in a public school cafeteria—the Spanish speakers sat clustered around the left end, the one Korean woman was in the middle, and the black and white patients were on the right. At the English side of the room, "The Price is Right" was going unwatched on a flatscreen.

The patients came from all over the city and state, many transferred directly from hospitals. Prior to their admittance, their families or caregivers filled out a questionnaire on their behalf. They assigned numerical values to the patient's eating ability, mobility, and propensity for "disruptive, infantile, or socially inappropriate behavior." The surveys were not profiles or biographies; they were for streamlining care. The nurses often learned the most about these patients from their obituaries.

Well? your correspondent asked his old man. *What do you think?*

The old man took a seat at the table. [He had no recollection of the conduct that had led him to this place: the wandering, the masturbating, the repetitive questioning, and the tics. He did those things because they were all he could think to do to bridge the moment-by-moment emptiness that yawned before and behind him.]

Some time ago, it was as though a switch had been flipped in his head. Rather than despair over his evanescing abilities, the old man insisted that he was capable of caring for himself. This was one of the great ironies of his disease. He wasn't denying the reality of his situation—he honestly couldn't remember that he was demented. Gone was the humiliation of being a burden. Gone was the taint of that gravest of sins: curbing someone else's freedom. Gone was his vision of himself as a jettisoned space cadet, floating farther out of radio contact and into soft oblivion.

As he saw it, he was about the same age as the man sitting next to him. [A man in the prime of his life. He felt fine. A little groggy, maybe, like he'd had three beers on his way home. Which-why was he not on his way home?]

Of this place? your correspondent persisted. *You like it here?*

The old man stood up to get away from the question. He made it halfway down the hall before a nurse caught up to him. She cinched him around his thin arms and pushed him toward his seat. [He tried to blurt an objection, but doing so felt like running to hop a train that was just out of reach. He tried to hit her, but his hands were clamped to his sides.] Your correspondent watched a free-floating state of distress blow across his old man's face, one that would long outlive the memory of what had caused it.

After lunch—nurses in surgical masks gossiping with one another while scraping food into the mouths of the more derelict—came quiet time, which to your correspondent was indistinguishable from the non-quiet time that had preceded it, save for the lights got turned off. Patients fell asleep where they sat, casket-style, their heads canted back. Those who stayed awake put a hand to their mouth, or temple, or chin, and looked into the distance.

Every now and then a nurse came by and plucked a patient from her chair, taking her to the bathroom or for a walk around the ward. An orderly wheeled in a cart stacked with board games and magazines. He sat down, flipped through his phone, got up, and wheeled the cart away.

It was hard for your correspondent to keep in mind that, ostensibly, these were people's loved ones. *What're their families doing right now?* he wondered. *Where are they, what's so important that this becomes acceptable?*

He wanted to judge them. But he could sympathize. How long had he dreamt of planting his old man in a (tasteful, respectful) home? Ho ho, be honest. How often had he pictured himself pulling a *Risky Business,* except the song he's dancing to is "I'm Coming Out," and instead of a suburban Chicago home, the thing he's dancing through is his rehydrated life?

Your correspondent knew that such a day would come. It comes for every one of the eleven million Americans who homecare their demented relations. The first two-thirds of the disease's arc are grueling if manageable. But then your loved one stops speaking, eating, or recognizing sound. You strain after them, but there's as much "loved one" in your loved one as there is ocean in a conch shell. The literature is telling: Dementia caregivers frequently struggle with clinical depression, and they die at a rate 63 percent higher than their unburdened peers.

It ruined you, caregiving. Emotionally and financially. For eight or twelve or 20 years, you poured yourself into a cracked, empty vessel. And for what?

Because, as much as people invoke the Golden Rule and all that, devotion was not something your correspondent was particularly trained (or expected) to practice. It's maybe not the most attractive thing to admit, but there it is. Giving himself over to another? Spending *his* days helping someone else get through *theirs?* Babies, maybe, sure. But with babies you got that snowballing sense of pride and joy. You got to watch a consciousness *you created* (!) countenance beauty and fellowship; you got to blissfully track her individual flourishing. And if you didn't fuck it up too bad, maybe one day you got to see her become a respected venture capitalist, one of the philanthropical stripe, who will soon repay you with a sleek pleasure-craft or chalet. A warm Thanksgiving, at least.

[Though it's not like *this* was how the old man had imagined going out. He, like anyone, had hoped that his life would more resemble a stock chart. Occasional hiccups, yes, but those would be offset by continual record highs. A diagrammed staircase to heaven: fulfilling work, travel, a loving spouse or two, some grandbabies. Then, the bubble suddenly bursts—a painless, collateral-damage-free kablooey—and that's all she wrote.]

Your correspondent would never tell another living soul, but—sometimes? He fantasized about knocking out his old man's teeth and burying the body unidentifiable. Then, at least, he would be to the world what he was already becoming to him:

a cold, anonymous skull. It would be an act of equitable mercy. Your correspondent's heart would finally stop flip-flopping like a hooked fish. He'd be returned to the stream of his life. And his old man would certainly find himself "in a better place." Anyplace and noplace at all seemed like better places.

And yet, even after a million such thoughts, your correspondent still took off running at the sound of his old man's raised voice. He still got up in there, no reservations, face to face with withered nethers, where he hummed soothing nonsense and wiped up clammy shit.

Would you care to try? his old man was asking him, holding out a large piece of the children's puzzle that a few patients were picking over on the table. The tenor of his question tracked upward, as though your correspondent was the new kid in school and his old man was feeling charitable. Too big for their wrists, the other patients' alarm bracelets rested against their hands like horseshoes around a stake.

A few hours later, after dinner was served and a far too jaunty version of "Swing Low, Sweet Chariot" attempted, your correspondent decided he'd seen enough. He led his old man to the elevator bank, supporting his hollow weight by holding his belt from behind. He reached under a taped-up sheet of printer paper and pressed the down arrow. Soon, the eighth-floor residents would be shepherded to the railed beds in their double rooms. They would sleep, or they wouldn't. The sun would come up on them, Groundhog Day unto death.

On the wall above the button was a list of the recently deceased. Three patients had expired here in the past month.

Their families—like millions more around the country—had paid about $219 per day, or $80,000 per year, to bury them preemptively.

What is it that we actually love, your correspondent wondered, *in those we claim to love?*

In the morning, with minimal fuss, he's able to get his old man aboard a 10:30 a.m. commuter train headed from Amsterdam Centraal to nearby Weesp, where the famed Hogewey complex is located. Your correspondent is suffering from the hot eyes and boiler-room skull that ride along with jet lag. But at the moment, he's more affected by either his competence or his good luck. Just being here with his old man is like drawing a short thread through the eye of a needle in one go.

Go our separate ways, his old man says, gazing out at the sloped dikes and drainage canals. *See what we see.*

The place they're zipping toward is renowned in the medical community for having completely reorganized itself according to the person-centered approach to caregiving. First popularized in the 1990s, this approach stresses the need for doctors, nurses, and loved ones to accept the demented person as he is *now*, not as he once was.

Hogewey sits at the edge of a bedroom community 15 minutes outside of Amsterdam proper. Five years ago, it was a nursing home like any other: a four-story tower rimmed with green space that was inaccessible to the ward-ridden patients. Following its government-funded, experimental reconstruction, though, Hogewey became a synecdoche of the world around it: an enclosed, open-air township with its own two-story apartment blocks, tulip-lined boulevards, and bright airy plazas.

From the outside, Hogewey's high walls are imposing; inside, there is a theater, pub, restaurant, grocery store, and salon—even a small park with a kidney-shaped pond. The 150 or so residents have the run of the place. They don't know they're in an assisted-living facility. They don't know that every one of the 240-plus people staffing Hogewey's shops and amenities are dementia-care professionals.

"Think of a traditional nursing home," asks Yvonne, a layered experience of scarves and thick blonde hair, one of Hogewcy's founders. She is speaking to a small crowd gathered for the English-language "study day," a $300 opportunity for the curious or desperate to see the cutting edge of dementia care. (Lately, Hogewey has been so swamped with outside interest that a public-information officer has been hired to coordinate multi-language "study days" and corporate visits.) Your correspondent and his old man are joined by a stooped, indubitably British psychologist who believes he can replicate Hogewey on the Isle of Man. Hovering around them is a dowdy social worker from the north of England, here to see if she can't smuggle ideas back into the monolithic National Health Service. Arriving via limo are two vampiric Finnish businesswomen. One is an entrepreneur; the other, her business manager. They have smelled blood.

"In that traditional nursing home, you wake up and you see a nurse in a nurse's uniform," Yvonne says, leading the group into Hogewey's restaurant. Here, your correspondent hands over his old man to a young aide in street clothes. *Your good friend's daughter,* he lies. He stops himself before he adds, *Go play.* [The old man walks off slowly but composedly, feeling as though there is an invisible stack of posture volumes on his head.]

"In that nursing home, you ask yourself, 'Where am I? What's wrong?'" Yvonne explains. "Then you have to be reminded where you are. Which you forget, but then you carry the anxiety with you." The restaurant is tastefully appointed with inset tangerine lighting, purple textiles, and a full bar. A few visitors are dining with their afflicted relatives. "The demented have support here that everything they do is OK," Yvonne says, presenting her guests with an array of fine milks. "We want to remove anxiety. No sense that they're in a wrong place, or that they've done something wrong, or people are only dealing with them because something is wrong with them. We want them to feel, 'I have a right to be here.'"

Like all Dutch nursing homes, Hogewey is publicly funded, and must make do with a per-patient budget of about $7,000 per month. The waiting list is long, even though Hogewey accepts only the most serious dementia cases. The reason there aren't more Hogeweys, Yvonne tells the group, is that doing so would require a radical upending of dementia-care organization and hierarchy. Governmental funding is drying up as it is, and new construction is certainly out of the question. The only way they can continue their experiment here, she admits, is if Hogewey remains a top-ten care center as reported by residents and their families in a biennial survey.

Surveys are crucial to the success of Hogewey. Prior to admission, a patient's family must fill out a deep personality questionnaire-cum-biography: What was their loved one's childhood like? Where did his or her interests and values lie? What was the story they told themselves *about* themselves? Depending on the answers to questions like these, the patient is added to a group apartment belonging to one of seven "lifestyles" reflecting contemporary demographics. There's the urban lifestyle group, the traditional (or blue-collar) group, the Asian, upper-class, cultural, "homey," and Christian groups.

"Small-scale living," Yvonne says, "with people you'd choose to live with if you could." Here, the demented are placed in a comfortable, familiar fiction. Only occasionally does a resident from one demographic shuffle over and knock on the door of another.

Yvonne walks the guests to apartment number 15, an upper-class home. The interior walls are covered in heavy green paper patterned with gold filigree. In the large living room, an ornate chandelier hangs above the overstuffed furniture. On it sit five ladies and one gentleman in fenestral glasses. All of them are staring blankly if contentedly at the guests; to your correspondent, they look like a line of guttering jack-o-lanterns. One of them waves. The Finns walk over to snap selfies with her.

The kitchen, normally joined to the living room in other groups' floor plans, is separated here by an ornate panel screen. Behind it, the two nurses assigned to the apartment are posing as servants, preparing dinner. One of them uncorks a bottle of wine.

"They are not being fooled," Yvonne says, opening a fluted armoire stacked with files and a computer for record-keeping. "We are making it so they have taken away from them the constant reminders that they are no longer normal, whatever that is."

She leads the group to the wing of bedrooms, opening the door to one. It is furnished in nice blonde wood and has a regular twin mattress. "We have never had a bedridden patient," Yvonne brags. "Except in the lead-up to death, for a week or two. It is not a part of dementia, being bedridden. It is a symptom of how we treat the old and infirm."

The study group leaves through the front door, which is never locked during the day. (It is locked at night, when the patients are monitored remotely via microphones hidden throughout each apartment.) "We have benches to sit on, tandem bikes to ride, places to socialize," Yvonne points out. "At an average nursing home, a patient gets 96 seconds of daylight per day."

The group ambles along the shopping district. It is laid with immaculate dark-red bricks, bricks like in a revitalized downtown, your correspondent thinks. Inside the travel agency, a volunteer is coordinating future day trips for patients. In the sconced pub, the card club is playing a kind of table shuffleboard. While the "cashier" keeps her eyes peeled, a few residents float through the grocery store, grabbing at gin and fresh vegetables. The physiotherapy department has its own storefront, as does the maintenance office, the window of which is displaying resident artwork. The salon houses the only freelance worker in the facility, the hairdresser, whose fretting over blue bouffants will be billed directly to patients' families. No currency is exchanged inside Hogewey.

Down a byway whisked with bare apple and pear trees, Yvonne escorts the group to a working-class home. "When it snows," she says, "and we clear paths through the snow, the demented will walk through the cleared paths. They will act as normal as you expect them to act."

The "traditional" apartment is hung themedly with washboards, hammers—all the manual tchotchkes. Your correspondent wonders what decorations his generation would get. (*Tablet computers? Debt certificates?*) In the living room are more men than women, and more mustaches than in the upper-class house. The staff is treating the demented like extended family or neighbors. A disguised nurse gives over dripping dishes to a woman whose hands dry them with a fluency that seems independent of her body. In the house workshop, a man cuts and pastes a collage, unpeels it, rearranges it again. The windows look out on Weesp, where schoolchildren are skipping home. Upon seeing them, one resident pushes herself out of an armchair and pads to the tempered glass. She gestures their way, rowing her arms as merrily as an oceangoing cruiser looking back on the dock.

At the conclusion of their visit, the guests are taken into Hogewey's theater, for fine cheeses. The British psychologist asks Yvonne what their plans for the future are. "Officials in Germany, Norway, Switzerland, and England have begun working with us to build similar facilities," she says. "They understand that you cannot appropriate just one part of our approach. You cannot take tricks. It won't work."

Into the theater wanders the old man. It's a small shock to see him alone, on the loose, totally vulnerable. As with a fumbled football, your correspondent feels impelled to dive after him. [Yet he moves placidly down the aisle, as if through a bit of deja-vu.]

"The dream," Yvonne goes on, "is to make mixed-use developments for *all* the people, not just the demented. We want everyone interacting. We get a lot of young people who visit

and say they wish to live here, too. They see it is different. It is like a real hamlet."

At this, your correspondent can't help but laugh. The answer to his old man's welfare-his own-ends up being something as seemingly, startlingly trite as, "It takes a village."

But for all the good that Hogewey does and represents—there's no going back to cooperative villages, where illness and death are allowed to stay in the picture, and leeway is collectively granted to the unwell. For one thing, illness and death are anathema to the selling of stuff. And the selling of stuff, the buying of stuff, the working of multiple jobs so your correspondent can do both—in short, participating in the consumer economy—*this* is the very definition of health in America. Mental and otherwise.

We'll get our Hogeweys eventually, your correspondent thinks. They will be bigger, and better, and more *American*, by God—and they will cater to our moneyed amnesiacs. Exclusively.

The rest of us broke-dicks, we'll have to get creative when it comes to finding a place for the demented in the plot of each day.

On their way out of Hogewey's front gate, your correspondent turns to his old man and says, *How about we hit the town, have your favorite—lamb chops—for dinner?* [The old man processes this as, *Wooden lamps are dimmer.* But seeping through him is a nebulous sense of comfort and relief. It's as though someone somewhere had stuck a needle in his voodoo doll, benignly so, in the exact right spot.]

He takes this young man's hand and squeezes it with something like tactile hunger.

Your correspondent coos, rolls the hotel blanket to his old man's chin. He is exhausted.

Returning from Hogewey, they got lost along the avenues bridging Amsterdam's concentric canals. Your correspondent became increasingly worried (and embarrassed) as his old man paid less and less mind to the bicycles and sniggering Continentals eddying around them. This was new, for on trips past, his old man had always refused to open a map, ask questions, appear in any way like he didn't know where he was going.

But amid the ease and banter on the street, he was wandering Magooishly, with a self-deprecating and self-orienting humor. The unfamiliar was demanding his focus, greedily occupying what remained of his consciousness. His dementia made all things new. He looked away, and the canal was gone. He looked back, and it was fresh and novel, flowing green glass.

Dikes! he exclaimed. *Dikes all over the place!*

Some mod and ethnically indeterminate young adults stopped to feign outrage over the perceived slur. Your correspondent pulled them aside and whispered, *I'm sorry, he has Alzheimer's. He's lost his mind.* They themselves apologized, commiserated. They asked, *Does he still recognize you?* They wanted to make sure that, *At least he knows your name, right?*

By asking if the old man recognized him, what the young people really wanted to know, whether they were aware of it or not, was, *Should we recognize him? As a person?*

Your correspondent began to feel a little bit bad for having brought his human hourglass *here,* to Amsterdam, the Disneyland of youthful self-actualization. The thick-haired Frenchwomen, the bros high and braying at the start of their Grand Tour—he did not want to be the one to break it to them that, dope as they are now, their lives *will* be breached by pain and ungovernability. They might be lucky enough to make it to retirement age (assuming that's still a thing) more or less free, autonomous, and self-directing—with no real obligation to any narrative other than their own. Then, *WHAMBO!* They or a loved one or a loved one's loved one will dement.

He did not want to say this. But he thought *somebody* should. Somebody should tell them that theirs will be an individual tragedy, albeit an individual tragedy that is replayed again and again. An entire First World of individual tragedies.

If he were a braver man, he would have rented a skiff and shouted it from the waterworks: *Peers! Children! History is irony on the move! Turns out that, by so bettering and extending our lives, we have re-achieved suffering!*

Instead, your correspondent leaned against the railing with his old man. He rubbed a widening spiral into his back. He thought on the phrase that was the wellspring of the rationalistic, capitalistic, Westernized world around him: "I think, therefore I am." According to that logic, this world is free to stop treating you as a "you" the moment that "you" forget who you are.

Alzheimer's, then, is more than a disease of the brain. It is a pandemic of selffiood.

If you believe that *you,* your *self,* is a singular inner possession—this cumulative state of you-ness, which you've cultured like a pearl—then dementia is a fate worse than death. It is watching yourself get shucked.

If, on the other hand, you believe that you are more the product of your chosen communities and relationships—that what *you* are is a loving husband plus esteemed teacher plus an even better friend—then what happens when your wife and pupils and old buddies stop visiting you in the home? Are you empty under all those layers, like a cartoon mummy?

If you can't hold onto what makes you *you,* and if other people can deny it, anyway—what's left? What was there to begin with?

It's almost too much to consider. Especially when whatever it is you happen to be feels just *right,* just *so.* And that's the thing. If you don't want to relate personally with the demented—cool. Your choice to make. If you don't want to think about them, much less live with them, you don't have to.

You don't have to *right now.* But maybe you should start considering what that might be like. Because, according to the numbers, it's looking more and more likely that you will become either a caregiver or care receiver. Possibly both. In either case, relationships will wither, selves will go to seed, and you will find yourself alone with an invalid. Your story won't be yours to tell anymore. You might come to think of your autonomy, your sovereignty, your very *self* as a figment of your imagination.

In the early hours of the morning, the old man wakes, certain that he has forgotten something. He walks into the bathroom and is puzzled by the new tiling and fixtures. He looks around, vaguely recognizing the space and its utility. He can't remember why he's come. He examines the many objects next to the sink. He picks up a green-handled thing with prickle thingies, squeezes a gooey something onto it. He looks into the mirror and is frozen with horror.

In place of a youngish man, thin-lipped and clear-eyed, he sees some wretched human ruin mimicking his every expression. It seems to be mocking him, his confused panic. Both the young man and the old one cry out.

Next thing he knows, his correct reflection is standing behind this uncanny geezer. He watches as the reflection wraps its arms around him. *I'm here,* the reflection is saying, holding the old man in place from behind. This reflection catches his eye and smiles.

He cannot comprehend this. And he will carry no memory of it. But in this moment, and for a few afterward, he detects something like a *presence.* The sort of full-body frisson that is felt only through what it undoes. Like sunshine burnt through cloud. Or the silence that comes after the coda but before the ovation.

Critical Thinking

1. Why is caring for someone with Alzheimer's disease so challenging?
2. Why are the numbers of cases of Alzheimer's disease expected to rise in the next 15 years?

Internet References

Alzheimer's Association
www.alz.org

Mayo Clinic
http://www.mayoclinic.org/diseases-conditions/alzheimers-disease/basics/definition/con-20023871

National Institutes of Health
http://www.nia.nih.gov/alzheimers/publication/alzheimers-disease-fact-sheet

Unit 8

UNIT

Prepared by: Eileen Daniel, *SUNY College at Brockport*

Health Care and the Health Care System

Americans are healthier today than they have been at any time in this nation's history. Americans suffer more illness today than they have at any time in this nation's history. Which statement is true? They both are, depending on the statistics you quote. According to longevity statistics, Americans are living longer today and, therefore, must be healthier. Still, other statistics indicate that Americans today report twice as many acute illnesses as did our ancestors 60 years ago. They also report that their pain lasts longer. Unfortunately, this combination of living longer and feeling sicker places additional demands on a health-care system that, according to experts, is already in a state of crisis.

Despite the clamor about the problems with our health-care system, if you can afford it, then the American health-care system is one of the best in the world. However, being the best does not mean that it is without problems. Each year, more than half a million Americans are injured or die due to preventable mistakes made by medical-care professionals. In addition, countless unnecessary tests are preformed that not only add to the expense of health care but may actually place the patient at risk. Reports such as these fuel the fire of public skepticism toward the quality of health care that Americans receive. While these aspects of our health-care system indicate a need for repair, they represent just the tip of the iceberg. Despite the implementation of the Affordable Care Act (Obama care), there are calls for the government to develop a better universal system that covers all. Many believe that universal coverage will not only insure all Americans but it will also help to reduce the cost of health care. A number of Americans also believe that costs continue to rise due to the blockage of price controls by the pharmaceutical industry. Laws that affect the way health care is provided and fewer regulations that impact market forces might reduce the overall cost of medical care and medications. While choices in health-care providers are increasing, paying for services continues to be a challenge as medical costs continue to rise. In addition, it appears that the uninsured have more health risks because they're more likely to be poor, smokers, less educated, obese, and unemployed.

Why have health-care costs risen so much? The answer to this question is multifaceted and includes such factors as physicians' fees, hospital costs, insurance costs, pharmaceutical costs, and health fraud. It could be argued that while these factors operate within any health-care system, the lack of a meaningful form of outcomes assessment has permitted and encouraged waste and inefficiency within our system. Ironically, one of the major factors for the rise in the cost of health care is our rapidly expanding aging population—tangible evidence of an improving health-care delivery system. This is obviously one factor that we hope will continue to rise. Another significant factor that is often overlooked is the constantly expanding boundaries of health care. It is somewhat ironic that as our success in treating various disorders has expanded, so has the domain of health care, often into areas where previously health care had little or no involvement.

Traditionally, Americans have felt that the state of their health was largely determined by the quality of the health care available to them. This attitude has fostered an unhealthy dependence upon the health-care system and contributed to the skyrocketing costs. It should be obvious by now that while there is no simple solution to our health-care problems, we would all be a lot better off if we accepted more personal responsibility for our health. While this shift would help ease the financial burden of health care, it might necessitate a more responsible coverage of medical news in order to educate and enlighten the public on personal health issues.

Article Prepared by: Eileen L. Daniel, *SUNY Brockport*

Deviated: A Memoir

A cautionary tale from the brave new world of health-care coverage

JESSE KELLERMAN

Learning Outcomes

After reading this article, you will be able to:

- Explain an insurance company's rationale for denying coverage based on a preexisting condition.

- Describe symptoms of a nasal deviated septum.

- Describe why surgery was required by the insurance company before issuing a policy.

Aside from a brief stint as a writing tutor during graduate school, I have managed to avoid respectable employment all my adult life. There was a time, after I earned my graduate degree and before I sold my first novel, when it looked like I might have to get an office job. I remember one interview with one stultifying prospective boss; it took him a half hour to describe the important tasks I would be called upon to perform, such as licking envelopes—a half hour I spent steadily withdrawing into a cocoon of self-pity, so that when he finally paused to ask if I was up for the challenge, I said, "Huh?" and wasn't called back.

I don't take my self-employment for granted. I commute 30 feet. I have the privilege to spend a great amount of time watching my son grow up. I have access to a supply of snacks rivaling that of a Silicon Valley start-up circa 1997. Still, there are drawbacks, most of them courtesy of the federal government. Some are minor, like having to pay estimated quarterly taxes, which for a writer with multiple contracts coming due at unpredictable times is a bewildering process akin to picking the next eight winners of the Kentucky Derby. More painfully, I am subject to the full amount of Medicare and Social Security tax, a burden more often shared with one's employer.

Until recently, though, I had never given much thought to one of the clearest benefits forfeited by the self-employed: simplified access to health insurance. I'd never given it much thought because for years I'd been covered by my wife's policy. Then she left her hospital job to work at home, and both of us were self-employed. The law entitled us to extend her coverage for an additional 18 months at the same rate paid by her former employer. After that, we knew, we were on our own. As a deadline, it seemed very abstract, and very far away. I don't remember hearing a ticking clock, anyway. Today I look back and speculate that its sound was smothered by red tape.

With our extension used up, we sat down to begin the paperwork. By *we,* I mean my wife, who took it upon herself to price out every plan under the California sun. Numbers were crunched, contingencies planned for. In the end we decided to reapply for coverage with the same provider. On some level, we had the idea that this would simplify things.

All was in *Ordnung,* or so it seemed, until the day we opened the mailbox to find a big fat envelope waiting for us. We tore it open like excited high schoolers awaiting SAT scores and unfolded the pages in search of our little plastic cards, the ones that would entitle us to stand before the gum-chewing receptionists at our local internal medicine clinic and declare, "Behold, I am a member of the working world, gainfully self-employed and nominally self-sufficient, evinced by the way I wield this card plus a $40 office visit co-pay."

There weren't any cards.

There was, rather, a lot of tiny black type.

"I'm approved," my wife said, squinting to read. "The baby's approved."

She frowned.

"You've been declined," she said.

I chuckled, mentally. Declined? Impossible. I was a healthy 33-year-old man with an unremarkable medical history. I took no medications other than the odd Claritin or Advil. I'd never broken a bone. I'd never had a hospital stay. At 17 I'd had my one and only surgery, performed under local anaesthetic, to remove a benign bone spur in my toe. I ate well. I exercised daily. And talk about blood work—oh, my blood work! It runs in the family. Many of my forebears on both sides lived well into their 90s. My 89-year-old grandmother recently complained to me that she can no longer play mah-jongg because "all my girls are dead." My 92-year-old grandmother does Israeli dance with a group of women half her age. Like my mother, who has a rare and beneficent gene variant, I have more good cholesterol than bad. A high triglyceride level is 200; 150–199 is borderline; lower than 150 is considered normal. Mine: 15.

"It's about your nose," my wife said, turning pages.

I instantly suspected anti-Semitism. "What about it?"

She showed me the page. In the interest of full disclosure, I suppose I ought to revise the rosy medical self-portrait a tad. One thing I have endured, from about fourth grade on, is insomnia. It gets better or worse depending on my stress level, and even when I do manage to fall asleep, I tend to wake up every three hours. The year that I spent abroad prior to college, learning in an Israeli yeshiva, was probably the roughest I ever had, sleepwise. At least once a week I was up all night, with the result that I rarely attended the regular 7 a.m. prayer service. Either I waited for the sunrise minyan, or I skipped services entirely and slept in. When I started writing full time, I embraced my inner night owl, often working until two or three in the morning and sleeping until nine.

A sour man with a badly patterned tie, Dr. K. regarded me distastefully from behind thick aviator glasses. He asked me what I did. I told him I wrote novels.

The arrival of my son forced me to get on his schedule. I could never quite manage it, though, and long after he had learned to sleep through the night, I would still spend hours at a stretch tossing and turning. Concerned that I might have apnea, I made an appointment with an ear-nose-and-throat man, whom I'll call Dr. K. I chose him because the practice he belonged to told me he had the first available opening. I've since learned that the person with the first available opening is seldom the person you want to see.

A sour man with a badly patterned necktie, he regarded me distastefully from behind thick aviator glasses. He asked me what I did. I told him I wrote novels. He asked if he had heard of any of them. I told him probably not. Then he shoved a wad of cotton soaked in topical anaesthetic up my nose. There was nothing gentle about the way he did this. Indeed, it seemed to be something of a game to him: *How much can I cram in there?* I shudder to imagine what the inside of his garage looks like. The anaesthetic still hadn't taken effect when he yanked the cotton out and impaled my face on a plastic scope. I gagged and choked. "Sorry," he said, smiling faintly. I tried to hold still while he rooted around up there, sighing and saying things like "hmm" and "yup." Finally he pointed to the live feed of my sinuses on the screen and turned to the terrified medical student standing in the corner, her notebook at the ready.

"Deviated septum," he said to her. She wrote it down. Then he flashed me a Bond villain smile. "*Severe.*"

I had three options. The first was a course of nasal steroids to reduce the swelling, although Dr. K. made it clear that this was a giant waste of time, strictly a formality to secure permission from my insurance company to proceed to option two: corrective surgery.

"What's option three?" I asked.

"You could try those little plastic thingies," he said, stroking the bridge of his nose. I couldn't afford to be laid out for a week

or more. I had a novel to write and a toddler to manage. I said I'd give the plastic thingies a shot. I could tell he was disappointed. "Suit yourself," he said, walking away to dictate his note into a pocket recorder.

My first few nights wearing Breathe Right Nasal Strips weren't all that different. Then I discovered that I had accidentally purchased the wrong size, the large ones, "for adults with larger noses." (Self-anti-Semitism?) Once I got hold of the small/mediums, my life literally changed overnight. For the first time in 20 years I slept seven straight hours. I called Dr. K.'s office and left a message saying I had the problem under control. And I did. The only apparent downside was that I developed, over the next few months, a semi-permanent red stripe across the bridge of my nose where the adhesive attached. It seemed a small price to pay. Every morning my wife would look at me and say, in the Jamaican accent of the guy from the beer commercials, "Reeeed Stripe."

We laughed the laugh of the young and able-bodied.

Back to the letter. "'Health history,'" my wife read. "'Deviated septum, surgery recommended. Should Jesse Kellerman wish reconsideration of our underwriting decision, he must, one, be sign-, symptom-, and treatment-free from the deviated septum, not a surgical candidate and no symptoms documented by your physician and no further treatment needed, and, two, meet the Medical Underwriting Guidelines in effect at the time of application.'"

It took a hard charge through several layers of voicemail and an hour on hold, but at last I found myself talking to the medical underwriting department.

"It's nice that they're employing the illiterate," I said.

"Here," she said. "Call them."

It took a hard charge through several layers of voicemail and an hour on hold, but at last I found myself talking to the underwriting department.

"You have failed to meet the underwriting criteria," the underwriter said.

"I realize that," I said. "My question is what I can do to qualify."

"You must be sign-, symptom-, and treatment-free—"

"But I *am* sign- and symptom-free. I wear those little plastic thingies. I pay for them myself."

"I understand, sir."

"So what's the problem, then?"

"You must be sign-, symptom-, and treatment-free, and not a surgical candidate, and if you meet the underwriting criteria at the time of application, you may qualify."

"That's what I'm trying to tell you. I feel fine."

"I understand."

"OK, so, just to be clear, here, if I get reevaluated and I'm OK, then I'll qualify."

"You must be—"

"Janet. Janet. Janet. May I call you Janet?"

"Sir."

"Janet, I understand that you have a script to follow. I understand that. I'm just trying to get some information here, like a normal person. And what I'm trying to understand, Janet, is what *else* I have to do to qualify, because, Janet, I *am* sign- and symptom-free."

"I understand that, sir, but until you are no longer a surgical candidate, and until you meet the underwriting criteria, we are declining to offer you coverage."

"My nose is shaped in a certain way. It's not going to change, magically."

"Sir."

"So as long as I have this nose, I'm always going to be a surgical candidate."

"Sir."

"The only way *not* to be a surgical candidate is to have surgery."

"Sir."

"But I don't want surgery. I don't need it. I'm *fine*. Janet, I promise you that I will not have surgery."

"I'm sorry, sir, but we can't offer you coverage based on your promises."

"Okay, well, what can I do to convince you?"

"You must be sign-, symptom-, and treatment-free, and not a surgical candidate, and if you meet the underwriting criteria at the time of application, you may qualify."

I paused. "Let's try another approach here."

"Sir?"

"Right now I'm covered by your company, right?"

"I don't know, sir. Are you?"

"Yes. I am. And I'm reapplying to be covered by your company."

"Sir."

"So you're telling me," I said, "that the only way for me to get new coverage is to no longer be a surgical candidate."

"If you meet the underwriting criteria at the time of application, you will qualify."

"Fine. Got it. So. I have the surgery, and now I meet the underwriting criteria, right?"

"I can't promise you that."

"*I'm not asking you to.*"

"There's no need to yell."

"I'm not asking you to promise me that. I'm asking you, Janet, my love, to follow me, please, down this theoretical path. OK? Let's say I get surgery. And I am no longer a surgical candidate. *And* I meet the underwriting criteria when I reapply. Then what happens?"

"Then you may be eligible for coverage."

"'May?'"

"Yes, sir, you may qualify."

"Okay. I 'may' qualify. Fine. Excellent. Super. Now answer me this. To not be a surgical candidate, I actually have to have this surgery. So let's say I decide to go for it. I'm gonna have this surgery. All right? So. Riddle me this, Janet: *Who's going to pay for it?*"

"I don't know, sir."

"You will. You will, Janet. *You* will pay for it, because you already *are* my insurance provider. Do you see what's happening here? You're incentivizing me to have an operation, which I neither need nor want, and which *you will pay for,* in order to *avoid* paying for that same operation in the future." I paused. "Janet?"

"Yes, sir," she said. "That sounds about right."

"And that doesn't strike you as odd?"

At last a hint of humanity crept into her voice. "I guess it does, a little."

"Well," I said. "As long as we're clear on that."

I had surgery. I had alternatives, of course. I could have bought into a pre-existing condition plan, or a HIPAA plan, either of which would have covered me and my bent septum. But these plans were extremely expensive, and when we amortized the cost of the operation over a year, it turned out to be cheaper to have it than not, even if I had to pay for it in full.

So, I had surgery.

I didn't go back to Dr. K. First, he creeped me out, and moreover he was booked. Everyone in San Diego was. I had to drive two hours north to Los Angeles to find someone who could operate soon enough for me to recover (and thereby qualify for the underwriting criteria) before our coverage ran out. I chose my parents' ENT. The walls of Dr. R.'s Beverly Hills practice were hung with the gold and platinum albums of pop stars whose nodules he had soothed. He booked me into a surgical center within 48 hours. My mother drove me over at five in the morning. I handed my credit card to a young woman who had no right to look that beautiful at that hour. She ran the card, and I signed for several thousand dollars.

"At least I'll get miles," I told my mother.

The surgery went well, and for the next few days I sat in bed and watched TV. When it came time to remove the packing from my nose, Dr. R. was good enough to come in on a Sunday morning.

The walls of Dr. R.'s practice in Beverly Hills were hung with the gold and platinum albums of pop stars whose nodules he had soothed.

"Don't blow, don't pick, don't futz with it at all," he said. I obeyed. Still, the incision kept on bleeding, so he had me return for a chemical cauterization. I drove back to San Diego with the smell of it in my nostrils. My wife met me at the door, scrutinizing me before she let me back in.

"I'm checking to see if you look different," she said.

"Do I?"

"No."

"Do I sound different?"

"You're bleeding," she said.

I ran to the bathroom. Sure enough, a little ruby droplet had formed near the inside corner of the left nostril—the one Dr. R. had just cauterized.

I called him.

"Don't futz with it," he said.

I didn't futz. Three days later, it was still bleeding.

"Come back in."

I drove to L.A. He cauterized the incision a second time.

"It has to scab and heal," he said. "Don't futz with it."

I drove back to San Diego. I didn't futz. It was hard not to; it itched like hell. And it was still bleeding.

"Come back in."

I got into the car.

An ENT's tools are either extremely sophisticated or else positively medieval, and I had discovered that Dr. R., for all his charm, shared Dr. K.'s enthusiasm for ramming larger-than-reasonable objects in my face. Before cauterizing the incision a third time, he pried the offending nostril open with pliers and gazed contemplatively into my sinuses.

"How's your breathing been?" he said.

"Pretty good," I said.

"Mm." He reached for the cauterization stick. "It's amazing, how the cartilage has a memory. It's curving back a bit. You can breathe, though?"

"Pretty well."

"Well, good enough."

The third cauterization took. The bleeding tapered off, and within a few weeks I was back to blowing my nose like normal. But in the interim, a new problem had arisen: The left nostril had turned shiny and crimson and tender to the touch. "It looks infected," my wife said.

I called my primary-care physician.

"He can see you in February."

"It's May."

"Do you want to see someone else?"

I saw an intern, who looked at my nose and wrote me a prescription for an antibiotic. It didn't work. I called the practice and spoke to a nurse, who told me I needed to come back in.

"I'm pretty sure it's one of those drug-resistant strains," I said. "You can't have them just write me a new prescription?"

"Not without seeing you first."

I went back in. A different intern looked at my nose.

"It's one of those drug-resistant strains," he said, writing me a new prescription.

Twice a day for the next seven days, I swallowed a pill the size of a ping-pong ball. The infection abated, and I stood victorious in front of the mirror, prodding my nose.

My wife entered with a torn envelope. "We've been approved."

"Great," I said. At that moment, it all seemed worth it. To celebrate, I reached for a tissue and blew my nose, expelling a massive quantity of bright red blood.

Eight months later, I've recovered, for the most part. The surgeon was right: Cartilage does have a memory. Every day I feel my septum curve a little bit more as it struggles to regain its original shape. After the surgery, flush with optimism, I threw away all my Breathe Right strips; I have since bought more, for use in the event of a cold or bad allergies, which render my nose just as obstructed as it ever was.

And so, some nights, I lie awake, gasping for air.

Critical Thinking

1. Why does an insurance company have the right to deny coverage based on a pre-existing condition?

2. What symptoms does a deviated septum produce?

Create Central

www.mhhe.com/createcentral

Internet References

American Medical Association (AMA)
  www.ama-assn.org
MedScape: The Online Resource for Better Patient Care
  www.medscape.com

JESSE KELLERMAN *is the author of four novels, including* The Genius *and, most recently,* The Executor. *His novel* Potboiler *will be published by Putnam in June. His April 2009* Commentary *article, "Let My People Go to the Buffet," was included in* The Best Spiritual Writing 2011.

Article

Prepared by: Eileen L. Daniel, *SUNY Brockport*

How Government Killed the Medical Profession

JEFFREY A. SINGER

Learning Outcomes

After reading this article, you will be able to:

- Explain how hospitals' reimbursements for their Medicare-patient treatments are determined.

- Understand how Diagnosis Related Groups incentivize hospitals to attach multiple codes in order to increase Medicare reimbursement.

- Describe how data accuracy is compromised with the coding system.

I am a general surgeon with more than three decades in private clinical practice. And I am fed up. Since the late 1970s, I have witnessed remarkable technological revolutions in medicine, from CT scans to robot-assisted surgery. But I have also watched as medicine slowly evolved into the domain of technicians, bookkeepers, and clerks.

Government interventions over the past four decades have yielded a cascade of perverse incentives, bureaucratic diktats, and economic pressures that together are forcing doctors to sacrifice their independent professional medical judgment, and their integrity. The consequence is clear: Many doctors from my generation are exiting the field. Others are seeing their private practices threatened with bankruptcy, or are giving up their autonomy for the life of a shift-working hospital employee. Governments and hospital administrators hold all the power, while doctors—and worse still, patients—hold none.

The Coding Revolution

At first, the decay was subtle. In the 1980s, Medicare imposed price controls upon physicians who treated anyone over 65. Any provider wishing to get compensated was required to use International Statistical Classification of Diseases (ICD) and Current Procedural Terminology (CPT) codes to describe the service when submitting a bill. The designers of these systems believed that standardized classifications would lead to more accurate adjudication of Medicare claims.

What it actually did was force doctors to wedge their patients and their services into predetermined, ill-fitting categories. This approach resembled the command-and-control models used in the Soviet bloc and the People's Republic of China, models that were already failing spectacularly by the end of the 1980s.

Before long, these codes were attached to a fee schedule based upon the amount of time a medical professional had to devote to each patient, a concept perilously close to another Marxist relic: the labor theory of value. Named the Resource-Based Relative Value System (RBRVS), each procedure code was assigned a specific value, by a panel of experts, based supposedly upon the amount of time and labor it required. It didn't matter if an operation was being performed by a renowned surgical expert—perhaps the inventor of the procedure—or by a doctor just out of residency doing the operation for the first time. They both got paid the same.

Hospitals' reimbursements for their Medicare-patient treatments were based on another coding system: the Diagnosis Related Group (DRG). Each diagnostic code is assigned a specific monetary value, and the hospital is paid based on one or a combination of diagnostic codes used to describe the reason for a patient's hospitalization. If, say, the diagnosis is pneumonia, then the hospital is given a flat amount for that diagnosis, regardless of the amount of equipment, staffing, and days used to treat a particular patient.

As a result, the hospital is incentivized to attach as many adjunct diagnostic codes as possible to try to increase the Medicare payday. It is common for hospital coders to contact the attending physicians and try to coax them into adding a few more diagnoses into the hospital record.

Medicare has used these two price-setting systems (RBRVS for doctors, DRG for hospitals) to maintain its price control system for more than 20 years. Doctors and their advocacy associations cooperated, trading their professional latitude for the lure of maintaining monopoly control of the ICD and CPT codes that determine their payday. The goal of setting their own prices has proved elusive, though—every year the industry's biggest trade group, the American Medical Association, squabbles with various medical specialty associations and the Centers for Medicare and Medicaid Services (CMS) over fees.

As goes Medicare, so goes the private insurance industry. Insurers, starting in the late 1980s, began the practice of using the Medicare fee schedule to serve as the basis for negotiation of compensation with the doctors and hospitals on their preferred provider lists. An insurance company might offer a hospital 130 percent of Medicare's reimbursement for a specific procedure code, for instance.

The coding system was supposed to improve the accuracy of adjudicating claims submitted by doctors and hospitals to Medicare, and later to non-Medicare insurance companies. Instead, it gave doctors and hospitals an incentive to find ways of describing procedures and services with the cluster of codes that would yield the biggest payment. Sometimes this required the assistance of consulting firms. A cottage industry of fee-maximizing advisors and seminars bloomed.

I recall more than one occasion when I discovered at such a seminar that I was "undercoding" for procedures I routinely perform; a small tweak meant a bigger check for me. That fact encouraged me to keep one eye on the codes at all times, leaving less attention for my patients. Today, most doctors in private practice employ coding specialists, a relatively new occupation, to oversee their billing departments.

Another goal of the coding system was to provide Medicare, regulatory agencies, research organizations, and insurance companies with a standardized method of collecting epidemiological data—the information medical professionals use to track ailments across different regions and populations. However, the developers of the coding system did not anticipate the unintended consequence of linking the laudable goal of epidemiologic data mining with a system of financial reward.

This coding system leads inevitably to distortions in epidemiological data. Because doctors are required to come up with a diagnostic code on each bill submitted in order to get paid, they pick the code that comes closest to describing the patient's problem while yielding maximum remuneration. The same process plays out when it comes to submitting procedure codes on bills. As a result, the accuracy of the data collected since the advent of compensation coding is suspect.

Command and Control

Coding was one of the earliest manifestations of the cancer consuming the medical profession, but the disease is much more broad-based and systemic. The root of the problem is that patients are not payers. Through myriad tax and regulatory policies adopted on the federal and state level, the system rarely sees a direct interaction between a consumer and a provider of a health care good or service. Instead, a third party—either a private insurance company or a government payer, such as Medicare or Medicaid—covers almost all the costs. According to the National Center for Policy Analysis, on average, the consumer pays only 12 percent of the total health care bill directly out of pocket. There is no incentive, through a market system with transparent prices, for either the provider or the consumer to be cost-effective.

As the third party payment system led health care costs to escalate, the people footing the bill have attempted to rein in costs with yet more command-and-control solutions. In the 1990s, private insurance carriers did this through a form of health plan called a health maintenance organization, or HMO. Strict oversight, rationing, and practice protocols were imposed on both physicians and patients. Both groups protested loudly. Eventually, most of these top-down regulations were set aside, and many HMOs were watered down into little more than expensive prepaid health plans.

Then, as the 1990s gave way to the 21st century, demographic reality caught up with Medicare and Medicaid, the two principal drivers of federal health care spending.

Twenty years after the fall of the Iron Curtain, protocols and regimentation were imposed on America's physicians through a centralized bureaucracy. Using so-called "evidence-based medicine," algorithms and protocols were based on statistically generalized, rather than individualized, outcomes in large population groups.

While all physicians appreciate the development of general approaches to the work-up and treatment of various illnesses and disorders, we also realize that everyone is an individual—that every protocol or algorithm is based on the average, typical case. We want to be able to use our knowledge, years of experience, and sometimes even our intuition to deal with each patient as a unique person while bearing in mind what the data and research reveal.

Being pressured into following a pre-determined set of protocols inhibits clinical judgment, especially when it comes to atypical problems. Some medical educators are concerned that excessive reliance on these protocols could make students less likely to recognize and deal with complicated clinical presentations that don't follow standard patterns. It is easy to standardize treatment protocols. But it is difficult to standardize patients.

What began as guidelines eventually grew into requirements. In order for hospitals to maintain their Medicare certification, the Centers for Medicare and Medicaid Services began to require their medical staff to follow these protocols or face financial retribution.

Once again, the medical profession cooperated. The American College of Surgeons helped develop Surgical Care Improvement Project (SCIP) protocols, directing surgeons as to what antibiotics they may use and the day-to-day post-operative decisions they must make. If a surgeon deviates from the guidelines, he is usually required to document in the medical record an acceptable justification for that decision.

These requirements have consequences. On more than one occasion I have seen patients develop dramatic postoperative bruising and bleeding because of protocol-mandated therapies aimed at preventing the development of blood clots in the legs after surgery. Had these therapies been left up to the clinical judgment of the surgeon, many of these patients might not have had the complication.

Operating room and endoscopy suites now must follow protocols developed by the global World Health Organization—an even more remote agency. There are protocols for cardiac catheterization, stenting, and respirator management, just to name a few.

Patients should worry about doctors trying to make symptoms fit into a standardized clinical model and ignoring the vital nuances of their complaints. Even more, they should be alarmed that the protocols being used don't provide any measurable health benefits. Most were designed and implemented before any objective evidence existed as to their effectiveness.

A large Veterans Administration study released in March 2011 showed that SCIP protocols led to no improvement in surgical-site infection rate. If past is prologue, we should not expect the SCIP protocols to be repealed, just "improved"—or expanded, adding to the already existing glut.

These rules are being bred into the system. Young doctors and medical students are being trained to follow protocol. To them, command and control is normal. But to older physicians who have lived through the decline of medical culture, this only contributes to our angst.

One of my colleagues, a noted pulmonologist with over 30 years' experience, fears that teaching young physicians to follow guidelines and practice protocols discourages creative medical thinking and may lead to a decrease in diagnostic and therapeutic excellence. He laments that "'evidence-based' means you are not interested in listening to anyone." Another colleague, a North Phoenix orthopedist of many years, decries the "cookie-cutter" approach mandated by protocols.

A noted gastroenterologist who has practiced more than 35 years has a more cynical take on things. He believes that the increased regimentation and regularization of medicine is a prelude to the replacement of physicians by nurse practitioners and physician-assistants, and that these people will be even more likely to follow the directives proclaimed by regulatory bureaus. It is true that, in many cases, routine medical problems can be handled more cheaply and efficiently by paraprofessionals. But these practitioners are also limited by depth of knowledge, understanding, and experience. Patients should be able to decide for themselves if they want to be seen by a doctor. It is increasingly rare that patients are given a choice about such things.

The partners in my practice all believe that protocols and guidelines will accomplish nothing more than giving us more work to do and more rules to comply with. But they implore me to keep my mouth shut—rather than risk angering hospital administrators, insurance company executives, and the other powerful entities that control our fates.

Electronic Records and Financial Burdens

When Congress passed the stimulus, a.k.a. the American Reinvestment and Recovery Act of 2009, it included a requirement that all physicians and hospitals convert to electronic medical records (EMR) by 2014 or face Medicare reimbursement penalties. There has never been a peer-reviewed study clearly demonstrating that requiring all doctors and hospitals to switch to electronic records will decrease error and increase efficiency, but that didn't stop Washington policymakers from repeating that claim over and over again in advance of the stimulus.

Some institutions, such as Kaiser Permanente Health Systems, the Mayo Clinic, and the Veterans Administration Hospitals, have seen big benefits after going digital voluntarily. But if the same benefits could reasonably be expected to play out universally, government coercion would not be needed.

Instead, Congress made that business decision on behalf of thousands of doctors and hospitals, who must now spend huge sums on the purchase of EMR systems and take staff off other important jobs to task them with entering thousands of old-style paper medical records into the new database. For a period of weeks or months after the new system is in place, doctors must see fewer patients as they adapt to the demands of the technology.

The persistence of price controls has coincided with a steady ratcheting down of fees for doctors. As a result, private insurance payments, which are typically pegged to Medicare payment schedules, have been ratcheting down as well. Meanwhile, Medicare's regulatory burdens on physician practices continue to increase, adding on compliance costs. Medicare continues to demand that specific coded services be redefined and subdivided into ever-increasing levels of complexity. Harsh penalties are imposed on providers who accidentally use the wrong level code to bill for a service. Sometimes—as in the case of John Natale of Arlington, Illinois, who began a 10-month sentence in November because he miscoded bills on five patients upon whom he repaired complicated abdominal aortic aneurysms—the penalty can even include prison.

For many physicians in private practice, the EMR requirement is the final straw. Doctors are increasingly selling their practices to hospitals, thus becoming hospital employees. This allows them to offload the high costs of regulatory compliance and converting to EMR.

As doctors become shift workers, they work less intensely and watch the clock much more than they did when they were in private practice. Additionally, the doctor-patient relationship is adversely affected as doctors come to increasingly view their customers as the hospitals' patients rather than their own.

In 2011, The New England Journal of Medicine reported that fully 50 percent of the nation's doctors had become employees—either of hospitals, corporations, insurance companies, or the government. Just six years earlier, in 2005, more than two-thirds of doctors were in private practice. As economic pressures on the sustainability of private clinical practice continue to mount, we can expect this trend to continue.

Accountable Care Organizations

For the next 19 years, an average of 10,000 Americans will turn 65 every day, increasing the fiscal strain on Medicare. Bureaucrats are trying to deal with this partly by reinstating an old concept under a new name: Accountable Care Organization, or ACO, which harkens back to the infamous HMO system of the early 1990s.

In a nutshell, hospitals, clinics, and health care providers have been given incentives to organize into teams that will get assigned groups of 5,000 or more Medicare patients. They will be expected to follow practice guidelines and protocols approved by Medicare. If they achieve certain benchmarks established by Medicare with respect to cost, length of hospital stay, re-admissions, and other measures, they will get to share a portion of Medicare's savings. If the reverse happens, there will be economic penalties.

Naturally, private insurance companies are following suit with non-Medicare versions of the ACO, intended primarily for new markets created by ObamaCare. In this model, an ACO is given a lump sum, or bundled payment, by the insurance company. That chunk of money is intended to cover the cost of all the care for a large group of insurance beneficiaries. The private ACOs are expected to follow the same Medicare-approved practice protocols, but all of the financial risks are assumed by the ACOs. If the ACOs keep costs down, the team of providers and hospitals reap the financial reward: surplus from the lump sum payment. If they lose money, the providers and hospitals eat the loss.

In both the Medicare and non-Medicare varieties of the ACO, cost control and compliance with centrally planned practice guidelines are the primary goal.

ACOs are meant to replace a fee-for-service payment model that critics argue encourages providers to perform more services and procedures on patients than they otherwise would do. This assumes that all providers are unethical, motivated only by the desire for money. But the salaried and prepaid models of provider-reimbursement are also subject to unethical behavior in our current system. There is no reward for increased productivity with the salary model. With the prepaid model there is actually an incentive to maximize profit by withholding services.

Each of these models has its pros and cons. In a true market-based system, where competition rewards positive results, the consumer would be free to choose among the various competing compensation arrangements.

With increasing numbers of health care providers becoming salaried employees of hospitals, that's not likely. Instead, we'll see greater bureaucratization. Hospitals might be able to get ACOs to work better than their ancestor HMOs, because hospital administrators will have more control over their medical staff. If doctors don't follow the protocols and guidelines, and desired outcomes are not reached, hospitals can replace the "problem" doctors.

Doctors Going Galt?

Once free to be creative and innovative in their own practices, doctors are becoming more like assembly-line workers, constrained by rules and regulations aimed to systemize their craft. It's no surprise that retirement is starting to look more attractive. The advent of the Affordable Care Act of 2010, which put the medical profession's already bad trajectory on steroids, has for many doctors become the straw that broke the camel's back.

A June 2012 survey of 36,000 doctors in active clinical practice by the Doctors and Patients Medical Association found 90 percent of doctors believe the medical system is "on the wrong track" and 83 percent are thinking about quitting. Another 85 percent said "the medical profession is in a tailspin." 65 percent say that "government involvement is most to blame for current problems." In addition, 2 out of 3 physicians surveyed in private clinical practice stated they were "just squeaking by or in the red financially."

A separate survey of 2,218 physicians, conducted online by the national health care recruiter Jackson Healthcare, found that 34 percent of physicians plan to leave the field over the next decade. What's more, 16 percent said they would retire or move to part-time in 2012. "Of those physicians who said they plan to retire or leave medicine this year," the study noted, "56% cited economic factors and 51% cited health reform as among the major factors. Of those physicians who said they are strongly considering leaving medicine in 2012, 55% or 97 physicians, were under age 55."

Interestingly, these surveys were completed two years after a pre-ObamaCare survey reported in The New England Journal of Medicine found 46.3 percent of primary care physicians stated passage of the new health law would "either force them out of medicine or make them want to leave medicine."

It has certainly affected my plans. Starting in 2012, I cut back on my general surgery practice. As co-founder of my private group surgical practice in 1986, I reached an arrangement with my partners freeing me from taking night calls, weekend calls, or emergency daytime calls. I now work 40 hours per week, down from 60 or 70. While I had originally planned to practice at least another 12 to 14 years, I am now heading for an exit—and a career change—in the next four years. I didn't sign up for the kind of medical profession that awaits me a few years from now.

Many of my generational peers in medicine have made similar arrangements, taken early retirement, or quit practice and gone to work for hospitals or as consultants to insurance companies. Some of my colleagues who practice primary care are starting cash-only "concierge" medical practices, in which they accept no Medicare, Medicaid, or any private insurance.

As old-school independent-thinking doctors leave, they are replaced by protocol-followers. Medicine in just one generation is transforming from a craft to just another rote occupation.

In the not-too-distant future, a small but healthy market will arise for cash-only, personalized, private care. For those who can afford it, there will always be competitive, market-driven clinics, hospitals, surgicenters, and other arrangements—including "medical tourism," whereby health care packages are offered at competitive rates in overseas medical centers. Similar healthy markets already exist in areas such as Lasik eye surgery and cosmetic procedures. The medical profession will survive and even thrive in these small private niches.

In other words, we're about to experience the two-tiered system that already exists in most parts of the world that provide "universal coverage." Those who have the financial means will still be able to get prompt, courteous, personalized, state-of-the-art health care from providers who consider themselves professionals. But the majority can expect long lines, mediocre and impersonal care from shift-working providers, subtle but definite rationing, and slowly deteriorating outcomes.

We already see this in Canada, where cash-only clinics are beginning to spring up, and the United Kingdom, where a small but healthy private system exists side-by-side with the National Health Service, providing high-end, fee-for-service, private health care, with little or no waiting.

Ayn Rand's philosophical novel *Atlas Shrugged* describes a dystopian near-future America. One of its characters is Dr. Thomas Hendricks, a prominent and innovative neurosurgeon who one day just disappears. He could no longer be a part of a medical system that denied him autonomy and dignity. Dr. Hendricks' warning deserves repeating:

"Let them discover the kind of doctors that their system will now produce. Let them discover, in their operating rooms and hospital wards, that it is not safe to place their lives in the hands of a man whose life they have throttled. It is not safe, if he is the sort of man who resents it—and still less safe, if he is the sort who doesn't."

Critical Thinking

1. What problems arose with the coding system from a doctor's perspective? A patient's?

2. Why has the persistence of price controls coincided with a steady ratcheting down of physician's fees?

Create Central

www.mhhe.com/createcentral

Internet References

American Medical Association (AMA)
www.ama-assn.org

Medicare.gov: the official U.S. government site for Medicare
www.medicare.gov

MedScape: The Online Resource for Better Patient Care
www.medscape.com

Article   Prepared by: Eileen Daniel, *SUNY College at Brockport*

Problems with Modern Medicine: Too Much Emphasis on Disease, Not Enough on Managing Risk

MACIEJ ZATONSKI

Learning Outcomes

After reading this article, you will be able to:

- Explain why medicine today is more about risk management than treating sick people.

- Understand the concept of defensive medicine.

- Understand that every abnormality does not develop into disease.

I am a doctor. A surgeon. I was taught to make sick people healthy and to make those who cannot be cured comfortable. I am lucky also. Major advances have benefited us all. We have learned how to put people to sleep during surgery; we have developed antibiotics to battle bacteria; we have started to transplant organs from the deceased. We have created technology that allows us to look into a living body and even observe metabolic processes on the cellular level in real time. We developed effective vaccinations and prevented millions from dying in accidents, from strokes, or from complications of chronic diseases. We have used modern scientific methods to analyze huge amounts of data, and we have managed to change the perception of medicine as a form of art and turn it into a hard science.

But it all happened at a price.

Nowadays, we try to improve our past discoveries, but we probably will need to wait for another breakthrough. In the meanwhile, our old discoveries are becoming available to increasingly larger numbers of people. And the more people we diagnose, the more diseases we find. But are doctors still making sick people healthy? Our definition of sickness and health is evolving but does not seem to catch up with current medical advances. We can detect cancers before they give us any symptoms. We scan, screen, and diagnose more and more individuals using the most advanced technology. But are we always helping our patients? Who actually benefits from early treatments? How many suffer from complications? How many are harmed, physically or emotionally? These are hard questions to answer, and we are looking into them.

We know that every advanced disease (cancer, for example) had to have a very early stage. It can start as a single mutation in our DNA. Historically, we were not able to pick those things early enough. The tumor had to be of a size that would be detectable with our fingers or eyes—and it often meant that it was too late for a cure. We have learned to look inside our bodies to identify tiny lumps that are invisible to the eye and impossible to feel or touch. Later came newer technologies that allowed us to spot abnormalities in tissues, cells, and even on the molecular level. We thought that this was good because every advanced disease had to start early. And the earlier we pick it up, the better the chances of survival.

Well, it is true to some degree. The problem is that we do not know if every detected pathology will become a real problem. Not all abnormalities develop into symptomatic diseases. We don't know which of them will. And we probably never will, as an attempt to investigate this issue would raise severe ethical issues.

Medicine today is not only about making sick people healthy. It is becoming a risk-management and quality-of-life improvement service. We need to needlessly treat hundreds of people with a mild hypertension to prevent a single death. Since not all people with hypertension die from its consequences, we have to treat a lot of people for one person to actually benefit. We don't know who this lucky person will be. It's like a lottery—lots of people have to play the game, so we can have one winner. Therefore, we treat everyone's "abnormal" findings. And this would be totally okay if there were no side effects from the treatment. If you play in a lottery you might lose just a few dollars. If you play with your life, the price to pay can be much higher.

The closer we look, the more "diseases" we find. Recently, National Health Service in the U.K. announced a nationwide "Health Check" program, where healthy people are encouraged to visit their doctors. Some lives will be saved. But how many people will be turned needlessly into patients? We don't know exactly, but the estimations are alarming.

It was easier to trust the doctors when we could see the results of their treatment immediately. But when doctors manage risks of possible (but not at all guaranteed) future problems, this undermines patients' trust in modern medicine. Treatments are often expensive and can make previously healthy people feel sick—both physically (from side effects) and psychologically (due to their changed perception of their own health).

Doctors don't give advice to their patients anymore. They give them options. We are told that this is good: it respects patients' autonomy, beliefs, and expectations. But it also takes a lot of responsibility away from doctors and leaves the decision regarding the treatment in the hands of the least qualified person. It's a part of the phenomenon called "defensive medicine." Doctors will always put their safety (and the financial safety of their families) first. This allows charlatans to thrive. Think about it: if you only prescribe sugar pills (such as homeopathy)—you can actually give any advice to your clients without putting yourself at risk, as each piece of advice is technically identical and risk-free. It's easy to actually advise a patient to take sugar pills, instead of presenting him or her with treatments, statistics, and decisions to make. If I knew enough to make a proper therapeutic decision, would I need to consult a doctor in the first place?

Don't get me wrong; I am not saying that the idea of offering a choice and providing information to patients is wrong. It's the best way we know. However, this great idea is flawed: after years of practicing medicine I would struggle to make a "good" decision myself. And if it's our life at stake, we tend to make irrational choices. There is a reason why many doctors admit that they would never consider treatments for themselves that they offer their patients. It is a complicated problem that might be impossible to solve in current legal and ethical realities.

Perhaps instead of battling homeopaths, it would be better to educate patients and doctors about the concept of medical risk-management (in the mathematical meaning). Understanding of statistics is poor among doctors and the general public—but in a world flooded with big data, basics of statistics (and its implications) should be a mandatory part of every primary school curriculum.

Are our expectations of modern medicine too high? We don't have a cure for loneliness, feeling down, lack of hope, or rejection. We don't even have a cure for most common diseases. We can "manage" certain conditions, reduce risks, prolong life. But we still cannot cure many illnesses. But neither can the "alternative medicine" shamans.

My impression is that we need to redefine our conception and definition of health and disease and introduce the concept of "risk-management of possible future health benefits." Perhaps skeptics can actually make a difference and lead the world into the changes that modern medicine needs. I invite the readers to share their ideas and opinions.

Critical Thinking

1. Why isn't it realistic or desirable to treat every symptom?
2. What are the risks of treating all abnormal findings?

Create Central

www.mhhe.com/createcentral

Internet References

American Cancer Society
http://www.cancer.org
Centers for Disease Control and Prevention
http://www.cdc.gov/vaccines

MACIEJ ZATONSKI, MD, PhD, is a surgeon and researcher working at BHR University Hospitals NHS Trust in the United Kingdom. He is a founder of Polish Skeptics Club and specializes in debunking unscientific therapies and claims in medicine. He is a leader of public understanding of science in Poland and is actively engaged in promoting evolution and evolutionary sciences.

Maciej Zatonski, "Problems with Modern Medicine: Too Much Emphasis on Disease, Not Enough on Managing Risk" from *Skeptical Inquirer* 30.1 (January/February 2014): 14–15.

Article   Prepared by: Eileen Daniel, *SUNY College at Brockport*

Still Unsafe

Why the American Medical Establishment Cannot Reduce Medical Errors

PHILIP LEVITT

Learning Outcomes

After reading this article, you will be able to:

- Explain major cause of preventable deaths in American hospitals.

- Understand why there was no drop in mortality from medical errors despite implication of the systems approach.

- Describe why many incompetent doctors are able to continue to practice medicine.

Every year, there are about 138,000 preventable deaths in hospitals throughout America. At least 30 percent of those deaths are the result of the actions of doctors who by any standards are incompetent.[1,2] Because it is easier to blame a system than an individual doctor, particularly if he or she is a peer, the medical establishment has chosen to attack the problem of preventable deaths by employing what it calls a systems approach. The theory behind such an approach, which was first widely instituted at the beginning of this century, is that if you standardize the delivery of health care in a hospital, you reduce the number of errors that can be made by fallible humans. Although such an approach has worked successfully in the airline and automobile industries, it has not caused any noticeable drop in the overall number of preventable deaths in American hospitals.

In 2007, I retired from neurosurgery after 32 years. During that time I had been the chief of staff of two hospitals in South Florida over a total period of five years. In those positions, I had responsibility for overseeing the professional and ethical conduct of roughly 1,800 doctors, about a tenth of those in the

state. It was nearly impossible to discipline any one of them who stepped out of line and endangered patients. A second important consideration was that I knew from daily experience that the systems methods that were put in place in my hospital and in nearly 80% of the hospitals in the country during the first decade of this century were unlikely to make a significant dent in the number of deaths due to caretakers' mistakes. Tactics such as checklists, time outs (where the nurses withhold the scalpel from the surgeon until he or she declares the name of the patient and the name and site of the operation), and labeling the correct extremity for surgery seemed merely to nibble around the edges of the identifiable hard core source of more deaths annually than automobile accidents—the inept doctors. I knew from direct experience and from sitting on numerous quality assurance committees for years and learning of their misadventures that they harmed many more patients than the occasional omission of typical systems tactics such as administering aspirin to a heart attack patient or giving preoperative antibiotics.

While researching the problem, I came upon two documents with overlapping authorship about harmful medical mistakes that contradicted each other. The first, published in the *New England Journal of Medicine,* were the Harvard Medical Practice Studies of 1991, based on data gleaned from scores of hospitals in New York State during the mid-1980s.[2,3] They are the gold standard dealing with "adverse events" a term meaning harm to patients as the result of medical management. "Adverse events" has almost completely replaced the much older term "iatrogenic mishaps" in the medical literature. "Iatrogenic" means doctor caused.

The Harvard Medical Practice Studies contained the results of screening by expert physician examiners of over

30,000 hospital charts for evidence of bad care. Nothing on that scale has been done since. The Harvard Studies analyzed, categorized, and put into easily scanned written tables the types of errors that resulted in significant harm to patients. Although follow-up studies that analyzed hospital charts have included enough patients to reach statistical significance—a venerable yardstick of scientific validity—they are still dwarfed in size and detail by the Harvard Studies.

The other document, which appeared in 1999, *To Err Is Human,* is a report written by a 19-person committee of the Institute of Medicine (IOM).[4] The IOM is a private scientific group that advises Congress and the public on matters of public health. *To Err Is Human* claimed to have as its scientific and factual basis the Harvard Medical Practice Studies. By projecting to the entire country the data from New York State in the Harvard Studies, it concluded that there were around 98,000 fatal adverse events in America's hospitals each year. Similar results have been echoed in two more recent studies published in 2010.[5,6] To Err Is Human did not contain any new facts. Its most significant and far-reaching impact was its recommendations for reducing medical errors. It concluded that the best way to do so was to apply the same general method used to reduce crashes of commercial airplanes, called the "systems approach." The authors, without scientific data arising from studies of hospitals and medicine, concluded *a priori* that most of the errors and deaths arose from faulty medical care delivery systems. It promised that if those systems were corrected that the number of deaths would drop by 50% in five years. The methods were started in 78% of American hospitals.[7] They included a variety of checklists that assured that a heterogeneous group of tasks were always carried out, such as giving aspirin and beta blockers to heart attack patients immediately upon admission to the hospital, polyvalent pneumonia vaccine to elderly patients upon discharge, and antibiotics to surgical patients within the hour before making the surgical incision.

Despite considerable change in how hospital medicine is practiced and with the vast majority of American hospitals participating, there was no drop in mortality from adverse events in the decade that followed the release of *To Err is Human.* Two research reports came out at the end of the last decade with very similar results. One of the studies was directed by the Inspector General of the U.S. Department of Health and Human Services, (HHS)[5] and the other, by a group from Harvard and Stanford medical schools.[6] The latter report was published in the November 2010 issue of the *New England Journal of Medicine*, the same time that the HHS report appeared on the Internet. In *To Err is Human,* the IOM estimated that 98,000 preventable deaths occurred based on data collected during the 1980s. During the period from the mid-1980s to mid-2000s, no other studies of a similar scope and resulting from an equally

rigorous methodology (a careful screening of hospital charts) were reported. In the Health and Human Services (HHS) report based on hospital chart review, 180,000 Medicare patients lost their lives. Its authors considered 44 percent—or 79,200 of the deaths—preventable. How does this compare with the numbers gleaned from the mid-1980s that were reported in *To Err is Human*? Given that Medicare admissions are somewhat less than half of all hospital admissions, the numbers are, sadly, comparable.

The Harvard-Stanford study looked at the inpatient charts of patients in all age groups in several hospitals in North Carolina. That state was chosen because compared to other states it "had shown a high level of engagement in efforts to improve patient safety," the authors said in their report. Those "efforts" involved the widespread use of systems tactics as championed by the authors of *To Err is Human*.[7] A typical example: every patient was given prophylactic antibiotics before surgery to prevent surgical wound infections. However, the use of these antibiotics was not only at the direction of the doctor; should he forget, a nurse was there to remind him. Another example involved the use of medication. A doctor could not prescribe penicillin to a patient without ascertaining whether the patient had any allergies to the medication. Regardless, the prescription was not filled until the pharmacist, checking with his or her pharmaceutical software, also confirmed that the patient, according to the software, had no allergies to penicillin. The system also enabled the pharmacist to double check the dose and the frequency prescribed by the physician. The nurse, a third party, also checked by asking the patient—even if the doctor already had—and double-checking the patient's chart. A system of checking and double-checking was in place, no matter how reliable or unreliable, renowned or unknown, the particular physician involved.

At the time of the scientific investigation, Dr. Christopher Landrigan, the senior author of the Harvard-Stanford study, estimated that about 96 percent of the hospitals in North Carolina and 78 percent of hospitals nationwide, were participating in the 100,000 Lives Campaign, an effort meant to save 100,000 lives a year in hospitals by putting in effect various systems approaches.[7] He and the rest of the authors of the study reasoned that if an improvement in patient outcomes were to be found, it would surely have occurred in North Carolina. Instead, the report found a much higher level of mortality from medical mishaps than expected. In doing their research, the authors of the Harvard-Stanford study continuously monitored adverse events—including deaths—and tabulated them by three-month periods over a span of six years. Their hypothesis was that the longer the systems approach was used, and the larger the number of systems methods employed, the more progressive the drop in the number of adverse events. In fact, the number of adverse events remained the same within the six-year period of the study. In 2002—the start of the study—the authors found 15 high severity harms per 100 admissions (with high severity harms defined as temporary harms requiring prolonged hospitalization, permanent harms, life-threatening harms, and death); in 2007, after the implementation of systems methods, they found exactly the same number.

Using the same method used in *To Err Is Human* and working with the data accumulated by the authors of the 2010 Harvard-Stanford article, one could project 215,000 deaths of patients in hospitals nationwide, of which 138,000 would be preventable. This number compares unfavorably to the 98,000 preventable deaths nationwide found in *To Err is Human,* a figure taken from 1984 before systems approaches were in place. If anything, the results were worse.

Dr. Landrigan, the lead author of the Harvard-Stanford paper and the director of Harvard's patient safety program, said, "We found that harms remain common, with little evidence of widespread improvement." Rather than looking for some other cause, Dr. Landrigan simply noted that the systems approach needed to be used more effectively. "Further efforts are needed to translate effective safety interventions into routine practice and to monitor health care safety over time."

A striking exception to these dismal results was the prevention of blood infections from central intravenous lines which the Centers for Disease Control and Prevention declared to be saving 3,000 to 6,000 lives a year during the same period as the Inspector General's and the Harvard-Stanford studies.[8] This occurred largely as the result of the efforts of Dr. Peter Pronovost of Johns Hopkins Medical School. However, those savings got swamped by all the other preventable deaths.

The failures of the systems approach were foreshadowed in the data of Harvard Medical Practice Studies. Table 7 of the second installment, which listed the types and numbers of adverse events shows that at least 61 percent of all adverse events could be laid at the feet of individual physicians and, according to the authors of the Harvard Medical Practice Studies, only 6 percent were attributable to systems problems.[2] The 61 percent comprised technical mishaps during surgery and other procedures and failure to order the correct diagnostic test. For verification in 2013, I asked one of the authors of *To Err is Human,* Dr. Joseph Scherger, about technical and diagnostic errors and he readily admitted that these were not amenable to systems fixes.[9] He could not reconcile for me his and his co-authors' great familiarity with the results of the Harvard Medical Practice Studies with the solution they proposed for saving lives, the systems approach. Neither could Dr. Lucian Leape of Harvard's School of Public Health, an author of both documents.[10]

The medical profession and its chief watchdogs—the state boards of licensure—had no trouble believing what was said in *To Err is Human.* In a joint statement in 2008, the medical boards of all 50 states and the provinces of Canada wrote that most medical errors were the result of faulty care delivery systems and not the fault of the individual physicians about whom they received complaints on a regular basis.[11]

The Deadly 2%

Based on information from the National Practitioner Data Bank, a federal data base which stores records of malpractice judgments, loss of licensure and hospital privilege revocations for all the doctors in the country, it is clear that a small number of doctors—about 2 percent—are responsible for half the cases in which a patient is seriously and unnecessarily harmed in the process of being treated. Dr. Robert Oshel, formerly the associate director for research and disputes at the Data Bank—he has since retired—confirms that the misdeeds of 2 percent of the physicians in practice during the last twenty years, from about 1990–2010, resulted in half of the money paid out in malpractice cases.[1] In other words, a very small number of doctors are responsible for a disproportionately large number of errors.

The distribution of error rates is not unique to hospitals in this country. Marie M. Bismark, a senior research fellow at the University of Melbourne, who is both a physician and a lawyer, found in a national sample of nearly 19,000 formal healthcare complaints lodged against doctors in Australia between 2000 and 2011, that "three percent of Australia's medical workforce accounted for 49 percent of complaints and one percent accounted for a quarter of complaints."[12]

Given such a small number of grossly incompetent doctors, it should be easy to identify and prevent them from practicing. Unfortunately, in most cases, they continue to practice. The average American hospital drops only one doctor from its staff every twenty years.[1] About 250 doctors lose their licenses each year, or 0.04 percent of the total number of practicing physicians, which is about 650,000.[1] At that rate, it would take 50 years to remove the most incompetent doctors—the 2 percent—from practice. Why do the vast majority of these doctors keep practicing? One reason is the pervasive leniency of the hospital peer review committees and state medical boards, the main institutions set up to deal with the problem.

This small number of incompetent physicians not only causes serious errors in terms of patient health; they also cost society a huge amount of money. Dr. Donald Berwick, the chief of Medicare and Medicaid from July 2010 to December 2011—he is currently a senior fellow at the Center for American Progress—estimated that $300 billion a year are spent on the waste that results from poor execution of care and on over treatment that subjects patients to care that is unsupported by science and that cannot possibly help them.[13] Giving unnecessary care is the favorite method of many less scrupulous physicians for padding their earnings.

What, then, is the solution to the large number of preventable deaths that happen each year specifically because of incompetent doctors? Combining the estimates of both Dr. Oshel and the Harvard Studies this number equals about 42,090—more than the average number of people who die from auto accidents each year.

The advocates of the systems approach try to avoid the issue of the incompetent doctor. They say we can reduce the number of preventable deaths by streamlining and routinizing the practice of medicine. However, that approach has not been successful in either reducing the number of preventable deaths or improving the practice of medicine.

Currently, hospitals do a poor job of disciplining incompetent doctors in spite of laws that exist to ferret them out. Alan Levine and Dr. Sidney Wolfe of Public Citizen, a nonprofit, lobbyist group based in Washington, D.C. and Austin, Texas, in examining the National Practitioner Data Bank, have found that although all hospitals are required by law to report serious disciplinary measures taken against a physician on their staff, 47% of American hospitals have never reported a single doctor.[14] Any practicing doctor of integrity will agree: it is highly doubtful that there are no incompetent doctors in 47% of American hospitals.

In addition, according to a separate report by the Inspector General of the Department of Health and Human Services (HHS), 26 states have laws requiring hospital administrations to report harms inflicted on patients to the state departments of health and state medical boards, but only 1 percent of adverse events are actually reported even in these states.[15] This data is critical to finding poorly performing doctors as, conservatively, 61 percent of adverse events are caused by the errors of individual physicians, not systems failures. Why don't hospitals do the required reporting? Stuart Wright, the deputy inspector general for HHS (for evaluations and inspections) wrote in his Memorandum Report to the Acting administrator of the centers of Medicare and Medicaid Services that this low rate of reporting is more likely the result of a hospital's failure to identify events rather than from its neglect to report known events.[15]

In fact, the opposite is true. Most hospital administrators know exactly who the incompetent doctors are and very rapidly learn of their mistakes. Elaborate mechanisms are set in place for reporting to the CEO on a daily basis so he or she does not get blindsided by doctors, nurses, or family members calling to complain. Once these poor outcomes are detected, however, hospitals are loath to act because both the hospital and the doctor become subject to fines, bad publicity and the loss

of licenses. Until hospitals have stronger incentives to report adverse events, most will do their utmost to avoid conveying the details to state authorities.

Two Modest Proposals

One obvious solution is to impose sufficiently high penalties—a fine of at least $250,000—on hospitals that fail to report to the state board doctors who commit disabling or fatal errors. If hospitals don't report errors, then how will any agency know to levy such a fine? Even when hospitals fail to report adverse events involving negligence, the state boards can and do find out about them through other sources: the patient, his or her family, attorneys, judges, or malpractice insurance companies. If the complaints made are deemed to be legitimate, then the doctor in question may lose his or her license. Therefore, the loss of a physician's license is the one crucial and indelible marker of medical negligence and adverse events. If it is found that a hospital has failed to report the incident that caused the physician to lose his license, the fine will be imposed. No CEO of any hospital could withstand the publicity associated with such a case, let alone the fine. The existence of such a law would affect all hospitals in a state, not just the ones investigated or fined. Because no one can predict what adverse event might lead to the revocation of a doctor's license, it is likely that many more events will be reported to the state. The second proposal concerns the 2 percent who cause half the damages to medical malpractice plaintiffs in America, a special group of repeat offenders. The identities of the 2 percent are a closely held secret of the National Practitioner Data Bank. It would take congressional action to disclose them. Publicity about the money, not to mention the lives lost, because of this small hardcore group of inept doctors, could sway public opinion. And to prevent these doctors from practicing, Congress could take away their participation in Medicare and Medicaid. Currently, few doctors other than those involved in Medicare or Medicaid fraud ever lose their right to participate.

These are not by any means the only solutions, but they at least seek to address the real source of the problem—the incompetent physician. The problem of the incompetent doctor is a constant, weaving throughout the history of modern medicine. Back in 1958, David Allman, president of the American Medical Association, exhorted the association's component bodies to root out bad doctors: "Any reluctance to reprimand an erring colleague does irreparable harm to our profession. Any use of a whitewash brush to sweep dirt under the rug imperils our disciplinary system. Any compromise with personal moral convictions damages the very character which makes a man or a woman a good doctor."[16] His words, however powerful, did not result in any notable action.

The irony is that the continuing tolerance for the incompetent physician is harmful not only to the public but also to the majority of hard working, competent physicians. The inept physicians drain huge amounts of money out of a vast system that also needs to reimburse the competent ones, tarnish the reputation of the profession as a whole, and create malpractice pitfalls for those doctors who work on the same patients with them. Lawyers are often obliged by circumstances and the law to sue doctors merely because their names appear in the hospital chart before the process of legal discovery clears the field of inappropriate defendants. This often takes years.

In the meantime, the inept doctors of America are still in place, sprinkled among the 5,700 hospitals of our country. They remain almost untouched by a so-called scientific systems approach that statistically has not succeeded in lowering or even maintaining the number of preventable deaths. So the silent casualties continue. More than a million patients will die because of medical error in the next decade. Until we confront the real problem, these unnecessary deaths will continue.

References

1. Oshel, R., 2012. Personal communication.
2. Leape L.L., T. A. Brennan, et al. 1991. "The nature of adverse events in hospitalized patients. Results of the Harvard Medical Practice Study II." *New England Journal of Medicine,* 324:377–384.
3. Brennan, T.A., L.L. Leape, et al. 1991. "Incidence of adverse events and negligence in hospitalized patients. Results of the Harvard Medical Practice Study I." *New England Journal of Medicine,* 324:370–376.
4. Kohn L.T., J.M. Corrigan, M. S. Donaldson (Eds.). 1999. *To Err is Human: Building a Safer Health System.* National Academy Press, Washington, DC.
5. Department Of Health And Human Services Office Of Inspector General: Adverse events in hospitals: national incidence among Medicare beneficiaries. November, 2010.
6. Landrigan C.P., G.J. Perry, et al. 2010. "Trends in rates of patient harm resulting from medical care." *New England Journal of Medicine,* 363:2124–2134.
7. Ibid., References 19 and 20: 19. North Carolina Center for Hospital Quality and Patient Safety. About us. (http://www.nc.qualitycenter.org/about.lasso. 20. Institute for Healthcare Improvement. A network that works! The 100,000 LivesCampaign nodes. Cambridge, MA: IHI, 2006. (http://www.ihi.org/IHI/Topics/Improvement/SpreadingChanges/ImprovementStories/ANetworkThatWorks100000LivesCampaignNodes.htm.)
8. Centers for Disease Control and Prevention. 2010.
9. Scherger, J. 2013. Personal communication.
10. Leape, L.L. 2011. Personal communication.
11. Federation of Medical Regulatory Authorities of Canada, Federation of State Medical Boards and Milbank Memorial Fund. 2008. *Medical Regulatory Authorities and the Quality of Medical Services in Canada and the United States,* 4.
12. Bismark, M.M., M. J. Spittal, et al. 2013. "Identification of doctors at risk of recurrent complaints: A National Study of Healthcare Complaints in Australia." *Quality and Safety in Health Care,* 1–9.
13. Berwick, D.M. and A.D. Hackbarth. 2012. "Eliminating Waste in US Health Care," *JAMA,* 307 No. 14, 1513–1516.
14. Levine, A. and S. Wolfe. 2009. "Hospitals Drop the Ball on Physician Oversight," *Public Citizen,* May 27: www.citizen.org/hrg
15. Wright S. 2012. "Memorandum Report." *Few Adverse Events in Hospitals Were Reported to State Adverse Events Reporting Systems,* OE1-06-09-00092, July 19.
16. Ameringer, C.F. 1999. *State Medical Boards and the Politics of Public Protection.* Johns Hopkins University Press, 35.

Critical Thinking

1. What are the primary reasons hospital CEOs do not report medical errors committed by incompetent doctors?
2. Are most medical errors caused by faulty delivery systems? Discuss.

Create Central

www.mhhe.com/createcentral

Internet References

Agency for Health Care Research and Quality
   http://www.ahrq.gov

American Hospital Association
   http://www.aha.org

Philip Levitt, "Still Unsafe: Why the American Medical Establishment Cannot Reduce Medical Errors" from *Skeptic* 18.4 (2013): 44–48.

Unit 9

UNIT

Prepared by: Eileen Daniel, *SUNY College at Brockport*

Consumer Health

For many people, the term *consumer health* conjures up images of selecting health-care services and paying medical bills. While these two aspects of health care are indeed consumer health issues, the term *consumer health* encompasses all consumer products and services that influence the health and welfare of people. A definition this broad suggests that almost everything we see or do may be construed to be a consumer health issue, whether it is related to products or discussions such as the concept of getting enough sleep or what foods will keep us healthy. In many ways, consumer health is an outward expression of our health-related behaviors and decision-making processes and, as such, is based on our desire to make healthy choices, be assertive, and be in possession of accurate information on which to base our decisions.

Consumer health encompasses all aspects of the marketplace related to the purchase of health products and services. It includes such things as buying a bottle of aspirin, a cough remedy, toothpaste, or exercise equipment and selecting a doctor, dentist, health insurance policy, book, website, or other source of information. Consumer health has both positive and negative components. On the positive side, it involves the facts and understanding that enable people to make medically and economically sound choices. Negatively, it means avoiding unwise decisions based on deception, misinformation, or other factors. Health information has become increasingly large and complex. Even well-trained health professionals can have difficulty sorting out what is accurate and significant from what is not. The media have tremendous influence. A multitude of radio, cable, and television stations broadcast health-related news, commentary, and talk shows. Thousands of magazines and newspapers carry health-related items, and many health-related books and pamphlets are published each year. Many of these books recommend unscientific health practices, as do countless websites, blogs, and other computerized information sources.

Fast-breaking news should be regarded cautiously. Many reports, although accurate, tell only part of the story. Unconfirmed research findings may turn out to be insignificant. The simplest strategy for keeping up to date is to subscribe to trustworthy newsletters and other review sources that place new information in proper perspective. Advertising should also be regarded with caution. Some advertisers use puffery, "weasel words," half-truths, imagery, or celebrity endorsements to misrepresent their products. Some marketers use scare tactics to promote their wares. Some attempt to exploit common hopes, fears, and feelings of inadequacy. Cigarette ads have used images of youth, health, vigor, and social acceptance to convey the opposite of what cigarette smoking will do to smokers. Alcohol ads stress fun and sociability and say little about the dangers of excessive drinking. Many ads for cosmetics exaggerate what they can do. Food advertising tends to promote dietary imbalance by emphasizing snack foods that are high in fat and calories, especially when marketing to children. Radio and television infomercials abound with promoters of health misinformation.

Overall, consumer health encompasses all aspects of the marketplace related to the purchase of health products and services. Although health care in America is potentially the world's best, many problems exist. Health information is voluminous and complex. Many practitioners fall short of the ideal and some are completely unqualified. Quackery is widespread. The marketplace is overcrowded with products, many of which are questionable. Rising costs and lack of adequate insurance coverage have reached crisis levels. Consumer protection is limited. Only well-informed individuals can master the complexity of the health marketplace. Intelligent consumers maintain a healthy lifestyle, seek reliable sources of information and care, and avoid products and practices that are unsubstantiated and lack a scientifically plausible rationale.

Article   Prepared by: Eileen Daniel, *SUNY College at Brockport*

Consumers Should Drive Medicine

David Goldhill on America's deadly, dysfunctional **health** care system

KMELE FOSTER

Learning Outcomes

After reading this article, you will be able to:

- Understand why turning patients into customers would help solve the problems of American health care.

- Explain why the United States spends so much on health care and lags behind other developed countries in health measurements.

- Understand how most health-care purchasing power is in controlled by insurance companies and not consumers.

In 2007, David Goldhill's father was admitted to a New York City hospital with pneumonia. Five weeks later, he died there from multiple hospital-acquired infections. "I probably would have been like any other family member dealing with the grief and disbelief," says Goldhill, a self-described liberal Democrat who now serves as CEO of the Game Show Network.

But then Goldhill read a profile of a physician named Peter Provonost, "who was running around the country with fairly simple steps for cleanliness and hygiene that could significantly reduce the hospital-acquired infection rate." Provonost had been having a hard time bringing hospitals aboard, which the TV executive found surprising.

"I had helped run a movie chain," Goldhill says, "and we had a rule that if a soda spilled, it had to be cleaned up in five minutes or someone got in trouble. And I thought to myself, if we can do that to get you not to go to the theater across the street, why are hospitals having such a hard time doing simple, cost-free things to save lives?"

That's how Goldhill first became interested in the economics of the American health care system. In 2009, he published a much-discussed feature story on the subject in the Atlantic under the provocative headline "How American Health Care Killed My Father." He has now expanded that article into a book.

In *Catastrophic Care* (Knopf), Goldhill decries a system of incentives that puts most health care purchasing power in the hands of insurance companies and bureaucrats, while cutting patients out of the equation. There's a direct link, he argues, between the way we pay for health care and the estimated 100,000 patients in the U.S. who die every year from infections they picked up in the hospital.

Reason TV contributor Kmele Foster sat down with Goldhill in October to discuss how turning patients into customers would go a long way toward solving the problems of American health care. An edited transcript of their conversation follows.

reason: In your book, the word incentives comes up a great deal.

David Goldhill: The fundamental argument I make is that removing us as the real consumer in health care and putting someone between us and providers—whether it's insurers, whether it's Medicare or Medicaid—has completely turned the incentives in the system on their head. What we see now is that the best way to make money in health care is to price high; provide excess service; be sloppy about safety; underinvest in service, which includes information technology; and lack the type of accountability we see in anything else.

reason: How did health care and health become synonymous?

Goldhill: You'll hear, "The United States spends so much on health care and lags behind other countries in health measurements." Well, we don't really measure the outcomes of health care. We measure how long we live, how vigorous we are through old age, how many of our children are born healthy. We measure those types of big things. Unfortunately, all of them have almost nothing to do with health care. The things that drive health are all lifestyle. Nutrition, exercise, stress, income, education, and public safety—all of these things drive health results far more than health care.

The most dangerous thing we do in health care policy is we imply that making sure that everyone has the maximum amount of health care is essential to health, when one could better argue that diverting 18 percent of our GDP into health care has made us significantly less healthy as a country. I always like to turn that little thing on its head and say, "You know what's amazing? No developed country's health seems to suffer, no matter how little it spends on health-care." It may be the least important factor in health, and yet it's the one we emphasize.

From there, a lot of things go wrong. From there, we have a system where much of the debate is about money: how do we pay for all the health care people? And we miss a big question: if we pay for health care in such a way that we take the individual out, are we going to subject people to excess care and excess treatment, which is a major cause of harm and injury and poor health in itself?

reason: There seems to be a real desire on the part of many Americans to not think about their health care costs.

Goldhill: The foundation of health care economics in this country is an article written by Kenneth Arrow. He said that health care can never be a normal industry because you'll buy whatever your doctor sells you. He's got all the expertise. You're desperate, you're sick, he's gonna tell you how not to be sick. You'll buy anything. There can't be any normal marketplace transaction.

So now, we never ask them what it costs, and we buy everything. It's almost what I would call Arrow's revenge, although I don't think he would take that very kindly.

There's a terrific website called the NNT.com. Every American should look at it before taking a pill or having a treatment. The NNT takes all the numbers that you see and translates it into a single number. How many people need to take this pill for one person to benefit? How many people need to have this operation? It's astonishing. I'm taking a statin for cholesterol. If you look at the NNT—admittedly, I'm contradicting my own point—it's a few people who benefit for every 100 who take it. And roughly the same number are hurt because of other risks that come from taking this pill.

It's extraordinary how removing the consumer from health care has caused us to buy everything. And because we've taken ourselves out, we've taken out the major incentive for keeping prices down. Health care should be unbelievably cheap, right? It's a capital-intensive, almost zero-marginal-cost business. Instead we've done everything we can to keep their prices high.

reason: Most of the conversation about controlling health care costs has centered around cost and not price.

Goldhill: The other day I was at a speech in which a politician said that if we could figure out a way to integrate care, we can reduce the number of MRIs performed and that will bring costs down. He and I were sitting next to each other afterward, and I said, "That doesn't bring costs down. The marginal cost of doing MRIs is zero. You already have the machine; you already have the technician. You're confusing price and cost."

In health care, we never talk about prices. We like to believe that somehow there's some force that actually determines what something costs that is independent of economics. That has been devastating to prices in health care.

There was a terrific piece in The New York Times about asthma drugs. Way into the story, toward the back, the reporter did a terrific job at looking at high prices in health care, and she recognized that these are prices, not costs. One thing that the asthma drug companies are determined to do is to avoid their drugs ever being sold over the counter. They want them sold on prescription, where the prices are high.

reason: Preventative care has been fundamental for folks who talk about controlling costs, that if we do more preventative care, that will bring down costs over time. What's your take on that? Is there much there?

Goldhill: Preventative care is an example of where the Affordable Care Act confused cost and price and visible cost. Preventative care was developing as a very competitive sector because under most people's high-deductible plans they were paying for most of their preventative care. You saw minute clinics growing all over the country—the drug stores in Walmarts and what have you. The reality is that the cost of performing most tests is almost zero. There are a lot of technologies out there that will bring it down close to zero and, more important, let you do it at home. Why? Well, they had a chance to succeed because you were paying for it.

The supporters of the Affordable Care Act think preventative care should be free. The problem with that is all that incentive to price preventative care cheaply went out the window the minute you said anybody who's insured should never have to pay a penny for preventative care. The incentive to keep prices down was gone.

It's an interesting example of what's happened in all of health care. Look at Medicare. In 1965, the average senior spent 10 percent of his or her income on health care and was paying for all of it. Fast forward almost 50 years. The average senior pays only 5 percent of their total health care costs; 95 percent is paid through Medicare. That 5 percent is now almost 20 percent of their income. They're no better off financially. The extremes are less; fewer people have extreme examples. But all you've done is you've enabled my disguise, my not knowing what something costs me, my crazy belief that someone else is really paying for it to allow the providers to push up prices.

reason: People might think that's because of all the technology in health care that technology is driving up the cost.

Goldhill: I once did a Google search seeing how many articles had been written in the previous year saying that technology had driven up the cost of health care. And then I tried to imagine how many of those articles were written on $400 laptops.

Technology does drive up the cost of anything—if you allow it to. If we said, "everybody should have a smartphone, but we know smartphones are expensive, so anything above $300 the government will pay for," well, your smartphone would be nuclear powered. It would have a can opener on it. It would do everything you can imagine. And technology will have driven up those costs in people's minds.

The issue with health care is: Do we have incentives for those technologies that bring down costs and prices? We don't. Do we have incentives for technology that seems to push up prices and costs to be adopted by providers? Yes. That's the difference. And that's what people miss.

The Reagan-era reform to bundle hospital payments had an enormous impact on hospital use in this country. Most people aren't aware of this, but the average stay per Medicare beneficiary in a hospital in terms of number of days has declined by 60 percent since then. In-patient care is totally transformed; most of it is short. What did the hospitals do in response? They cut their prices because demand declined by 60 percent? No. They invested it in things that push up their costs. So hospitals now say to Medicare, "Our costs are now seven times what they were 30 years ago. And the prices you pay us are now five times." That's not what other industries would have done.

If you go into a typical hospital, you see less information technology than you do at your Jiffy Lube. It's not because Congress pushed Jiffy Lube to adopt information technology; it's because they want to save money. Hospitals never had an incentive to save money. They had the opposite incentive. And that's why technology seems to be pushing up prices.

reason: What are the best and worst attributes of the Affordable Care Act?

Goldhill: The best part of the Affordable Care Act is basing Medicaid on income levels. One of the great dysfunctions of the Medicaid program is that it becomes the favored disease or condition program as opposed to what it needs to be, which is a safety net for those

Americans who can't afford health care. I don't like the way Medicaid functions, but I think the idea of saying, "look, this is about helping people who can't afford health care, period," is a real positive. If we're going to have a safety net, it should be structured more simply.

Unfortunately, the rest of the Affordable Care Act is the opposite of simple. It takes a system that's already way too complex, way too hard for normal consumers to navigate through, and makes it ever more complicated. I don't think there's a lot of genuine market incentives in the Affordable Care Act. I think the people who wrote it think there are. I think most of them are so constricted, so narrow, and so manipulated—I think the exchanges are a good example of this—that we are as likely to see them depress competition and all the benefits that competition brings as to enable competition.

The ACA was most interested in insurance: expanding the amount of insurance coverage in both the number of people covered and the type of coverage itself. There are obviously positives in that. Unfortunately, the American system of insurance, both public and private, is unique in that it has no brake. The principle here is that any care you need should be paid for by your private or public insurance. No other country on earth does this.

reason: You certainly don't see that in places where there's single-payer insurance policies. They have to stop at some point.

Goldhill: Somebody somewhere gets to say no. And by the way, I don't think this is fixable. It's one of the reasons I think you have to have a greater role for the consumer; in the United States, the consumer is the only one who has the recognized authority to say no.

reason: What would a system that works look like?

Goldhill: I would like to see a straightforward, simple, truly universal safety net. It would insure against what insurance can actually do well without distorting the market, which is catastrophic care. We need to protect people from health care catastrophe. You can be born with it. You can destruct suddenly at any point in life.

Beyond that, we really need to unleash in health care those forces that work in everything else. Competition, incentives for innovation, incentives for value, need to satisfy a customer, and need to be accountable to a customer. And the only way to do that is to take some of the $3 trillion we're going to spend on health care and give it back to the places it came from. Give it back to the individuals.

reason: Is that catastrophic coverage necessarily run by the government?

Goldhill: It doesn't have to be, but I think there's an argument for being single-pool. I think the more you limit it to catastrophe, the more efficiently it can be run. I think it needs to be single-pool because as we have found in insurance here, there is no way for a private insurer not to game insurance. And if you're going to make it tax-benefited, if you're going to make it the default way for people to pay for any part of health care, you are going to unfortunately incent for-profit behavior and skimming, which is really what our health care industry and insurance industry are, and we have difficulty relying on it.

I'm very attracted to what Singapore has done. Singapore has a very large environment for government health care. But it does one thing that no other developed country does. It says at every point of purchase that the individual is the customer. The effect is transformative. Not just on price, but on service and safety.

Singapore spends under 4 percent of GDP on health care, making it by far the lowest in the developed world. What's even more interesting is the average Singaporean—and this is a country with roughly the same income per person as the United States—is estimated to have enough in his health savings account after 20 years of the system to pay for 11 hospitalizations.

reason: Any good news on the horizon?

Goldhill: I think there is. I actually think we see it with our own employees here. We now have a significant percentage of our work force that really thinks about the price, the cost to them, of actually buying health care.

And we're starting to see new business models. We're starting to see new technologies take advantage of the fact that we have price-conscious consumers. This is an enormous benefit. It may end up being the biggest accidental result of the Affordable Care Act. To get subsidies on the exchanges, for companies to possibly offer insurance for less than the Cadillac tax [on high-end health plans], we're going to see more and more cost sharing.

On the island of health care, people are focused on, "Oh my God, does that mean somebody might not get health care they need?" In the real economy, what we know is going to happen is that, as you get a scale of cost- and value-motivated consumers, you then have a reason for providers and for business models to seek them out. There are tons of technologies in health care that would save cost.

You want to look at simple health care? Go to a clinic that serves the undocumented or go to a concierge practice that serves the rich. The undocumented and the rich benefit from two things. They're both the only customer. There's no one behind them. They both opted out, either voluntarily or involuntarily, of the insurance system. And what do we see there? Simple, straightforward, price-conscious care.

We're going to see that in more of our economy. People say all the time, "Where are the Bill Gateses? Where are the Steve Jobses? Where are the FedExes? Where are the Walmarts?" Well, there's never been enough scale and customers to build those business models that emphasize value, true innovation, service, and accountability. I think we're going to get to a point where enough people pay the first $2,000 or $2,500 or even $10,000 out of pocket that the Steve Jobs of health care comes along. He's soon going to have a big enough market to actually build a better product and offer better service and that's going to be great for health care.

We're already seeing hospitals advertise for safety. We're seeing cancer care centers advertise on service, convenience, and comfort. In health care, these are all seen as waste. State-of-the-art health care can be a commodity. That would be a great thing. Differentiated on service and accountability and value? We could get there. We'd get there in opposition to public policy, but it wouldn't be the first time that has happened.

"It's extraordinary how removing the consumer from health care has caused us to buy everything."

"In health care, we never talk about prices. We like to believe that somehow there's some force that actually determines what something costs that is independent of economics."

Critical Thinking

1. What are the reasons hospitals have little incentive to save money?
2. How will preventive care bring down medical costs?

Create Central

www.mhhe.com/createcentral

Internet References

Centers for Disease Control and Prevention
http://www.cdc.gov

Fair Health Consumer Costs
http://fairhealthconsumer.org

Article   Prepared by: Eileen L. Daniel, *SUNY Brockport*

Bed Bugs: The Pesticide Dilemma

REBECCA BERG

Learning Outcomes

After reading this article, you will be able to:

- Explain the risks, if any, associated with infestation with bed bugs.

- Describe why the number of bed bugs is increasing.

- Describe how bed bugs have become pesticide-resistant.

"Six different companies have now found them in movie theaters," said Michael Potter, professor of entomology at the University of Kentucky.

Potter works with pest control companies and their customers all over the country. Asked where bed bugs are cropping up, he rattled off a list that included everything from single-family homes to hospitals, libraries, schools ("obviously dormitories," he noted), and modes of transportation. The problem is particularly daunting in apartment buildings since people frequently move in and out with all their belongings.

"It's bad and getting worse," he said. "It's almost like an epizootic or a pandemic where somebody coughs and six more people get it."

He is not alone in sounding the alarm.

"I don't think we've hit anywhere near the peak," observed Jack Marlowe, president of Eden Advanced Pest Technologies. Eden Commercial I.P.M. Consultant Cody Pace, who was on the same call, added that before World War II, one in three homes were infested with bed bugs. "People dealt with it, and it was part of life. . . . I hope it doesn't get to the point where we're all just living with bed bugs."

A Logistical Nightmare

They are small. They can hide in any crack or crevice. (Think furniture joints, floorboards, baseboards, box springs, picture frames, closets full of clothing, personal belongings of almost any sort.) The early stages of infestations are hard to spot.

They can spread from room to room through duct work or false ceilings. They can be transported from venue to venue on clothing and belongings.

Their eggs are even smaller and almost transparent. They are attached to surfaces by means of a sticky substance.

You can't reduce infestations the way you might with cockroaches, by cleaning up food scraps, depriving them of shelter, and putting out bait. "You *are* their meal," said Elizabeth Dykstra, public health entomologist for the Zoonotic Disease Program of the Washington State Department of Health (WDOH).

And, she said, they can survive up to 18 months without a meal.

They have a history of developing resistance to pesticides. Potter and colleagues' research has shown widespread resistance to the pyrethroid insecticides that are currently the standard treatment (Romero, Potter, & Haynes, 2007).

They have idiosyncratic tastes—they're attracted by the heat and carbon dioxide that sleeping people generate, and they will feed only through a membrane. That means significant logistical challenges for trapping and baiting. (A Rutgers University Web page provides information on devising traps out of cat food bowls and dry ice—but only for diagnostic purposes. See njaes.rutgers.edu/pubs/publication.asp?pid=FS1117.)

None of the experts *JEH* spoke with saw any prospect of the bed bug problem spontaneously lessening in coming years.

Solutions from the Last Time Around

For half a century now, most Americans haven't had to worry about bed bugs. The problem previously reached its height in the 1920s and 1930s. Bed bugs had spread from port areas to major cities and eventually reached less populated rural areas.

Through the '40s and '50s, populations of the pest declined, primarily because DDT was widely available. Consumers could, for instance, buy DDT bug bombs in grocery stores. By the time bed bugs began developing resistance to DDT—which, inevitably, they did—organophosphates like diazinon and malathion were being used to clear up remaining infestations.

Larry Treleven, whose family has been in the pest control business for 84 years, said that his father and grandfather used to fumigate used furniture in their vaults. State laws required that the furniture be tagged as fumigated before it could be resold.

It was a different way of life, according to Potter. When people traveled, they knew to check their beds. When children came back from summer camp, their clothes and bedding had to be checked. He wondered whether people these days are prepared to exercise that kind of vigilance.

"And," he said, "people have a lot more clutter today, a lot more *stuff*. Which makes bed bug elimination more difficult."

Today, the hazards of pesticide treatment are also more widely recognized. Pesticide treatment options have narrowed for other reasons. DDT, for instance, is now illegal in the United States (U.S. Environmental Protection Agency [U.S. EPA], 1972). Besides, toward the end of the last epidemic, it had lost much of its effectiveness because bed bugs had developed resistance to it. Then other chemicals such as lindane and the organophosphates diazinon and malathion were used to mop up.

The Propoxur Proposal

On October 21, 2009, Matt Beal, acting chief of the Plant Industry Division of the Ohio Department of Agriculture (ODA), submitted a Section 18 request to the U.S. Environmental Protection Agency (U.S. EPA). The request was for an emergency exemption that would allow a pesticide called propoxur to be used by pest control professionals for treatment of bed bugs.

"For reasons nobody fully understands," Potter told *JEH*, "Ohio is really getting hammered."

Mystery Pesticide

Propoxur is a carbamate pesticide with a murky regulatory history. Currently it is used in some ant and cockroach baits, insecticidal strips, shelf paper, and pet collars. Although it is also labeled for use as a crack-and-crevice spray in food-handling establishments, U.S. EPA does not currently permit its use in locations where children may be present. That means no use in residential buildings and hotels.

But there's a loophole: products that were already in the channels of trade when current prohibitions went into effect may still be labeled for now prohibited uses. Strictly speaking, Beal said, use of those products is still legal. "The label is the law," as Jennifer Sievert, public health advisor for the WDOH Pesticide Program, put it. Indeed, because some of the labels allow consumers to use the product indoors, the permission that ODA is seeking (which would make propoxur available only to pest control professionals) would actually be *more* restrictive than the law as it now stands. That circumstance, according to Beal, has been a factor in the choice of propoxur for the Section 18 exemption request.

Of course, legality is not synonymous with safety. In 1988, U.S. EPA considered conducting a Special Review of propoxur "because of the potential carcinogenic risks to pest control operators and the general public during indoor and outdoor applications and risks to occupants of buildings treated with propoxur products" (U.S. EPA, 1997a, 1997b). In 1995, the agency decided *not* to initiate the Special Review because "the uses which posed the greatest concern had been eliminated through voluntary cancellation or label amendment" (U.S. EPA, 1997b). And in 2007, at the request of the registrant, it issued a final order terminating indoor use, according to the U.S. EPA document *Risk Management Decisions for Individual N-methyl Carbamate Pesticides* (U.S. EPA, 2007).

Sievert interprets that history to mean that propoxur was withdrawn because of evidence suggesting it was not safe. Potter interprets the withdrawal as a business decision; he believes that the cost of refuting challenges to its safety would have been more than the product was worth to its manufacturers. Either way, there are now some gaps in the data on health effects.

U.S. EPA has placed propoxur in Toxicity Category II (the second-highest category) for oral exposure and Toxicity Category III for dermal and inhalation exposures. Propoxur is also classed as a "probable human carcinogen."

Why Propoxur?

A couple of years ago, Potter and colleagues at the University of Kentucky decided to test some older insecticides and compare their efficacy to that of pyrethroids. They tested propoxur and chlorpyrifos (an organophosphate) on five populations of bed bugs collected from the field. Four of those populations had proved to be highly resistant to pyrethroids. Both pesticides killed 100% of all populations within 24 hours—"and frankly," Potter told *JEH*, "within an *hour.*"

Ohio is not making its request in a vacuum. Beal has worked on this issue not only with Potter, but also with the Association of Structural Pest Control Regulatory Officials (ASPCRO). There were also some preliminary conversations with U.S. EPA, he said, and "there's a multitude of other states awaiting this decision."

What about the safety concerns? Beal told *JEH*: "Basically, our role here is that we have a serious situation at hand. . . . We feel that it's a reasonable request to ask the agency to take a look at this. Certainly I'm not a toxicologist, I'm not a physician. I'm in the area of pesticide regulation. So we felt it was a reasonable request."

Does that mean ODA is putting this request out as an open question to U.S. EPA? In other words, the gist is not: We think it's safe, and we definitely want to use it? Rather, the gist is: Will you check this out and see if it's safe?

"Exactly," Beal said. "That's what the process is."

What if U.S. EPA says no, it's not safe? Is there a plan B?

"That is an interesting dilemma," he said. "Then we stand back and we keep talking amongst the ASPCRO states. We talk with the professional management folks—the pest management professionals—and try to see if there are any other avenues for us to go down. Fortunately, we're not at that point right now."

Contra

Early this year, Dykstra and Sievert submitted the following comment to U.S. EPA: "We do not support the proposed health exemption request from the Ohio Department of Agriculture to use the pesticide propoxur . . . to treat indoor residential single or multiple unit dwellings, apartments, hotels, motels, office buildings, modes of transportation, and commercial industrial buildings to control bed bugs." They cited research showing that the pesticide "remains detectable in indoor air weeks after initial application" and that "use of propoxur exposes the developing fetus in pregnant women to the chemical."

Carbamate pesticides, of which propoxur is one, are neurotoxins. Like organophosphates, they inhibit cholinesterase,

Propoxur and the Regulatory Process: Information from U.S. EPA

In response to *JEH*'s request for an interview, U.S. EPA sent the following written statement about the regulatory history of propoxur and the process the agency is following in determining whether to grant ODA's Section 18 request:

Section 18 of Federal Insecticide, Fungicide, and Rodenticide Act (FIFRA) authorizes EPA to allow an unregistered use of a pesticide for a limited time if EPA determines that an emergency condition exists. EPA's review process for a Section 18 includes determining whether the use meets the applicable safety standard as well as whether the unregistered use meets the criterion of being an emergency. See www.epa.gov/opprd001/section 18/for more information.

Propoxur is currently registered for use as follows:

- Indoor sprays in commercial buildings including food handling establishments to control roaches, ants, beetles, bees, etc. Labels explicitly exclude sprays in locations where children may be present (so no use in hotels, residential buildings, libraries, daycare facilities, schools). In food handling establishments, the use is restricted to crack and crevice application. Note that products in the channels of trade currently before the most recent labeling requirements may still be labeled for indoor residential use.
- Granular and gel baits for ants and cockroaches, some enclosed in bait stations.
- Impregnated insecticidal strips and shelf paper, to control cockroaches, bees, wasps, ants, etc.
- Pet collars to control fleas and ticks. Some are combination products with other active ingredients.

Information about historical use/regulation is available in the Propoxur Reregistration Eligibility Decision (1997), which can be accessed at www.epa.gov/pesticides/reregistration/propoxur/.

of Environmental Health. Children are not small adults, he reminded *JEH;* their neurological pathways are developing. "There's so much going on there biologically that *isn't* happening in full-grown adults, and they are much more sensitive. That's the primary population that we're trying to protect."

But the fact that propoxur is classed as a probable carcinogen is of concern for people of any age.

Dykstra and Sievert think pest control professionals should pursue alternative treatments. Such treatments might not, Dykstra acknowledged, completely eliminate the problem. But they would reduce it to tolerable levels.

"Instead of poisoning yourself or your children or whoever lives in the house," Sievert said. "That's really being played down here by propoxur proponents. In fact, there's basically no mention of it, that I can see."

Other Options

Marlowe of Eden Advanced Pest Technologies told *JEH* he is not a "fan" of the Ohio request: "From a *business* standpoint, it seems like we're headed in the wrong direction, to use a product like that around people's beds and in their bedrooms." Pesticides in sleeping quarters, he noted, are a potential liability for a company: "Even if it was made available to us, I'd probably stay with some of the other, lighter chemistries that we already have in the toolbox."

Eden uses steam heat to kill bed bugs, in combination with cedar oil and some other essential oils. Since these methods kill bed bugs only upon direct contact, Eden also applies diatomaceous earth to cracks, crevices, and any area bed bugs might be likely to crawl across. Diatomaceous earth abrades the exoskeleton, so that bodily fluids leak out and the insect eventually dries up.

Everyone agreed that diatomaceous earth is effective and that it shares an important advantage with propoxur: the ability to act residually. That is, it will act on any bugs not killed by direct-contact treatments, as well as on any bugs that get reintroduced after a treatment. A drawback, however, is that it works slowly. Potter also noted that application is tricky because it requires an extremely fine dusting, and applicators are not readily available to consumers. Pest control professionals have to be called in, and that means expense. Of course, the same would also be true of propoxur.

Another alternative, used by Treleven's company, Sprague Pest Solutions, is volumetric heating, which involves "superheating" an entire room to around 140F. Probes are used to ensure that the internal temperatures of objects in the room also reach temperatures high enough to kill the bugs. In addition, Sprague has dogs trained to sniff out any bed bugs that might remain. Unfortunately, this approach is expensive. The cost of equipping a single pest control team with a heater and generator approaches $50,000, and the setup and breakdown work make treatment an all-day, labor-intensive affair. Treleven estimated that treating a 1,700 square foot townhouse could cost a couple thousand dollars. Any conjoined units might then also have to be treated. Room-by-room treatment of multi-unit buildings could be a daunting prospect.

although poisoning with carbamates is more easily reversed with treatment, and there is a "greater span between symptom-producing and lethal doses," according to Reigart and Roberts's *Recognition and Management of Pesticide Poisonings* (Reigart & Roberts, 1999). Serious overexposure can cause death by cardiorespiratory depression. Early symptoms include malaise, sweating, muscle weakness, headache, dizziness, and gastrointestinal symptoms. Other symptoms of acute toxicity are coma, hypertension, trouble breathing, blurred vision, lack of coordination, twitching, and slurring of speech.

The biggest concern is with chronic (or acute) exposure to small children and developing fetuses, according to Wayne Clifford, who manages the Pesticide Illness and Zoonotics Disease Surveillance and Prevention program in WDOH's Office

Treleven does recommend heat, combined with diatomaceous earth and canine detection, as a first, best treatment choice. But, he said, "If they can't afford the heating and the alternatives and things, it would be nice to have propoxur. I mean, I'm not going to lie to you. Because it is an alternative that would work."

Conclusion

In the case of bed bugs, none of the options are ideal. All can take a bite, figuratively speaking, out of someone's life.

Let's start with pesticides. Cancer risk, developmental detriments, and central nervous system effects can all subtract from longevity, fruitfulness, and life satisfaction. According to U.S. EPA's *R.E.D. Facts,* a reference dose (RfD) of 0.004 mg/kg/day is not expected to cause adverse effects over a 70-year lifetime (U.S. EPA, 1997). But as Clifford of WDOH put it, "there is not really a safe level of exposure to a carcinogen," because effects are cumulative and people may have exposures from other sources, such as residue on food. Propoxur treatments in areas where people sleep could entail extended exposures, especially since the pesticide has been demonstrated to volatilize in the air and be absorbed into the blood weeks after application (Whyatt et al., 2003).

But absent an effective pesticide, the need for relentless vigilance just as assuredly takes a bite out of life. Potter told *JEH* that he's had residents call him in tears when infestations have persisted after months of vigilant laundering and vacuuming. Added to the many stresses contemporary Americans already face, that kind of constant pressure can have a cumulative effect. Nor is money a negligible concern: the need for repeated expensive treatments can further contribute to financial insecurity—which in turn has its own, well-documented, health impacts.

Individual consumers could well come to different conclusions depending on personal circumstances, and making propoxur available could add to their choices.

But there are a couple of problems with casting this issue as a straightforward risk-benefit decision for individuals.

First, the impacts of neurotoxins on developing brains are difficult to sort out, much less document and quantify—which doesn't mean they're not happening. As Colborn writes: "Unlike obvious birth defects, most developmental effects cannot be seen at birth or even later in life. Instead, brain and nervous system disturbances are expressed in terms of how an individual behaves and functions, which can vary considerably from birth through adulthood" (2006, p.10).

Second, there's the question of whose risk and whose benefit. It's one thing for homeowners to weigh risks and benefits on their own and their families' behalf. Apartment buildings and other rental properties represent a different scenario. How many landlords, given the choice between repeated expensive heat treatments and a quick, inexpensive treatment with a U.S EPA approved pesticide, can be expected to choose the former? Perhaps a few. But it seems likely that in most cases, the decision will be a foregone conclusion. In the end, apartment dwellers could be subject, involuntarily and perhaps unknowingly, to extended exposures.

Nobody *JEH* interviewed thinks propoxur holds all the answers. ODA's exemption request is just a way of looking for something to, as Beal said, "help us through this critical time right now that we're seeing until something else further down the road can be developed to try to take care of the problem."

But will something else be developed "down the road"? Or will propoxur simply become the default treatment—at least until bed bugs develop resistance to it, too?

References

Colborn, T. (2006). A case for revisiting the safety of pesticides: A closer look at neurodevelopment. *Environmental Health Perspectives,* 114(1), 10-17.

Reigart, J.R., & Roberts, J.R. (1999). *Recognition and management of pesticide poisonings* (5th ed.). Washington, DC: U.S. EPA. Retrieved March 3, 2010, from www.epa.gov/pesticides/safety / healthcare/handbook/Chap05.pdf

Romero, A., Potter, M.F., & Haynes, K.F. (2007, July). Insecticide-resistant bed bugs: Implications for the industry. *Pest Control Technology.* Retrieved April 6, 2010, from www.pctonline.com /Article.aspx?article%5fid=37916

U.S. Environmental Protection Agency. (1972). *DDT ban takes effect.* Retrieved April 5, 2010, from www.epa.gov/history/topics /ddt/01.htm

U.S. Environmental Protection Agency. (1997a). *Reregistration eligibility decision (RED): Propoxur.* Retrieved April 5, 2010, from www.epa.gov/oppsrrd1/REDs/2555red.pdf

U.S. Environmental Protection Agency. (1997b). *R.E.D. facts: Propoxur* (U.S. EPA document # EPA-738-F-97-009). Retrieved April 5, 2010, from www.epa.gov/oppsrrd1/REDs /factsheets/2555fact.pdf

U.S. Environmental Protection Agency. (2007). *Risk management decisions for individual N-methyl carbamate pesticides.* Retrieved April 3, 2010, from epa.gov/oppsrrd1/cumulative /carbamate_ risk_mgmt.htm#propoxur

Whyatt, R.M., Barr, D.B., Camann, D.E., Kinney, P.L., Barr, J.R., Andrews, H.F., Hoepner, L.A., Garfinkel, R., Hazi, Y., Reyes, A., Ramirez, J., Cosme, Y., & Perera, F.P. (2003). Contemporary-use pesticides in personal air samples during pregnancy and blood samples at delivery among urban minority mothers and newborns. *Environmental Health Perspectives,* 111(5), 749–756.

Critical Thinking

1. What are the risks, if any, associated with bed bug bites?
2. How can bed bugs be eliminated?

Create Central

www.mhhe.com/createcentral

Internet References

Environmental Protection Agency
    www.epa.gov
World Health Organization
    www.who.org

Article   Prepared by: Eileen Daniel, *SUNY College at Brockport*

How Not to Die

Angelo Volandes's low-tech, high-empathy plan to revolutionize end-of-life care.

JONATHAN RAUCH

Learning Outcomes

After reading this article, you will be able to:

- Understand why the U.S. medical system was built to treat anything that might be treatable, at any stage of life—even when there is no hope of a cure, and when the patient, if fully informed, might prefer quality time and relative normalcy to intervention.

- Explain why unwanted treatment seems especially common near the end of life.

- Understand why unwanted medical treatment is a by-product of two strengths of American medical culture: the system's determination to save lives and technology.

D
r. Angelo Volandes is making a film that he believes will change the way you die. The studio is his living room in Newton, Massachusetts, a suburb of Boston; the control panel is his laptop; the camera crew is a 24-year-old guy named Jake; the star is his wife, Aretha Delight Davis. Volandes, a thickening mesomorph with straight brown hair that is graying at his temples, is wearing a T-shirt and shorts and looks like he belongs at a football game. Davis, a beautiful woman of Guyanese extraction with richly braided hair, is dressed in a white lab coat over a black shirt and stands before a plain gray backdrop.

"Remember: always slow," Volandes says.

"Sure, hon," Davis says, annoyed. She has done this many times.

Volandes claps to sync the sound. "Take one: Goals of Care, Dementia."

You are seeing this video because you are making medical decisions for a person with advanced dementia. Davis intones

the words in a calm, uninflected voice. *I'll show you a video of a person with advanced dementia. Then you will see images to help you understand the three options for their medical care.*

Her narration will be woven into a 10-minute film. The words I'm hearing will accompany footage of an elderly woman in a wheelchair. The woman is coiffed and dressed in her Sunday finest, wearing pearls and makeup for her film appearance, but her face is vacant and her mouth is frozen in the rictus of a permanent *O.*

This woman lives in a nursing home and has advanced dementia. She's seen here with her daughters. She has the typical features of advanced dementia. . .

Young in affect and appearance, Volandes, 41, is an assistant professor at Harvard Medical School; Davis, also an MD, is doing her residency in internal medicine, also at Harvard. When I heard about Volandes's work, I suspected that he would be different from other doctors. I was not disappointed. He refuses to let me call him "Dr. Volandes," for example. Formality impedes communication, he tells me, and "there's nothing more essential to being a good doctor than your ability to communicate." More important, he believes that his videos can disrupt the way the medical system handles late-life care and that the system urgently needs disrupting.

"I think we're probably the most subversive two doctors to the health system that you will meet today," he says, a few hours before his shoot begins. "That has been told to me by other people."

"You sound proud of that," I say.

"I'm proud of that because it's being an agent of change, and the more I see poor health care, or health care being delivered that puts patients and families through—"

"We torture people before they die," Davis interjects, quietly.

Volandes chuckles at my surprise. "Remember, Jon is a reporter," he tells her, not at all unhappy with her comment.

"My father, if he were sitting here, would be saying 'Right on,'" I tell him.

Volandes nods. "Here's the sad reality," he says. "Physicians are good people. They want to do the right things. And yet all of us, behind closed doors, in the cafeteria, say, 'Do you believe what we did to that patient? Do you believe what we put that patient through?' Every single physician has stories. Not one. Lots of stories."

"In the health-care debate, we've heard a lot about useless care, wasteful care, futile care. What we"—Volandes indicates himself and Davis—"have been struggling with is unwanted care. That's far more concerning. That's not avoidable care. That's *wrongful* care. I think that the most urgent issue facing America today is people getting medical interventions that, if they were more informed, they would not want. It happens all the time."

Unwanted treatment is American medicine's dark continent. No one knows its extent, and few people want to talk about it. The U.S. medical system was built to treat anything that might be treatable, at any stage of life—even near the end, when there is no hope of a cure, and when the patient, if fully informed, might prefer quality time and relative normalcy to all-out intervention.

In 2009, my father was suffering from an advanced and untreatable neurological condition that would soon kill him. (I wrote about his decline in an article for this magazine in April 2010.) Eating, drinking, and walking were all difficult and dangerous for him. He ate, drank, and walked anyway because doing his best to lead a normal life sustained his morale and slowed his decline. "Use it or lose it," he often said. His strategy broke down calamitously when he agreed to be hospitalized for an MRI test. I can only liken his experience to an alien abduction. He was bundled into a bed, tied to tubes, and banned from walking without help or taking anything by mouth. No one asked him about what he wanted. After a few days, and a test that turned up nothing, he left the hospital no longer able to walk. Some weeks later, he managed to get back on his feet; unfortunately, by then he was only a few weeks from death. The episode had only one positive result. Disgusted and angry after his discharge from the hospital, my father turned to me and said, "I am *never* going back there." (He never did.)

What should have taken place was what is known in the medical profession as The Conversation. The momentum of medical maximalism should have slowed long enough for a doctor or a social worker to sit down with him and me to explain, patiently and in plain English, his condition and his treatment options, to learn what his goals were for the time he had left, and to establish how much and what kind of treatment he really desired. Alas, evidence shows that The Conversation happens much less regularly than it should and that, when it

does happen, information is typically presented in a brisk, jargony way that patients and families don't really understand. Many doctors don't make time for The Conversation, or aren't good at conducting it (they're not trained or rewarded for doing so), or worry their patients can't handle it.

This is a problem because the assumption that doctors know what their patients want turns out to be wrong: when doctors try to predict the goals and preferences of their patients, they are "highly inaccurate," according to one summary of the research, published by Benjamin Moulton and Jaime S. King in *The Journal of Law, Medicine & Ethics*. Patients are "routinely asked to make decisions about treatment choices in the face of what can only be described as avoidable ignorance," Moulton and King write. "In the absence of complete information, individuals frequently opt for procedures they would not otherwise choose."

Though no one knows for sure, unwanted treatment seems especially common near the end of life. A few years ago, at age 94, a friend of mine's father was hospitalized with internal bleeding and kidney failure. Instead of facing reality (he died within days), the hospital tried to get authorization to remove his colon and put him on dialysis. Even physicians tell me that they have difficulty holding back the kind of mindlessly aggressive treatment that one doctor I spoke with calls "the war on death." Matt Handley, a doctor and an executive with Group Health Cooperative, a big health system in Washington state, described his father-in-law's experience as a "classic example of overmedicalization." There was no Conversation. "He went to the ICU for no medical reason," Handley says. "No one talked to him about the fact that he was going to die, even though outside the room, clinicians, when asked, would say 'Oh, yes, he's dying.'"

"Sometimes you block the near exits, and all you've got left is a far exit, which is not a dignified and comfortable death."

"Sometimes you block the near exits, and all you've got left is a far exit, which is not a dignified and comfortable death," Albert Mulley, a physician and the director of the Dartmouth Center for Health Care Delivery Science, told me recently. As we talked, it emerged that he, too, had had to fend off the medical system when his father died at age 93. "Even though I spent my whole career doing this," he said, "when I was trying to assure as good a death as I could for my dad, I found it wasn't easy."

If it is this hard for doctors to navigate their parents' final days, imagine what many ordinary patients and their families face. "It's almost impossible for patients really to be in charge," says Joanne Lynn, a physician and the director of the nonprofit

Altarum Center for Elder Care and Advanced Illness in Washington, D.C. "We enforce a kind of learned helplessness, especially in hospitals." I asked her how much unwanted treatment gets administered. She couldn't come up with a figure—no one can—but she said, "It's huge, however you measure it. Especially when people get very, very sick."

Unwanted treatment is a particularly confounding problem because it is not a product of malevolence but a by-product of two strengths of American medical culture: the system's determination to save lives and its technological virtuosity. Change will need to be consonant with that culture. "You have to be comfortable working at the margins of the power structure within medicine, and particularly within academic medicine," Mulley told me. You need a disrupter, but one who can speak the language of medicine and meet the system on its own terms.

Angelo Volandes was born in 1971, in Brooklyn, to Greek immigrants. His father owned a diner. He and his older sister were the first in their family to go to college—Harvard, in his case. In Cambridge, he got a part-time job cooking for an elderly, childless couple, who became second parents to him. He watched as the wife got mortally sick, he listened to her labored breathing, he talked with her and her husband about pain, death, the end of life. Those conversations led him to courses in medical ethics, which he told me that he found abstract and out of touch with "the clinical reality of being short of breath; of fear; of anxiety and suffering; of medications and interventions." He decided to go to medical school, not just to cure people but also "to learn how people suffer and what the implications of dying and suffering and understanding that experience are like." Halfway through med school at Yale, on the recommendation of a doctor he met one day at the gym, he took a year off to study documentary filmmaking, another of his interests. At the time, it seemed a digression.

On the very first night of his postgraduate medical internship, when he was working the graveyard shift at a hospital in Philadelphia, he found himself examining a woman dying of cancer. She was a bright woman, a retired English professor, but she seemed bewildered when he asked whether she wanted cardiopulmonary resuscitation if her heart stopped beating. So, on an impulse, he invited her to visit the intensive-care unit. By coincidence, she witnessed a "code blue," an emergency administration of CPR. "When we got back to the room," Volandes remembered, "she said, 'I understood what you told me. I am a professor of English—I understood the words. I just didn't know what you meant. It's not what I had imagined. It's not what I saw on TV.'" She decided to go home on hospice. Volandes realized that he could make a stronger, clearer impression on patients by showing them treatments than by trying to describe them.

He spent the next few years punching all the tickets he could: mastering the technical arts of doctoring, credentialing

himself in medical ethics, learning statistical techniques to perform peer-reviewed clinical trials, joining the Harvard faculty and the clinical and research staff of Massachusetts General Hospital. He held on to his passion, though. During a fellowship at Harvard in 2004, he visited Dr. Muriel Gillick, a Harvard Medical School professor and an authority on late-life care. Volandes "was very distressed by what he saw clinically being done to people with advanced dementia," Gillick recalls. "He was interested in writing an article about how treatment of patients with advanced dementia was a form of abuse." Gillick talked him down. Some of what's done is wrong, she agreed, but raging against it would not help. The following year, with her support, Volandes began his video project.

The first film he made featured a patient with advanced dementia. It showed her inability to converse, move about, or feed herself. When Volandes finished the film, he ran a randomized clinical trial with a group of nine other doctors. All of their patients listened to a verbal description of advanced dementia, and some of them also watched the video. All were then asked whether they preferred life-prolonging care (which does everything possible to keep patients alive), limited care (an intermediate option), or comfort care (which aims to maximize comfort and relieve pain). The results were striking: patients who had seen the video were significantly more likely to choose comfort care than those who hadn't seen it (86 percent versus 64 percent). Volandes published that study in 2009, following it a year later with an even more striking trial, this one showing a video to patients dying of cancer. Of those who saw it, more than 90 percent chose comfort care—versus 22 percent of those who received only verbal descriptions. The implications, to Volandes, were clear: "Videos communicate better than just a stand-alone conversation. And when people get good communication and understand what's involved, many, if not most, tend not to want a lot of the aggressive stuff that they're getting."

Even now, after years of refinement, Volandes's finished videos look deceptively unimpressive. They're short, and they're bland. But that, it turns out, is what is most impressive about them. Other videos describing treatment options—for, say, breast cancer or heart disease—can last upwards of 30 minutes. Volandes's films, by contrast, average six or seven minutes. They are meant to be screened on iPads or laptops, amid the bustle of a clinic or hospital room.

They are also meant to be banal, a goal that requires a meticulous, if perverse, application of the filmmaker's art. "Videos are an aesthetic medium; you can manipulate people's perspective," Volandes says. "I want to provide information *without* evoking visceral emotions." Any hint that he was appealing to sentiments like revulsion or fear to nudge patients toward a certain course of treatment would discredit his whole project, so Volandes does all he can to eliminate emotional cues. That is why he films advanced-dementia patients dressed and groomed to the nines. "I give them the nicest image," Volandes told me. "If with the nicest image we show a huge effect, you can imagine what it would be like if they really saw the reality."

The typical video begins with Davis explaining what the viewer is about to see, stating plainly facts that doctors are sometimes reluctant to mention. She says, for example: *People with advanced dementia usually have had the disease for many years and have reached the last stage of dementia. They are nearing the end of life.* The video cuts to a shot of a patient. Then Davis outlines the three levels of care, starting with the most aggressive. Over footage of CPR and mechanical ventilation, she explains that in most cases of advanced dementia, CPR does not work, and that patients on breathing machines are usually not aware of their surroundings and cannot eat or talk. Then she describes limited care and comfort care, again speaking bluntly about death. *People who choose comfort care choose to avoid these procedures even though, without them, they might die.* She concludes by recommending The Conversation.

It seems a minor thing, showing a short video. As, indeed, it will be, if it happens only occasionally. I didn't get my head around the scale of Volandes's ambition until I understood that he wants to make his videos ubiquitous. His intention is not only to provide clearer information but, more important, to trigger The Conversation as a matter of medical routine. "We're saying, 'You're not doing your job if you are not having these conversations in a meaningful way with patients and their families,'" he tells me. "If every patient watched a video, there's standardization in the process. That's why I call it subversive. Very few things in medicine can change the culture like that."

Routine use, however, is far, far away. According to Volandes, only a few dozen U.S. hospitals, out of more than 5,700, are using his videos. I spoke with physicians and a social worker at three health systems that are piloting them, and all were very enthusiastic about the results. Volandes is particularly hopeful about a collaboration with the Hawaii Medical Service Association, the state's dominant health-insurance provider, which is piloting the videos in hospitals, nursing homes, and doctors' offices. Officials say that they hope to expand use statewide within three years. Right now, though, Volandes's videos have a limited reach.

The problem is not his product but the peculiar nature of the market he wants to push it into. His innovation is inexpensive and low-tech, and might avert misunderstanding, prevent suffering, improve doctor-patient relationships, and, incidentally, save the health-care system a lot of money. He goes out of his way not to emphasize cost savings, partly because he sees himself as a patients'-rights advocate rather than a bean counter, and partly because it is so easy to demagogue the issue, as Sarah Palin did so mendaciously (and effectively) in 2009, when she denounced end-of-life-care planning as "death panels." Anyone who questions medical maximalism risks being attacked for trying to kill grandma—all the more so if he mentions saving money. For all its talk of making the health-care system more rational and less expensive, the political system is still not ready for an honest discussion. And the medical system has its own ways of fighting back.

Volandes works on his videos ceaselessly. He has curtailed his medical practice and his teaching responsibilities, both of which he misses, and last year gave more than 70 speeches evangelizing for the video project. In an effort to batter the medical establishment into submission with the sheer weight of scientific evidence, he has conducted 13 clinical trials using videos to depict different diseases and situations, and he has seven more studies in the pipeline. He says he gets by on three or four hours of sleep a night. The project has taken over his house. Davis would like her living room back; there are floodlights and a big gray backdrop where her paintings should be.

Volandes thinks he can sustain this pace for perhaps five years—by which time he hopes to have revolutionized American medicine. Davis tries to dial back his expectations, but he resists. "Not when I have nurses and doctors use words like *torture* as often as they do," he says. "In order to make a change, you've got to be ambitious. If not, then just publish and get your tenure and move on."

Volandes has entrepreneurial OCD: the gift, and curse, of unswerving faith in a potentially world-changing idea.

During my visit, I realized that I had encountered Volandes's type before, but in Silicon Valley. Volandes has entrepreneurial obsessive-compulsive disorder: the gift, and curse, of unswerving faith in a potentially world-changing idea.

It is not a huge exaggeration to say that obsessive entrepreneurs, from Cornelius Vanderbilt to Steve Jobs, made America great. It is also not a huge exaggeration to say that health care, more than any other nongovernmental sector, has made itself impervious to disruptive innovation. Medical training discourages entrepreneurship, embedded practice patterns marginalize it, bureaucrats in medical organizations and insurance companies recoil from it. And would-be disrupters are generally disconnected from patients, their ultimate

an advisory panel was to be convened to address whether a NIOSH investigation was even necessary.

In notes from a later conference call, Baumrind is quoted as saying that the trip was postponed because of concern about the department's obligation to respond to NIOSH's recommendations.

For a few weeks, de Perio and state officials, including Baumrind, frantically searched for a new "sponsor" to call NIOSH in. The heads of the prison-guard unions—representatives of the very people the workplace-safety study was intended to protect—declined or ignored the request. California's independent public health department felt it was not appropriate to take the helm "in light of concerns that without full engagement from CDCR, the request would not lead to a successful outcome."

Then, in June 2009, the corrections department shuttered its own Office of Risk Management. In the four years after the CDCR canceled the workplace health and safety study, three correctional officers died of valley fever.

"We had the opportunity to have a quality study performed at no cost to California," MacLean wrote in an email to the director of the California Department of Public Health a few weeks later. "Cocci morbidity and mortality will continue regardless of our choice to ignore it. I think it's a sad comment on the state of public health in California."

In July 2013, lawyers representing several inmates at Pleasant Valley State Prison filed a class action lawsuit against the state. The suit alleged, among other accusations, that the CDCR and the state failed to protect and care for inmates vulnerable to cocci at several Central Valley prisons. The treatment that incarcerated valley fever patients received—and the system's unwillingness, for seven long years, to exclude at-risk inmates from the endemic prisons—constituted negligence, and was tantamount to cruel and unusual punishment, violating the Eighth Amendment. This wasn't the first time a prisoner had sued over valley fever. In 2009, a former inmate of the federal penitentiary in Taft, a small town at the southern end of the Central Valley, sued the federal government for "recklessly" exposing him to cocci. The feds settled and agreed to pay him $425,000.

The 2013 lawsuit listed case after case of prisoners with valley fever receiving subpar care. According to state reviews of inmate deaths, in 2008 a 26-year-old inmate told a prison nurse that he'd lost 10 pounds in the past month and suffered from chest pain and a constant cough. He was referred to a physician, but no appointment was made for him. Two weeks later, he submitted a request for care, writing, "Emergency. I would like to see the doctor ASAP." There is no record of a response from the clinic. Ten days later, he was 20 pounds lighter. After he was finally sent to a local hospital, doctors confirmed he had advanced cocci, but the infection had progressed too far to treat. The man died of renal and respiratory failure 10 days later.

In 2009, prison health care providers failed to evaluate two prisoners; one had lost 56 pounds and suffered from consistent fever, cough, and chest pain. One had not been prescribed anti-fungal medication for two months. They both died soon after.

In 2010, when a 68-year-old inmate had a recurrent case of valley fever, doctors didn't consult with a specialist until the man was near death. At a local hospital, a unilateral "do not resuscitate/do not intubate" order was written by physicians. There are no records showing that the inmate, who died a few days later, was consulted.

In 2011, specialists failed to recognize that a 42-year-old HIV-infected man diagnosed with pneumonia had in fact been suffering from disseminated valley fever. He died.

In 2012, a 45-year-old black man told prison doctors he'd lost 20 pounds in the past six months. The attending physician checked a box on his medical chart indicating that the man was at high risk for valley fever, but no testing was done for the disease. Three months later, after precipitous weight loss, the man entered the clinic in an altered mental state—a clear sign of meningitis—and was finally diagnosed with cocci. He died the next month.

Dr. John Galgiani, a professor at the University of Arizona and one of the world's leading experts on valley fever, later wrote in a review that the prison medical system's response to the cocci outbreak was unacceptable, noting that the medical staff in the middle of the endemic zone was slow to recognize the signs of valley fever, particularly in African Americans, even years after the outbreak began. "As a result," wrote Galgiani, "needless suffering and death were inflicted on these men."

Arthur Jackson, a black inmate at Pleasant Valley, caught valley fever in 2011. "Two years after contracting this disease, I suffer from loss of vision, severe and often debilitating headaches and joint pain, weight loss, fatigue, and numerous other ailments for which I am consistently denied treatment," he wrote to me. "I often wonder if this disease were to have affected all races alike, would the response of prison officials have been the same or would more have been done to protect and treat us?"

"Living with valley fever in prison is simple," Pleasant Valley inmate LaCedric Johnson wrote to me. "You live every day like the last till you die." Johnson, who was convicted of carjacking and assault, contracted the disease in 2011. He's experienced lung damage, fever, chills, sweats, headaches, aching joints, severe weight swings, fatigue, sleeplessness, and loss of concentration. Like Eteaki, he was prescribed Diflucan. "Who gives a fuck," he wrote, "if a few thousand inmates are housed in a prison built on soil that contains a fungus in the ground that kills African Americans at a high rate?"

As the inmates' case winds its way through federal court, much of it will likely revolve around whether officials should have removed inmates from prisons in the hyperendemic area sooner. A key goal, attorneys say, is to force the state to cover the health care costs of former inmates who contracted valley fever in prison. One study found that many long-term valley fever patients, like Eteaki, spend tens of thousands of dollars on care, on top of the cost of hospital visits.

And while the prison system argues that it didn't know how bad the problem was—or didn't have the capacity to handle it—the attorneys say that doesn't wash. Nazareth Haysbert, one of the lawyers involved, told me, "It's a special irony that the US and California would knowingly confine US citizens, albeit prisoners, to the same areas—known to cause deadly outbreaks of cocci—from which they had removed Nazi prisoners of war mere decades earlier."

I n October 2013, I called Eteaki and asked how he was doing. Things had been looking up for a while—with regular doses of Diflucan, he gained back some weight, went to work full time, and even began taking some community college classes. But when he stopped taking his Diflucan because he couldn't afford it, the disease invaded his right index finger. His doctor recommended amputation to stop the fungus from spreading; a side benefit would be that he'd qualify for disability, which would pay for the Diflucan. Eteaki was despondent. "I'm doing welding," he said. "How can I work without my finger?"

That November, I visited Pleasant Valley myself. By that time, all the African American and Filipino inmates were gone—more than a year after the receiver urged CDCR to transfer prisoners whose racial or ethnic backgrounds put them at high risk for valley fever, the department finally complied. Officials took me on a show-and-tell tour. I saw what court-mandated steps had been taken to help halt the spread of the cocci spores. I saw new ventilators, door seals, and informational signs about the dangers of dust inhalation. I was told CDCR would start screening all inmates for valley fever with a new skin test, in January 2015.

Eteaki had told me about his cousin Johnny Kalekale, who'd robbed a liquor store at gunpoint a few years earlier and was now serving a multiyear sentence. It was Johnny's younger brother, Mosese, who'd died of valley fever that he contracted at an Arizona construction site. Eteaki told me that Johnny had just been transferred to Pleasant Valley, sent to fill one of the vacancies left by the black and Filipino inmates—Pacific Islanders were not included in the transfer order. Johnny says he had told the transfer committee that his brother had died from valley fever, but this had changed nothing. (CDCR maintains he did not advise it of his brother's death.)

I wanted to meet Johnny, but I wasn't allowed to interview specific inmates. I was, however, allowed to wander the yard and talk to random prisoners. I met an older man, Nicolas Moran, who said that he'd had valley fever for several years but the doctors were refusing to treat his latest outbreak. He was in pain, he said. He begged me to tell his story. "We're human beings too," he said. "What's the difference between us?"

I sent Johnny Kalekale a letter. In his reply from Pleasant Valley, he wrote, "I honestly felt like they were sending me to my death...I won't let my wife bring my kids, for fears they might catch it...I know I've done things to end up here, but I hope I don't leave this world because of VF."

Critical Thinking

1. Why is Valley Fever so prevalent in the United States?
2. What organs are most affected by Valley Fever?

Internet References

Centers for Disease Control and Prevention
   http://www.cdc.gov/features/valleyfever/
Mayo clinic
   http://www.mayoclinic.org/diseases-conditions/valley-fever/basics/definition/con-20027390

Article

Prepared by: Eileen L. Daniel, *SUNY College at Brockport*

Brain Cancer Cases Shot Up in This Florida Town—Is a Defense Contractor to Blame?

Families in this South Florida town point to two companies as the source of the contamination that caused their children's disease.

SHARON LERNER

Learning Outcomes

After reading this article, you will be able to:

- Discuss the causes of pediatric brain cancer in Acreage.

- Identify the causes of groundwater contamination in Acreage.

A pixielike girl with big blue eyes and straight brown hair, Hannah Samarripa began experiencing headaches and fatigue in the middle of eighth grade. By the time the spring dance rolled around, Hannah didn't have the strength to paint her own toenails. Her mother, Becky Samarripa, did it for her, and then drove Hannah to school and waited outside, knowing she'd be able to put in only a brief appearance. The teenager's mysterious decline continued on to limping, vomiting, incontinence, and—perhaps her most disturbing symptom—occasional fits of barking laughter that sounded so strange and demonic, her father wondered whether she was on drugs. Then, in the summer before ninth grade, while her family was visiting a Civil War memorial on the coast of Alabama, Hannah collapsed.

Still, it was a full six months later, when a doctor spotted her brain tumor during an eye exam—literally seeing the growth through the lens of Hannah's eye—that the 14-year-old got the diagnosis and then the surgery that saved her life.

When Hannah got sick in 2007, her mother had no idea that, just a few blocks away in the Acreage—their lush South Florida community—other children had also suffered through the same awful symptoms. Had she known about Jessica Newfield, who was close to her daughter's age and had been ill for many months before being diagnosed; Joey Baratta, who developed two tumors before dying at age 20; or little Jenna McCann, who got sick at age 3, perhaps she'd have gotten Hannah's tumor diagnosed sooner.

But it would take all of the afflicted families years to connect the dots among their tragedies.

When becky heard from her pastor that another child in their congregation had been diagnosed with a brain tumor, she reached out to the boy's parents, arranging to meet them in the waiting room of Miami Children's Hospital. While Hannah was recovering from her brain surgery, and the boy—a 5-year-old named Garrett Dunsford—was undergoing his own, the parents started talking.

At the time, neither Jennifer Dunsford nor Becky Samarripa considered that her child's illness might be part of something larger. "I figured it was a weird coincidence," says Dunsford, a sharp-witted mother of three with glasses and shoulder-length brown hair. Like Samarripa, Dunsford was consumed with her own crisis—first, Garrett's loss of the use of his left hand and arm; then, his misdiagnosis (Garrett's doctor thought he had a sore elbow); and after his brain tumor was discovered, the failure of surgery to completely remove it.

But a few months later, Dunsford learned that another student in the local elementary school had been diagnosed with a brain tumor, which made four children with brain cancer that she knew about, all living within two miles of one another. This odd fact kept troubling her, and at the suggestion of Garrett's neurologist, she e-mailed the Florida Department of Health about it. The department responded by sending forms that she was encouraged to share with anyone she encountered in the area who had cancer, asking about the specifics of their diagnoses, their ages and their addresses.

By May 2009, Jennifer Dunsford had developed a database documenting dozens of cancers in children and adults throughout the neighborhood. She had also gotten together with the mothers of other sick children, including Tracy Newfield, Becky Samarripa and Kaye McCann, as well as a few concerned friends and relatives, to see how they might get to the bottom of what was going on in the Acreage. "We were moms and wives and grandmothers on a mission," remembers Newfield, who describes herself as both "this little housewife" and—as she would come to see herself over the years of struggle that followed—someone who, if necessary, could become "your worst enemy."

Less than twenty miles inland of west Palm Beach, the Acreage functions as that city's country cousin. In contrast to the smooth pavement and careful landscaping of coastal West Palm, the Acreage has a wild, almost jungly feel. Shaggy cabbage-palm and cypress trees flank the neighborhood's sandy, unpaved roads. The smallest plots are more than an acre, and many are larger, so houses are a good distance from one another. Because the Acreage is unincorporated, the city doesn't provide services—even water. Instead, most homeowners rely on private wells.

Many of the young families in the Acreage were drawn there by its relative lack of development. When she first moved to the area, Becky Samarripa was charmed by the sight of horses trotting by and people fishing in the canals that crisscrossed the neighborhood. She explains why she came: "I wanted my children to play in the dirt and enjoy nature and breathe the fresh air." Tracy Newfield also liked the community's spaciousness, which allowed ample storage for her family's boat and Jet Skis. And Joey Baratta, who moved to the Acreage with his mother and stepfather in 2004, when he was 15, spent much of his time there riding his ATV and working on his parents' land, which abutted one of the area's many canals.

Jenna McCann, too, liked the outdoors. In the fall of 2004, the little girl often played in the grass of her yard with her two dogs. During the next year, while Jenna was undergoing cancer treatment, both dogs developed tumors and died. Jenna was a strong-willed, generous and ultimately prescient child, according to her mother, Kaye. After Jenna got sick, Kaye and her husband, David, began making kid-size surgical scrub caps with cars and animals on them. When Jenna was near death, she told her mother she wanted to take her caps to the hospital so the other kids could use them after she was gone. "She knew and somehow understood and was OK with it," Kaye McCann said recently. When she died, Jenna was 4 years old.

In June of 2009, a local reporter got hold of one of the forms Dunsford was sending around and wrote a story about her efforts. Soon after, the state announced that it would undertake an official cancer-cluster investigation—a rare step, given the high expense and low likelihood of finding any statistically significant increase.

Half a year later, on a mild evening in early 2010, state officials called a town meeting at the local high school to tell the community what the investigation had found. Seminole Ridge High is a big school, and its ample, stucco-walled auditorium can hold hundreds of people, as it does for the pep rallies before Hawks games. Still, the crowd was standing-room-only on this night. As they anxiously eyed the array of health officials lined up on the stage, the Acreage's residents got the news that none of them wanted.

The Centers for Disease Control and Prevention (CDC) defines a cancer cluster as a "greater-than-expected number of cancer cases that occurs within a group of people in a geographic area over a period of time." Yet because elevated numbers of any disease can occur by chance, and because cancer is relatively rare—and it's incredibly difficult to determine if rare events occur by chance—the vast majority of investigations into suspected clusters don't confirm them.

Some in the room knew the long odds, having followed the pediatric brain-cancer scare in the neighboring town of Port St. Lucie a few years earlier. Like most other suspected clusters, that one had failed upon investigation to clear the statistical bar. So they were shocked to hear the health officials explain that the community was definitely experiencing a cluster of pediatric brain tumors, as well as elevated rates of all cancers at all ages.

Typically, each year, one in 30,000 to 40,000 children in the United States is expected to develop a brain tumor; but the Acreage, with a population of 39,000, had four pediatric brain-tumor cases between 2005 and 2007. Though the investigation turned up thirteen brain tumors in Acreage kids between 1994 and 2007, the official cluster consisted of just three girls, all of whom were diagnosed with brain cancer between 2005 and 2007. Based on the calculations in the report from the Florida Department of Health, a girl's chance of getting a brain tumor in the Acreage was five and a half times what it was in the rest of Florida. And that scary figure didn't include the four additional Acreage children who were diagnosed with brain tumors the following year, 2008. Nor did it account for the fact that many of the cases were clumped in the northern part of the study area, which meant that the concentration of cancer in that particular spot was even higher there than what the Health Department had found in the larger area. Indeed, some of the children with cancer had lived just 1,000 feet from one another.

Tracy Newfield cried when she first heard the news. Becky Samarripa, too, was shaken by the cluster designation, which seemed to confirm her worst fear: that something in their surroundings was making them sick. Still, mixed in with an overwhelming sadness, Samarripa felt a sliver of hope that the Acreage was on its way to finding—and eliminating—whatever carcinogens were lurking in the environment.

Kaye McCann, also in the auditorium, was more pessimistic. Since Jenna's death in 2006, Kaye had become less trusting. That night, she found herself wondering whether health officials would ever find out what had caused her daughter's cancer—or whether they would even try.

Kaye's doubts proved well-founded just a few days later, when Dr. Alina Alonso, director of the Palm Beach County Health Department, told reporters that her agency wasn't planning to do any soil testing or other investigation into the causes of the cluster beyond interviewing families. Alonso emphasized the many questions about the causes of cancer: "diet soda, cellphones, and microwave ovens may play a role," she said, concluding that "it doesn't seem practical or reasonable to start searching blindly." Instead, Alonso said, the health agency would focus on raising awareness of the signs and symptoms of brain cancer to increase early detection.

Alonso argues that tracking down environmental causes of cancer is not her agency's forte. When it comes to cancer, "we're more on the prevention side," she told me when I met with her in Palm Beach this past April. "That's where public health does its best job." She felt that the high number of pediatric brain tumors in the Acreage was most likely due to chance rather than any environmental cause (she also noted that the rate was no longer elevated).

Alonso was surely aware of how daunting a task it would be to pinpoint and prove the cause of the increase. In fact, by current standards, conclusively blaming a chemical culprit for a cancer cluster is so difficult that only 3 of 428 cluster investigations conducted in the United States since 1990 have established a link between pollution and illness.

"The epidemiological tools are too crude," explains Richard Clapp, an epidemiologist who has been involved in dozens of investigations into possible disease clusters in his career.

Given the expense and labor involved, health departments are often loath even to attempt to track down the causes of clusters. "They don't walk, they *run* in the opposite direction of these kinds of things," says Clapp. "If they do have to do an investigation, they have to find the funds for it or have to get the Legislature to appropriate funds. Then they have to say, 'Well, we don't even know that this is cause and effect'—in which case, people feel like they got nothing."

So it's to the credit of those who pushed for a more thorough look at the Acreage—including then-Governor Charlie Crist and Senator Bill Nelson—that an investigation into the possible causes of the cluster was launched at all. The process involved, at various points, the CDC, the state and Palm Beach County departments of health, and the Florida Department of Environmental Protection (FDEP). The agencies tested water from over seventy private wells and several of the canals that ran through the area, as well as soil samples from thirty-five homes, for more than 200 chemicals.

As the results of those studies trickled out, the community found itself divided into two distinct camps. One, composed primarily of families of the children stricken with cancer, focused on the fact that the research had identified several contaminants above FDEP cleanup levels, including radium-226, benzene and a variety of other commonly occurring carcinogens. Though nothing stood out as the obvious cause, they felt that such findings should have prompted further testing.

The other camp focused on the good news, such as the FDEP's pronouncement that the local drinking water was "generally good," as the letter accompanying the water-testing results put it, reassuring residents that "in general, residential property in the Acreage is safe for families to enjoy outside activities in their yards."

Much of the information released by the Health Department during this period was open to interpretation. To a lay audience, the scientific documents were indecipherable. The results of radon testing appeared as strings of letters and numbers, and the soil-testing report was essentially a 500-page compendium of test values and chemical names.

So reactions in the community were decidedly mixed when, in November 2010, with the battery of state and local studies having rendered their results, the Acreage investigation was officially closed. Many parents of the children with cancer were angry and frustrated, but other residents felt relief. Though it was unclear whether probing for answers would ever solve the cancer mystery, there was no question that all the attention to the risks of living in the Acreage had carried a steep financial cost.

By that time, home prices in the Acreage had fallen to about half their peak in 2006. Some of that drop was due to the nationwide crash that followed the housing bubble, but the news of the cancer cluster clearly played a role. In August, the Federal Housing Authority began advising appraisers that the cluster might affect properties in the neighborhood, a move that made it very difficult to get a mortgage there. Some who were unable to sell simply walked away from their homes.

Without a clear culprit for the cancers, some residents began blaming the families of the sick for the crisis. Tracy Newfield, who had been vocal in asking for an investigation, started receiving prank calls about the cluster and had her mailbox knocked over several times. Someone threw a rock at her house, breaking her glass porch light.

Becky Samarripa felt the hostility, too. On one occasion, her car got egged. On another, two of her children, then toddlers, were shot with a paintball gun while they played in her backyard. "None of this stuff had ever happened before," Samarripa says. "I felt like people were looking at me saying, 'She's the evil one who wants to ruin everything.' "

Much of the mudslinging took place online. Within six months of the cluster designation, five community-run websites had sprung up and just as quickly devolved into nastiness. Some online commenters went so far as to accuse the affected families of "just plain lying." As one poster put it, "Using your child's illness as a platform is repulsive."

Jen Dunsford, who created the Acreage Cancer Study website and had posted a picture of Garrett in the hospital with his head bandaged, was particularly savaged. "The Dunsfords created all this fear," resident Michelle James told *The Palm Beach Post.* Eventually, the family moved to Tennessee, but even now the comments still sting. "People said stuff like 'The Dunsfords are gold diggers, and they used their son's tumor as an excuse to go after a big company and get dollars,' " Dunsford remembers.

The entire story might have ended there, in 2010, if attorneys hadn't taken up where public-health officials left off. Erin Brockovich, who inspired the eponymous film about her fight against polluted water in California, had taken on some of the affected families as clients. And a local firm began representing several of the cases.

The Acreage suits—which now include at least thirteen individual personal-injury and wrongful-death cases, and two class-action suits over the loss of real-estate value—are no easy moneymakers. The history of such litigation doesn't paint a hopeful picture for the plaintiffs, who include Jessica Newfield; Garrett's parents, Jennifer and Greg Dunsford; and Joyce and Bill Featherston, the mother and stepfather of Joey Baratta.

Only two personal-injury and wrongful-death lawsuits involving cancer clusters in the United States have yielded any financial reward for plaintiffs. And both were so grueling that they left the "victors" unsure whether the effort had been worth it. The suit over whether several companies had caused a cluster of leukemia cases in children in Woburn, Massachusetts, chronicled in the book (and later movie) *A Civil Action,* was incredibly lengthy, costly and labor-intensive, and the plaintiffs walked away with relatively small settlements. After years of litigation, their attorney, Jan Schlictmann, was left temporarily bankrupt, homeless, and personally devastated.

The case in Toms River, New Jersey, documented in Dan Fagin's Pulitzer Prize–winning book *Toms River: A Story of Science and Salvation,* took place over ten years and was similar to the Woburn case in both its underwhelming financial payoff and the monumental public and private effort that led to it. The epidemiological investigation of the cluster took five years to conduct and cost taxpayers more than $10 million. "One of Toms River's legacies is that public-health agencies are quite uninterested in pursuing these investigations, which are very expensive, very difficult to resolve conclusively, make a lot of people angry, and make life difficult for politicians," Fagin told me.

Perhaps because of all these obstacles, in September 2011, Brockovich's firm withdrew from the Acreage case, leaving the local law firm of Searcy, Denney, Scarola, Barnhart & Shipley to represent the families of at least seven children and five adults who had developed tumors and brain cancer.

Definitively proving the cause of a cluster is so difficult because we live amid so many carcinogens. Unequivocally laying the blame on one often requires showing that no other was involved. "Experimental science tries to understand the relationship between x chemical and y outcome in a controlled setting," says Madeleine Scammell, an assistant professor of environmental health at the Boston University School of Public Health. "Whatever you find, there will be people who doubt the veracity of your findings because we don't live in an experimental setting, and you can never control all of the factors that might have contributed to that disease occurrence."

In the Acreage, there were many possible hazards to consider. Workers dressed in protective gear sometimes sprayed pesticides in the citrus groves that abut Seminole Ridge High, even as teenagers practiced on nearby sports fields in shorts and T-shirts. Then there were the rumors that the area had been a dumping ground before the Acreage was developed. Who knew what had been in the water that might be coming back to haunt residents? And the air was often filled with smoke, which came from both the burning of sugar cane and the fires on the banks of nearby Lake Okeechobee.

Yet to Mara Hatfield, the attorney from the local firm who spent the most time on the Acreage cases, the unusual cancer cluster was likely caused by an unusual pollutant. Hatfield, who had grown up in the area and had young children of her own, was familiar with the rumors of pollution and pesticides in the Acreage—and throughout South Florida. "There are a lot of communities down here built on that," says Hatfield. "But not a lot of communities with brain-tumor clusters."

The one kind of contamination that distinguished the Acreage, according to Hatfield, was ionizing radiation, which was not just an established cause of brain cancer but also the by-product of local industry.

Though Becky Samarripa chose not to get involved in any litigation, the radiation theory makes sense to her. The Samarripas left the Acreage in 2010. But when they lived there, Becky's husband, who worked as a customs official, wore a radiation-detecting gun belt for his job and stored it in the closet. Periodically, the belt would start beeping in the middle of the night. "After a while, we realized it was going off when our water was regenerating from our well," says Samarripa, who worried over the fact that Hannah's bedroom was closest to the well.

Hatfield and her colleagues at the law firm traced the radio-active contamination in the Acreage to two companies with operations in the area. One is the local mining company Palm Beach Aggregates, which has mined limestone for road construction for more than two decades using a dredging process that contributed naturally occurring radiation to the local water system. ("Naturally occurring" means that the radioactive substances originated in the soil, water or other natural materials, but may have been concentrated by industrial activity.) At various points, contaminated water escaped the dredging pits and seeped into the canal and groundwater in the Acreage, according to the plaintiffs' complaint.

Palm Beach Aggregates did not respond to a request for comment for this article, and in court documents has vehemently denied causing any environmental harm.

The mining company had already been caught up in a related environmental scandal. In 2003, Palm Beach Aggregates sold its used mining pits to the South Florida Water Management District, the local government agency that oversees water usage, for $217 million. The deal, which helped land two county commissioners in prison for fraud (a consultant advising the agency, it turned out, was being paid by the mining company), stipulated that Palm Beach Aggregates couldn't be held legally responsible for any contamination of water in the used pits. In its eagerness to close on the deal, Palm Beach Aggregates minimized the hazards posed by its pits and allowed the radiation problem to escalate, according to the plaintiffs' lawyers in the Acreage case.

But Hatfield's radiation theory also involves the operations of another, far larger company: Pratt & Whitney, one of the "big three" airplane-engine manufacturers in the world, whose local industrial site was separated from the homes of the sick children in the Acreage by a swampy preserve.

In 2011, Hatfield's firm filed its first suit against both Palm Beach Aggregates and Pratt & Whitney, accusing the companies of creating the pollution, including radiation, that caused Joey Baratta's death.

At the opening of pratt & whitney's South Florida campus in 1958, the chairman of the county commission said that "Pratt & Whitney's coming to this site is considered the largest single industrial accomplishment so far in Palm Beach County." Since then, Pratt and its parent company, United Technologies, have received tens of millions of dollars in tax breaks from the county and state to encourage it to keep its operations—and jobs—in Florida.

Today, Pratt & Whitney has more than $10 billion in defense contracts, and United Technologies is the sixth-biggest Pentagon contractor. Pratt & Whitney designs and manufactures engines for airplanes, rockets, and even the space shuttle. With its engines for fighter planes such as the F-22 Raptor, Pratt & Whitney's products power air forces in twenty-two countries.

Isolation was clearly part of the reason that Pratt originally chose its location in Florida. The company's 7,000 acres of swampland are bordered on the south by a 60,000-plus-acre wildlife preserve. At least at first, the land to the south of that was uninhabited—and, since much of it was underwater, largely uninhabitable. The company was seeking privacy because some of its projects were classified. As retired engineer Robert Abernethy reminisced at a 2004 reunion of Pratt employees who had worked on the J58 engine, "In late 1957, Pratt & Whitney had two top-secret—'black'—engine projects that were to use poison fuels! Not a good idea in the middle of Connecticut … how about the middle of the Everglades?"

One of those projects, known by its code name "Suntan," was an engine to be powered by liquid hydrogen, which was later scrapped in part because of the danger of explosion. Pratt was taking other risks, too. Consider Abernethy's 2004 description of his work on the J58 engine: "We built a huge swimming pool with a tall tower to centrifuge the poison out of the exhaust." (When recently deposed by attorneys in the Acreage case, Abernethy said he had trouble recalling any "poison fuel.")

In court filings, Pratt & Whitney has denied the use of poison fuel, calling charges that it contaminated the Acreage "completely speculative." But while the company's attorneys dismissed their opponents' theories, Pratt & Whitney hasn't offered much explanation of its operations: it resisted requests to do water and soil testing on its property and declined to answer several of the opposing lawyers' questions on the grounds that they related to classified matters of national security.

So the plaintiffs' attorneys have been constructing their case based on the defense contractor's well-known history of involvement with projects that involve radioactive materials. Since so many of its operations are top secret, it is difficult to disprove the company's claims that it has never worked on nuclear planes or spacecraft in Florida. But documents from the 1960s through the '90s show that Pratt & Whitney had licenses to use at least a dozen radioactive substances, including radium D and E, thoriated nickel and cesium-137, in Florida. The plaintiffs' lawyers also unearthed company correspondence indicating that some of these radioactive materials wound up outside of their proper storage places. In court filings, Pratt & Whitney denied having any "contaminations" beyond "properly stored chemical compounds."

In fact, there is a clear documentary record, stretching across many decades, of Pratt & Whitney contaminating its Florida environs with a variety of toxic materials, both radioactive and nonradioactive. According to a 1985 Department of Environmental Regulation update, the company had soil on its property that contained PCBs—chemicals that have been linked to brain cancer—at more than 200 times the maximum level now allowed even in fenced-off, nonresidential areas. PCBs were also found in fish that swam in ponds on the company's grounds, at more than 7,000 times the safe level set by the Environmental Protection Agency (EPA) for human consumption.

Jet fuel, which was the suspected cause of another cancer cluster in Fallon, Nevada, may also have played a role at the Acreage. A mixture of chemicals that can cross the blood-brain barrier and cause cancer in mice, jet fuel was found at the Pratt & Whitney facility in Florida. According to a 1983 report, there were three plumes of jet fuel totaling some 53,000 gallons beneath the company's property, and a layer on top of the groundwater in certain places as well.

In 1978, the same year the Acreage Homeowners Association formed and began constructing a system of canals to make the area habitable, the company admitted to health officials that 2,000 gallons of trichloroethylene (TCE), a carcinogenic solvent, had leaked into the groundwater and surface water on its campus. After the company shut several of the wells that supplied water to its workers, it commissioned a study by the University of Miami to look into the possible health effects of the contamination. The research found that, between 1967 and 1980, the average death rate from cancer among the company's employees had shot up from 13 per 100,000 workers to 122—a roughly ninefold increase. When the study came out, a Pratt & Whitney vice president called the university's research "full of crap," according to a report in *The Palm Beach Post*. Then, two years later, another study was published concluding that cancer rates among the company's workers were not elevated.

A similar back-and-forth ensued when Pratt & Whitney hired epidemiologists to investigate a possible cancer cluster in its North Haven, Connecticut, jet-engine plant, where an unusual number of workers had died from an especially lethal form of brain cancer called glioblastoma—the same kind that Joey Baratta and Debora Craig, another Acreage plaintiff, had. The company trumpeted the results of a ten-year investigation that found "no statistically significant elevations in the overall cancer rates among the workforce" throughout the state. However, though the study did not find an association with workplace exposures, it did confirm the elevated brain-cancer rate at the North Haven plant.

Throughout the 1980s, the EPA was preparing to designate Pratt & Whitney's South Florida location as a federal Superfund site, which would have required detailed public disclosure of the contamination and the various steps that would be taken to remediate it. The designation would have also alerted people in the area—and those considering moving there—to the potential for environmental danger. And, most important, it would have ensured a higher level of enforcement than the state was likely to provide.

In response, the company waged a fierce, years-long battle against the Superfund designation—and, in 1985, it won that fight.

Since then, the Florida Department of Environmental Protection has overseen the cleanup of the area, a process that has involved the removal of many tens of thousands of tons of contaminated soil and thousands of gallons of fuel from the groundwater. But the details of the process aren't public. Though the FDEP says that Pratt & Whitney is in compliance, it also says there are still twenty-five hazardous-waste sites being remediated, and the cleanup—which began in 1985—is today only 77 percent complete.

Meanwhile, the government's investigation into the Acreage cancer cluster provided some evidence for the theory that radiation was behind it. Water testing in the affected homes turned up several radioactive contaminants. Hatfield and her boss, Jack Scarola, ordered further testing of the soil and water. In August 2013, the results showed some extremely high levels of radioactive contamination, including non-naturally occurring radioactive substances—the kind that can only be produced by a man-made nuclear reaction.

To the attorneys' assertion that Pratt & Whitney was the only possible source of the radiation, Pratt's lawyers replied that it could have come from other sources, such as the Chernobyl disaster, through which nuclear radiation "has been spread world-wide."

The plaintiffs' attorneys notified both the state and county health departments of their findings in September of last year and urged them to begin larger-scale testing. Yet neither agency did so. Instead, the Palm Beach County Health Department told Hatfield to direct further contacts to its lawyer.

"Once the lawyers get involved, then the lawyers have to talk," the county's Alina Alonso explained to me.

So Hatfield and Scarola took their test results to the media. Their press conference last August yielded a few local stories, and one unintended consequence: Judge Joseph Marx, who was presiding over Joey Baratta's case, ordered the attorneys not to speak about the case with the press. He claimed that further press coverage could bias jury selection. Interviews for this article with Hatfield and her firm's plaintiffs were conducted before the gag order went into effect in September. Also citing the gag order, Pratt & Whitney declined to answer questions for this article, stating only that "Pratt & Whitney's position is documented in its court filings related to the Acreage."

There are many factors that make it easy for a company to pollute with impunity. In *Deceit and Denial: The Deadly Politics of Industrial Pollution*, historian David Rosner describes how plastics and chemical manufacturers avoided regulation in part by making their own economic interests seem synonymous with those of the country. In Pratt & Whitney's case, no fancy PR was necessary: its product is already understood to be not just airplane and rocket engines but also national security itself. And being part of the defense industry carries weight not just in the court of public opinion but also in a court of law.

"Judges tend to be, historically, extremely deferential to anything relating to national security, especially if it involves the military," says Stephen Dycus, a professor at Vermont Law School and the author of *National Defense and the Environment*. Dycus notes that it's not uncommon for defense-related companies to resist providing information because of military sensitivity, as Pratt & Whitney has done in the Acreage case.

Although the Defense Department (which utilizes some 30 million acres of land) and its contractors are subject to the same environmental laws as everyone else, the difficulties of prosecuting such cases means that they can—and often do, according to Dycus—get away with contaminating the environment. This constitutes a huge problem, though one that, he says, seems to spur little outrage.

"If Al Qaeda sent a team of sleeper cells to poison our groundwater and release toxic materials into the air, people would go nuts. It would be an act of war," Dycus notes. "But if we do it to ourselves in the name of national security, in preparation for war, that seems to be sort of OK."

Pratt & Whitney has not only identified itself with the country's security but has enhanced its public image by embracing the fight against cancer and the cause of protecting the environment. It's a gold-level sponsor of the American Cancer Association's local "Relay for Life" fundraiser, and its chief executive was a vice chair of the group CEOs Against Cancer. It helped start the P2 Coalition of Palm Beach County ("P2" is short for "pollution prevention") in 1994, along with the Palm Beach County Health Department, other local businesses and the Jupiter Chamber of Commerce. P2 began as a friendly collaboration based on "the good working relationship between the regulatory community and industry," as one internal document put it. The group's efforts extend to sponsoring green-themed events, such as elementary-school poster contests on environmental topics and Earth Day "Peace Jams."

But the defense contractor and the county were less keen about publicizing contamination on the company's property. In 2000, when Pratt & Whitney was considering leaving its Florida site, it entered into discussions with Palm Beach County about selling some of its land as a site for drinking wells. But after two assessments of the plot in question found "ubiquitous" contamination, the deal quietly fell through. Though the parcel was on the part of the company's property nearest the Acreage, this never came up during the cluster investigation. (It did come up in the litigation, but the company's lawyers dismissed it as a "red herring.")

Meanwhile, Pratt & Whitney enjoys close ties with regulators. One state regulator who was involved in the process that spared the company from the Superfund designation went directly to work for Pratt & Whitney after those negotiations.

The tangle of allegiances between the company and local officials was on display in 2009, when the Acreage Community Focus Group was founded, supposedly to address residents' concerns about the cluster. Within a few months, some of the participants felt they were being pressured to stop pursuing questions about water contamination. "They wanted us to move on and say our water was fine," recalls Tracy Newfield, who was a member of the group.

Newfield's mistrust, and that of others in the group, grew when they realized that the group's chair—who seemed particularly eager to put the questions of contamination to rest—was a former Pratt & Whitney employee. "He was introduced to us as an engineer," Newfield says. "He left out the fact that he was an engineer for Pratt & Whitney." While the frustrated participants resigned in protest, another member of the group, who had expressed doubts about environmental factors in the cluster, later received a nice surprise: a letter from the Florida Department of Health commending his efforts and offering help in finding funding for his projects.

It will likely take years for the lawsuits against Pratt & Whitney to be resolved. In the meantime, after so much bitterness, the subject of the cancer cluster has become almost taboo in the Acreage. When I asked Jess Santamaria, the Palm Beach County commissioner representing the Acreage, whether there was ever a cancer cluster there, he told me he doesn't know: "I'm not an expert." And when I called Michelle Damone, a local politician who helped set up the Acreage Community Focus Group, to discuss the cancer cluster, she told me that she will "never utter those two words," because "they drive a stake into the heart of my community."

The remaining residents of the Acreage now live with excruciating uncertainty about what caused the cancers here. "I think about it every day," says one resident, who didn't want to give her name lest she be pilloried for believing in the cluster. Even though her children are healthy, she said her life was forever changed by that announcement four years ago. "I'm usually a very rational person, but that night I put on a pair of shoes that belong to someone with OCD. Every day since, I've woken up with a pit in my stomach, worrying about my children. I think about it every time I open up the freezer and we're out of store-bought ice."

This woman was one of several who told me they fought often with their husbands about leaving the Acreage. She wants so desperately to remove her children from the possible harm there that she keeps a bag packed in her bedroom and thinks about leaving daily. "I feel a panic for my kids' health. It's always with me—we're out to dinner or whatever, and you hear 'Tick, tock.'" Her husband refuses to leave, though, because they are three years from paying off their mortgage and, if they sold the house, would lose so much money that they couldn't afford to buy another.

For many of the families whose children developed cancer, there was simply no question of staying. The Samarripas moved to Alabama, where Hannah, now 20 and in college, is flourishing, according to her mother. Perhaps because her tumor was only partially removed by the surgery, or perhaps because she now has fluid in her skull, she still suffers from severe headaches, vomiting, and peripheral eye damage. She can't see some colors and has difficulty with organization and telling time, according to her mother. But she is also a musical girl who enjoys life and loves to sing.

Garrett Dunsford, too, is both thriving and living with the ongoing health effects of his cancer. Now 12, he has auditory processing problems, memory issues, and dyslexia, which were all diagnosed after his cancer. And he's particularly prone to headaches. But he also has a special outlook on life that his mother treasures—and thinks may have resulted from his trauma. "He doesn't value things at all," is how Dunsford described Garrett recently, adding that he's become the "family comforter. He'll ask for something and say, 'I appreciate that you bought me that, but let's go snuggle.' He values spending time with people."

The ordeal was also a turning point for Jennifer Dunsford. The family moved to Tennessee and sold their Acreage home through a short sale in 2011. Because of the damage to their credit, they haven't been able to buy another, Jennifer told me. But that's not her focus. "We have learned what's truly important in life, and it's definitely not a house," she says.

The McCanns left as well and are now living in the mountains of North Georgia with their two children. Kaye McCann says she doesn't miss Florida—only Jenna, who is still buried there. McCann ultimately found it too painful to be around the group of Acreage parents pursuing the cause of their children's cancer because most of their children survived. "In one sense, I would not go through what they're going through every day of their lives, wondering if [regular testing for cancer] is going to come back positive," she says. "But on the other hand, I envy them every day of their lives." The loss of her daughter has only become harder over time. She enjoys her family, her job, and her small town. "But when the low times do hit, each time it hits a little bit harder and lasts a little bit longer."

McCann knows that even if the puzzle of the Acreage cluster is finally solved, it wouldn't bring Jenna back. Still, she fervently hopes that someone can find "whatever it is that's made kids sick, stop it, and help clean it up." She is now exploring the possibility of moving Jenna's grave near their home in Georgia.

The Newfields are one of the few directly affected families to stay in the Acreage. While Jessica, now 20, is attending college, Tracy has been spearheading the creation of the Garden of Hope, a place in the Acreage where people can go to honor their loved ones who have had cancer. The Newfields also recently installed a sophisticated water-filtration system for their well, though Tracy recently discovered that Jessica had bought and stashed away bottled water.

For its part, Pratt & Whitney is staying, too. In November 2012, the company announced plans to add 230 jobs at its Florida campus over the next eight years and to invest $63 million in its facilities there. The deal is being financed with some $4.4 million in public incentives, including $3.4 million from the state and $1 million from Palm Beach County.

Critical Thinking

1. What is the relationship between groundwater contamination and pediatric brain cancer?
2. What are the risk factors for brain cancer?

Internet References

American Cancer Society
  www.cancer.org

Environmental Protection Agency
  www.epa.gov

Article   Prepared by: Eileen L. Daniel, *SUNY College at Brockport*

Public Health Issues to Watch in 2015

Jane Esworthy

Learning Outcomes

After reading this article, you will be able to:

- Describe the major public issues for 2015.

- Be aware of the regulations imposed on electronic cigarettes.

- Understand the growing epidemic of prescription drug abuse.

Infectious disease outbreaks, electronic cigarettes, prescription drug abuse, motor vehicle injuries, and marijuana possession are just a few of the hot topics expected to impact state health departments and public health in 2015. The U.S. healthcare industry is undergoing a large transformation and important decisions about health and healthcare are occurring at the state level. This year, our national healthcare expenditures are projected to hit $3.2 trillion, or $10,000 per person. As public health issues dominate the nation, health departments are predicting that many ongoing and emerging health threats are expected to make headlines this year.

"Each year, state legislatures across the country consider numerous proposals that have implications for the public's health," says Andrea Garcia, ASTHO's director of state health policy. "This year, given the national attention focused on the public health system's response to Ebola and the measles outbreak, we can expect states to address gaps and strengthen their laws to address future health threats."

Infectious Disease Outbreaks and Response

Since the first confirmed imported case of Ebola hit the United States in September 2014, and with the most recent multi-state measles outbreak affecting 17 states, state health departments are increasing efforts to prevent and control infectious disease outbreaks. In late 2014, several state legislatures met to discuss state health departments' ability to respond to infectious disease outbreaks; some states, however, rely heavily on federal funding for this work. Since the United States is facing ongoing budget pressures, states may need to provide their own funding to help control infectious diseases.

Recently, infectious disease outbreaks have sparked controversies, particularly isolation and quarantine policies regarding Ebola cases. Meanwhile, the current measles outbreak has ignited a vaccination debate. Given the attention to state isolation and quarantine policies, some states are evaluating existing powers and considering changes to their state laws, including employment protections for infected individuals and their caretakers. In addition, the current measles outbreak raises concerns because vaccination rules vary across states. All states require vaccinations, but there are some exemptions for individuals with weakened immune systems, allergies to ingredients, and previous negative reactions, in addition to religious and philosophical reasons.

Electronic Cigarettes

Electronic cigarettes (e-cigarettes) continue to be a controversial issue across states, and many will consider new regulation approaches in 2015. Some states will consider requiring child-safe packaging for e-cigarette cartridges and solutions, while others are considering taxing the products. Many e-cigarette users disagree with these tax proposals, arguing that the devices are healthier than traditional cigarettes. New Hampshire will propose adding e-cigarettes to its clean indoor air laws, and Texas will consider prohibiting their use in schools. ASTHO has developed an issue brief that highlights the emerging issues that states face with regards to e-cigarettes.

"This is going to be one of the most introduced and debated topics in state legislatures this year, especially the tax issue," says Max Behlke, analyst for the National Conference of State

Legislatures. With the popularity of e-cigarettes growing, more states are more likely to look to the new devices for revenue, according to The Pew Charitable Trusts.

Prescription Drug Abuse, Misuse, and Overdose

Prescription drug abuse is a growing epidemic in the United States. An estimated 2.4 million Americans have used prescription drugs nonmedically, according to results from the 2010 National Survey on Drug Use and Health. In 2014, ASTHO Past-President Terry Cline launched the ASTHO President's Challenge to reduce the nonmedical use of and unintentional overdose deaths involving controlled prescription drugs 15 percent by 2015. Forty-six states took the pledge to help reduce prescription drug abuse and deaths.

This year, states will continue to address this public health problem by establishing immunity for individuals who seek medical assistance for victims of overdoses, expanding access to the opioid antagonist naloxone, and requiring opioid education and addiction counseling for patients who are prescribed Schedule II or III controlled substances for chronic pain for extended periods. With $20 million in new funding in 2015, CDC will dramatically expand its work on this issue and provide more resources to states on the front lines of the epidemic.

Motor Vehicle Injuries

Motor vehicle injuries are a top cause of death among children in the United States. In 2012, more than 2.5 million Americans went to the emergency department, and almost 200,000 were hospitalized for crash injuries, according to CDC. To keep people safe and costs down, a number of states are considering bills related to motor vehicle injuries. In particular, California, Kentucky, North Carolina, and South Carolina are considering bills that require ignition interlock devices on all vehicles for individuals convicted of a DUI.

California is considering a bill requiring motor vehicle drivers to secure all children under the age of 2 in rear-facing child safety seats. Utah will consider a primary seatbelt law, and several states will consider repealing their motorcycle helmet laws. New Mexico will consider a bill to create a fatal injury diagnosis fund, which would require individuals to pay for motorcycle validating stickers indicating whether the operator is required by law to wear a helmet.

Critical Thinking

1. What controversies arose from the recent measles epidemic?
2. Why are more regulations needed for electronic cigarettes.
3. Why are new measures being proposed to increase motorist's safety?

Internet References

Centers for Disease Control and Prevention
www.cdc.gov/

National Highway Traffic Safety Administration
www.nhtsa.gov/

Food and Drug Administration
www.fda.gov

Giving ADHD a Rest: with Diagnosis Rates Exploding Wildly, Is the Disorder a Mental Health Crisis — or a Cultural One? by Kate Lunaue

221

Article　　　　　　　Prepared by: Eileen Daniel, *SUNY College at Brockport*

Giving ADHD a Rest: with Diagnosis Rates Exploding Wildly, Is the Disorder a Mental Health Crisis—or a Cultural One?

KATE LUNAU

Learning Outcomes

After reading this article, you will be able to:

- Discuss whether the ADHD epidemic is a mental health crisis or a cultural and/or social one.

- Explain why the rate of children diagnosed with ADHD is so much higher in North Carolina than California.

- Understand some of the causes of ADHD misdiagnoses.

Any visitor to North Carolina and California will know that the two states have their differences. The former is a typically "red state"; California is staunchly "blue." Each has certain geographic, ethnic and cultural peculiarities, different demographic makeup, family income levels, and more. Yet perhaps the most surprising divide, one many wouldn't expect, is that North Carolina appears to be a hotbed for attention deficit hyperactivity disorder, or ADHD—especially when compared to California. A child who lived in North Carolina instead of California in 2007, according to U.S. academics Stephen Hinshaw and Richard Scheffler, was 2½ times more likely to be diagnosed.

In their forthcoming book *The ADHD Explosion,* Hinshaw and Scheffler—a psychologist and health economist, respectively, at the University of California at Berkeley—examine the causes behind the startling and rapid rise in diagnosis rates of ADHD, a neurobehavioural disorder that has somehow become epidemic. In the U.S., more than one in 10 kids has been diagnosed; more than 3.5 million are taking drugs to curb symptoms, from lack of focus to hyperactivity. While ADHD typically hits middle-class boys the hardest, rates among other groups are steadily rising, including girls, adults, and minorities. Kids are being tested and diagnosed as young as preschool. In North Carolina, as many as 30 percent of teenage boys are diagnosed. Scheffler says, "It's getting scary."

According to psychologist Enrico Gnaulati, who is based in Pasadena, California, ADHD is now "as prevalent as the common cold." Various factors seem to be driving up the numbers, factors that extend from home to school to the doctor's office and beyond. "So many kids have trouble these days," says longtime ADHD researcher L. Alan Sroufe, professor emeritus at the University of Wisconsin at Madison. "I doubt it's a change in our genetic pool. Something else is going on."

A closer look at the case of North Carolina and California may be instructive. According to Hinshaw and Scheffler, North Carolinian kids between the ages of four and 17 had an ADHD diagnosis rate of 16 percent in 2007. In California, it was just over 6 percent. Kids with a diagnosis in North Carolina also faced a 50 percent higher probability they'd get medication. After exhaustively exploring demographics, health care policies, cultural values, and other possible factors, they landed on school policy as what Scheffler calls "the closest thing to a silver bullet."

Over the past few decades, incentives have been introduced for U.S. schools to turn out better graduation rates and test scores—and they've been pushed to compete for funding. North Carolina was one of the first states with school accountability laws, disciplining schools for missing targets, and rewarding them for exceeding them. "Such laws provide a real incentive to have children diagnosed and treated," Hinshaw and Scheffler write: kids in special education classes ideally get the help they need to improve their test scores and (in some areas) aren't counted in the district's test score average.

The rate of ADHD diagnosis varies between countries; as Hinshaw and Scheffler have shown, it even varies significantly within countries. This raises an important question: is the ADHD epidemic really a mental health crisis, or a cultural and societal one?

ADHD is a "chronic and debilitating mental disorder," Gnaulati says, one that can last a lifetime. It's believed to affect between 5 and 10 percent of the population, and boys still seem especially prone. (Nearly one in five high school boys have ADHD, compared to 1 in 11 girls, according to the U.S. Centers for Disease Control and Prevention.) Kids with ADHD can have a hard time making and keeping friends. In one study of boys at summer camp, Hinshaw found that after just a few hours, those with an ADHD diagnosis were far more likely to be rejected than those without one. The disorder can persist into adulthood, raising the risk of low self-esteem, divorce, unemployment, and driving accidents; even getting arrested and going to jail, according to a report from the Centre for ADHD Awareness Canada.

In fact, the brains of people with ADHD are different. They're short on receptors for the neurotransmitter dopamine, and their brain volume looks to be slightly smaller. But no medical test or brain scan can yet give a definitive diagnosis. The gold standard comes from the *Diagnostic and Statistical Manual of Mental Disorders*, or DSM, from the American Psychiatric Association. The latest version of this "bible of psychiatry," released in May, lists nine symptoms of inattention (making careless mistakes on homework; distractibility; trouble staying organized), and nine of hyperactivity or impulsivity (interrupting others; climbing when it's inappropriate; and excessive talking, to give some examples). They'll sound familiar to anyone who's spent time with kids. "Every child is to some extent impulsive, distractible, disorganized, and has trouble following directions," says Gnaulati, author of *Back to Normal,* an investigation of why what he calls "ordinary childhood behaviour" is often mistaken for ADHD.

The DSM specifies that a child should be showing many symptoms consistently, in two or more settings (at home and at school, for example), a better indication that he isn't just acting out because of a bad teacher, or an annoying sibling. "Studies

show that if you stick to the two-informant requirement, the number of cases falls by 40 percent," says Gnaulati. Surprisingly often, the diagnoses seem to be hastily given, and drugs dispensed.

It was once thought that stimulants affected people with ADHD differently—calming them down, revving up everyone else—but we now know that's not the case. Virtually everybody seems to react the same in the short term, Sroufe says. "They're attention-enhancers. We've known that since the Second World War," when they were given to radar operators to stay awake and focused. Those with true ADHD show bigger gains, partly because their brains may be "underaroused" to begin with, write Hinshaw and Scheffler. (About two-thirds of U.S. kids with a diagnosis get medication; in Canada, it's about 50 percent.) Stimulants have side effects, including suppressing appetite, speeding up the heart rate, and raising blood pressure. Kids who take them for a long time might end up an inch or so shorter, according to Hinshaw and Scheffler's book, because dopamine activity interferes with growth hormone. And those who don't need them will eventually develop a tolerance, needing a greater and greater quantity to get the effect they're after.

"Brain doping" is by now a well-known phenomenon among college and university students across North America. Many students don't see stimulant use as cheating: one 2012 study found that male college students believe it's far more unethical for an athlete to use steroids than for a student to abuse prescription stimulants to ace a test. "Some red-hot parents want to get their kid into Harvard, Berkeley or Princeton," Scheffler says. "They're going to need a perfect score, so they're going to push." With an ADHD diagnosis, students can seek special accommodations at school, like more time on tests including the SAT, a standardized college entrance exam. With parents, students, and even school boards recognizing the potential benefits that come with diagnosis, ADHD is occurring with increasing frequency among groups other than the white middle class, where rates have typically been highest: according to Hinshaw and Scheffler, African American youth are now just as likely, if not more, to be diagnosed and medicated.

Drug advertisements could also be driving rates of diagnosis upward. Hinshaw and Scheffler describe one ad from Johnson & Johnson, maker of the stimulant Concerta, which shows a happy mother and a son who's getting "better test scores at school" and doing "more chores at home," the text reads. "The message is clear: the right pill breeds family harmony," they write. Sometimes, another underlying health problem will be mistakenly diagnosed as ADHD. In his new book, *ADHD Does Not Exist,* Richard Saul documents 25 conditions that can look like ADHD; most common are vision and hearing issues. "Until you get glasses, it's very hard to understand what [the teacher] is speaking about if you can't see the board," he says.

"Same with hearing." Conditions ranging from bipolar disorder to Tourette's syndrome can also be mistaken for ADHD, Saul writes. Despite the strongly worded title of his book, he believes that 20 percent of those diagnosed are "neurochemical distractible impulsive" and have what we'd term ADHD. The rest are being misdiagnosed, and as a result, he says, "the right treatment is being delayed."

Sleep deprivation is another big cause of misdiagnosis. "It's paradoxical, but especially for kids, it does create hyperactivity and impulsivity," says Vatsal Thakkar of New York University's Langone Medical Center. Given mounting academic pressures, and the screens that populate virtually every room, many kids simply aren't getting enough downtime. A child's relative immaturity can factor in, too. In 2012, a study in the Canadian Medical Association Journal found that the youngest kids in a classroom were more likely to have an ADHD diagnosis, and to be prescribed medication. Those born in December are nearly a full year younger than some of their peers, a big difference, especially in kindergarten. (In the U.S., half of all kids with ADHD are diagnosed before age six.)

Gnaulati, who has a son, worries the deck's been stacked against boys, who are more prone to blurt out an answer, run around the classroom, or otherwise act out. "During the kindergarten years, boys are at least a year behind girls in basic self-regulation," he says. Gnaulati notes that school teachers, pediatricians, and school psychologists are all more likely be female—which he argues could be a contributing factor. "In a sense," he writes, "girl behaviour has become the standard by which we judge all kids."

In Canada, we don't track ADHD diagnosis rates as closely as in the U.S. But the rate of diagnosis does look to be picking up here, and elsewhere, too. A study by Hinshaw and Scheffler compared the use of ADHD drugs to countries' per capita gross domestic product. "Richer countries spend more [on ADHD medications]," Scheffler says. "But some countries still spend more than their income would predict." They found that Canada, the U.S., and Australia all had a greater use of these drugs than GDP suggests. A 2013 paper in the British Journal of Medicine notes that Australia saw a 73 percent increase in prescribing rates for ADHD medications between 2000 and 2011. The Netherlands had a similar spike—the prevalence of ADHD, and the rate at which ADHD drugs were prescribed to kids, doubled between 2003 and 2007.

Peter Conrad of Brandeis University, outside Boston, is studying how the DSM definition of ADHD (which we use in Canada) has been exported around the globe, leading to more kids diagnosed and treated. "Until the late '90s, most diagnosis in Europe was done under the World Health Organization's International Classification of Diseases," which is much more strict, he notes. (The ICD, for example, required symptoms of inattention, impulsivity, and hyperactivity, while an older version of the DSM required only two.)

European countries began to adopt the DSM definition, a response to the fact that so much research on ADHD comes out of the U.S.—and the DSM began to be seen as the standard. "France and Italy still have low rates," says Conrad, "partly because they don't use the DSM." A 2013 study from the University of Exeter found that U.K. kids were much less likely than those in the U.S. to be diagnosed with ADHD, which may be due to tougher criteria, or to parents' resistance to medicating their kids. Even so, other countries are catching up. According to Hinshaw and Scheffler, the use of ADHD medication is rising over five times faster around the world than in the U.S.

Many of the same pressures that motivate diagnosis in the U.S. are at play in Canada, although in different ways. Given the tight job market and increasing academic demands, students are under more pressure to succeed than ever. And while our school test results aren't tied to funding like in the U.S., "high-stakes testing" is increasingly important, says Elizabeth Dhuey, a University of Toronto economist who studies education.

For one thing, it's a point of pride for schools. Results from Ontario's EQAO standardized test are reported in the media and used to rank and compare institutions. ("EQAO: How did your school fare in Ontario's standardized tests?" reads one 2012 Toronto Star headline.) What constitutes an "exceptionality" and triggers special services also varies between provinces. In Newfoundland, ADHD has been an "exceptionality" for the past two decades; in Ontario, it isn't considered a special category, but ADHD students can access special education and other extra help on a case-by-case basis. And in B.C., school districts can get supplemental funding for students with ADHD, according to the ministry of education.

These pressures aren't abating—if anything, many are getting stronger—and so, it seems likely we haven't yet reached peak ADHD. Scheffler and Hinshaw raise the possibility that, within the decade, ADHD rates in the U.S. might reach 15 percent or higher; and that as many as four-fifths of those diagnosed could have a prescription.

The hope lies in finding better scientific markers—a definitive test that could confirm true cases of ADHD, and those who will benefit most from treatment, including medication. Otherwise, we're facing the prospect of a generation of kids living with a serious mental health diagnosis, and quite possibly taking powerful drugs long term into adulthood, with all the potential side effects they entail. Whatever is contributing to ADHD's startling rise, it's clear that this isn't a contagious disease kids are swapping on the playground. In many cases, we're giving it to them.

Critical Thinking

1. How are the brains different between individuals with and without ADHD?

2. Why are so many ADHD diagnoses done so hastily resulting in medications dispensed?

Create Central

www.mhhe.com/createcentral

Internet References

Centers for Disease Control and Prevention
http://www.cdc.gov/ncbddd/ADHD

National Institutes of Mental Health
http://www.nimh.nih.gov/health/topics/attention-deficit-hyperactivity-disorder-adhd/index.shtml

Kate Lunau, "Giving ADHD a Rest: With Diagnosis Rates Exploding Wildly, Is the Disorder a Mental Health Crisis-or a Cultural One?" from *Maclean's* 127.8 (March 3, 2014).